# AN ATLAS OF
# CARDIOLOGY

# AN ATLAS OF

# CARDIOLOGY

## ELECTROCARDIOGRAMS
## AND CHEST X-RAYS

## NEVILLE CONWAY

### MB, FRCP

*Consultant Cardiologist*
*Southampton University Hospitals*
*and Wessex Regional Health Authority*
*Senior Lecturer in Cardiology*
*The Medical School, Southampton*

WOLFE MEDICAL PUBLICATIONS LTD

Copyright © Neville Conway, 1977
Published by Wolfe Medical Publications Ltd, 1977
Printed by Sackville Press Ltd, Billericay
ISBN 0 7234 0401 1

General Editor, Wolfe Medical Books
G Barry Carruthers, MD(Lond)

AN ATLAS OF CARDIOLOGY is a companion volume to
*A colour atlas of Cardiac Pathology.* Other books
in that series already published include:

*A colour atlas of Human Anatomy*
*A colour atlas of Haematological Cytology*
*A colour atlas of General Pathology*
*A colour atlas of Oro-Facial Diseases*
*A colour atlas of Ophthalmological Diagnosis*
*A colour atlas of Renal Diseases*
*A colour atlas of Venereology*
*A colour atlas of Dermatology*
*A colour atlas of Infectious Diseases*
*A colour atlas of Ear, Nose & Throat Diagnosis*
*A colour atlas of Rheumatology*
*A colour atlas of Microbiology*
*A colour atlas of Forensic Pathology*
*A colour atlas of Paediatrics*
*A colour atlas of Histology*
*A colour atlas of General Surgical Diagnosis*
*A colour atlas of Physical Signs in General Medicine*
*A colour atlas of Tropical Medicine & Parasitology*
*A colour atlas of Histological Staining Techniques*
*A colour atlas and textbook of Oral Anatomy*

Some further titles now in preparation:
*A colour atlas of Gynaecological Operations (6 volumes)*
*A colour atlas of Oral Medicine*
*A colour atlas of Diabetes Mellitus*
*A colour atlas of Bone Diseases*
*A colour atlas of Eye Tumours*
*A colour atlas of Eye Surgery*
*A colour atlas of the Liver*

The series of Wolfe Medical Atlases brings together
probably the world's largest systematic published
collection of diagnostic colour photographs.
For a full list of Atlases in the series, including
details of our surgical, dental and veterinary
Atlases, plus forthcoming titles, please write to
Wolfe Medical Publications Ltd, 3–5 Conway Street,
London W1.

# ACKNOWLEDGEMENTS

Naturally, I owe an enormous debt to the cardiographers, cardiac technicians, and radiographers of the various hospitals in which I have worked. I cannot name them individually but ask them to accept my sincere thanks for their goodwill, patience, and skill. I also wish to thank my many colleagues at the Western Hospital, Southampton, in the Southampton University Hospitals, and in the Wessex region for their generous permission to use material from their cases. Once again it is impossible to list them all but I am particularly grateful to Drs J Cruikshank, I Hyde, A M Johnson, D Mullan, R J McGill, and G Sterling, and to Messrs I K R McMillan and T Kalloway for individual contributions of great interest. The axis diagram in **39** was prepared in the then Wessex Regional Centre for Medical Illustration; all other illustrations were prepared and photographed personally. David Whitcher of the Teaching Media Centre, Southampton University Medical School, prepared the prints of the x-ray section, and I am very grateful to him for his unstinted energy and expertise.

TO MY WIFE

# PREFACE

Any examination of the heart without an electrocardiogram and a chest x-ray in at least one projection is not only incomplete; it is almost certainly inaccurate. This atlas, therefore, in combining the illustration of these two aspects of the basic cardiac assessment, is intended as a clinical benchbook to assist undergraduates, family doctors, and physicians (both in training and established) at the bedside. It is not directed at the specialist. To satisfy the obviously diverse requirements of so wide a readership is not as difficult as it seems, for a book of this kind can, and should, be used as a ready reference rather than as a formal text. The key lies in the index, which has been made as comprehensive as possible and will enable the more experienced to avoid the elementary material needed by relative newcomers to the subject.

With this philosophy in mind, the captions concentrate on describing what is seen in, and may be deduced from, the illustrations themselves, and this means that, in a few areas of electrocardiography in which complex electro-physiological investigations are necessary to arrive at a complete diagnosis (e.g. of an arrhythmia) traditional teaching has been perpetuated at a time when these techniques are furnishing conclusive evidence of the fallibility of the surface electrocardiogram in isolation. However, the practicalities are that such procedures are unavailable outside specialised centres and likely to remain so for they require cardiac catheterisation, and they are totally unfamiliar to non-cardiologists; moreover, electrocardiograms have to be interpreted as they are taken. That said, it may seem inconsistent to have included a handful of angiograms and films of catheters within the heart, but these simply underline visual points on the plain x-ray more neatly than explanatory diagrams.

The material covered and the problems on interpretation raised are based on many years' experience of teaching and practising clinical cardiology. As is only sensible, common conditions have been given more space than uncommon ones, but some rarities have been included to add spice and stimulate interest. Normal appearances are illustrated, as far as this can ever be done. The neonatal and infant period receives only brief mention, for it is a considerable subject in its own right and, outside paediatric cardiological circles, unlikely to be of sufficient interest to merit the extensive illustration adequate coverage would require.

Subjects have been dealt with as syndromes or diseases as seemed most expedient, the avoidance of needless repetition being the over-riding consideration. No natural logic is claimed for the result, nor for the classification or order in which topics appear. Inevitably arbitrary decisions have been taken when lesions fall into more than one category. Once again, the answer to any problems of cross-reference or differential diagnosis should be available in the index.

# CONTENTS

PART 1: ELECTROCARDIOGRAMS

Introduction

| | |
|---|---|
| Normal electrocardiograms | 1–30 |
| Recording faults | 31–38 |
| Mean QRS axis | 39–53 |
| P wave | 54–59 |
| Sino-atrial arrhythmias | 60–70 |
| Atrioventricular junctional rhythm | 71–80 |
| Extrasystoles | 81–122 |
| Parasystole | 123–125 |
| Bradycardia | 126–129 |
| Supraventricular tachycardia | 130–163 |
| Wolff–Parkinson–White syndrome | 164–172 |
| Ventricular tachycardia | 173–189 |
| Ventricular fibrillation and cardiac arrest | 190–198 |
| Atrial flutter | 199–214 |
| Atrial fibrillation | 215–235 |
| Heart block | 236–278 |
| Pacing | 279–293 |
| Ventricular hypertrophy | 294–319 |
| Bundle branch block, hemiblock, multifascicular block | 320–353 |
| Myocardial ischaemia | 354–379 |
| Myocardial infarction | 380–413 |
| Pericarditis | 414–418 |
| Miscellaneous conditions | 419–446 |
| Some diagnostic patterns of congenital heart disease | 447–453 |

PART 2: CHEST X-RAYS

Introduction

| | |
|---|---|
| Normal appearances and common influences on heart size | 454–496 |
| Enlargement of individual cardiac chambers | 497–504 |

Pulmonary evidence of heart failure            505–517

Coronary disease                               518–534

Pericardial disease                            535–546

Primary myocardial disease                     547–553

Aortic valve disease                           554–573

Mitral valve disease                           574–605

Tricuspid and multivalvar disease              606–617

Pulmonary embolism and pulmonary hypertension  618–625

Congenital heart disease                       626–677

Diseases of the thoracic aorta                 678–717

Pacing                                         718–729

Miscellaneous conditions                       730–752

INDEX

# PART 1

# ELECTROCARDIOGRAMS: INTRODUCTION

The approach to this section has been pragmatic. The emphasis has been placed on pattern recognition, though the theoretical basis of this is mentioned wherever it seems secure. Vectorial analysis has been avoided, for it is unfamiliar to most students and general physicians. Specific diseases are illustrated when the pattern they produce is distinctive, but not otherwise, so that, for instance, hypertrophic cardiomyopathy is singled out but no attempt is made to demonstrate individually the many causes of congestive cardiomyopathy. By a like token there is, for example, no separate section on digitalis-induced dysrhythmias, though the drug is mentioned whenever a particular rhythm could reasonably be attributed to it (e.g. junctional rhythm in atrial fibrillation, or multiform ventricular ectopics). The greatest problem has been how far to include the electrocardiograms of young children, which differ so much from appearances later in life. The result is a compromise; they are illustrated briefly but no more—to go further would be beyond the purpose of a book such as this.

# NORMAL ELECTROCARDIOGRAMS

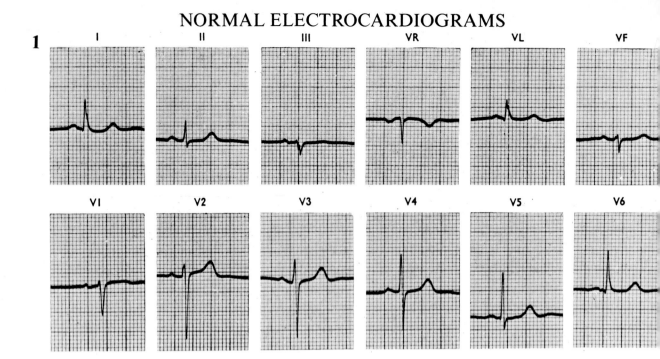

**1** **Normal electrocardiogram, horizontal heart.** The complex in VL resembles that in V6 while the complex in VF resembles that in V1.

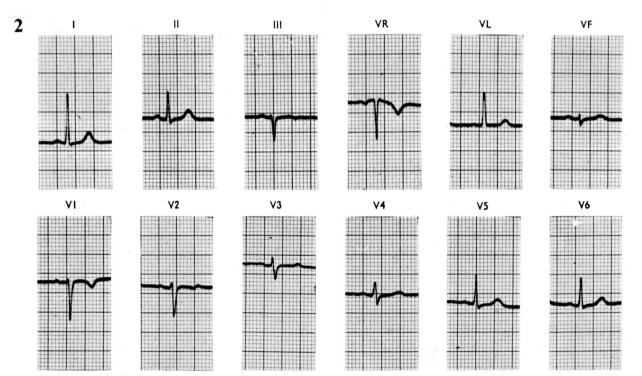

**2** **Normal electrocardiogram, semi-horizontal heart.** The complex in VL resembles that in V6 but the complex in VF is of low voltage and strongly resembles neither V6 nor V1.

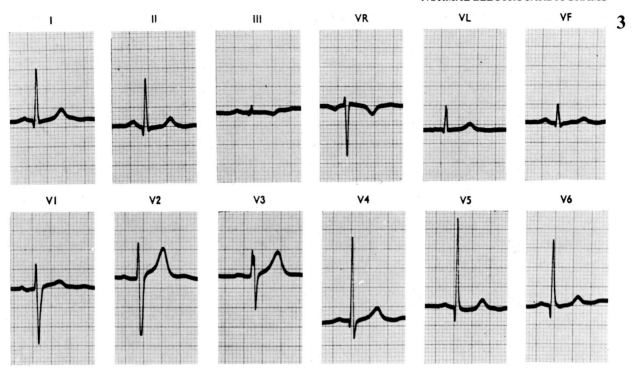

**3 Normal electrocardiogram, intermediate position.** The complexes in VF and VL are similar in shape and both resemble that in V6.

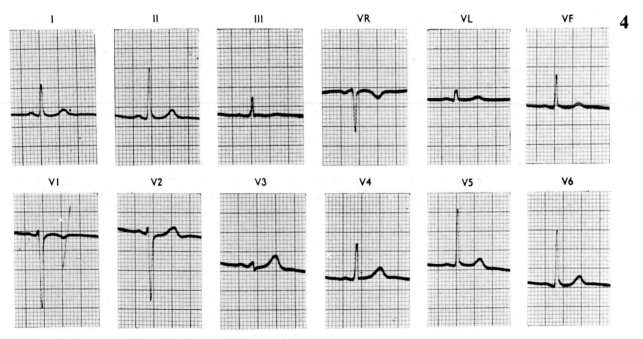

**4 Normal electrocardiogram, semi-vertical heart.** The complex in VF resembles that in V6 but the complex in VL is of low voltage and strongly resembles neither V1 nor V6.

For another example, see **6**.

**5**

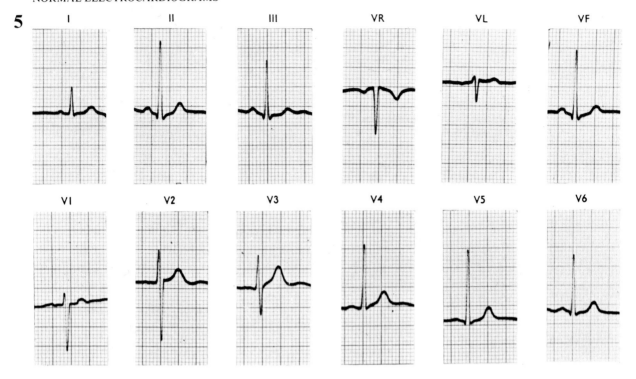

**5 Normal electrocardiogram, vertical heart.** The complex in VF resembles that in V6 while the complex in VL resembles that in V1.

**6 Normal electrocardiogram, clockwise rotation.** The term refers to the position of the transitional zone in the chest leads—i.e. the point at which the QRS complexes become equiphasic and change from a dominantly negative to a dominantly positive deflection. The imaginary viewpoint is from beneath the diaphragm and the transitional zone is conceived as moving around the chest wall—hence the name. The usual place for this alteration in QRS is V3 or V4. In clockwise rotation it is V5 or farther to the left. The result is that the maximum height of R wave is no longer seen in V5 but is shifted into V6, or V7, if this is recorded. An S wave is seen in V6.

**7 Normal electrocardiogram, anticlockwise rotation.** See **6**. The transitional zone is shifted into the right chest leads—here, V2 and V3—and the maximum height of R wave is found to the right of V5—here, V4. The S wave disappears from V5.

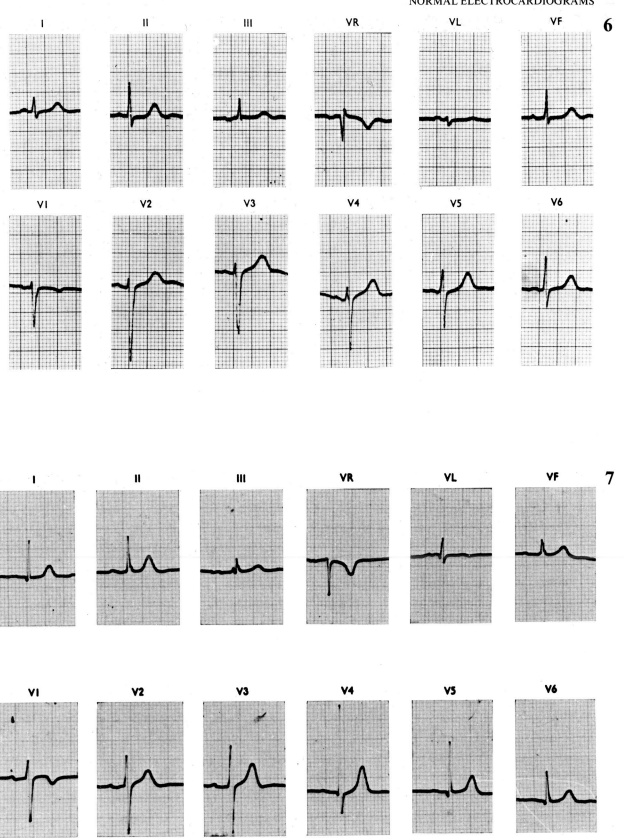

**8**

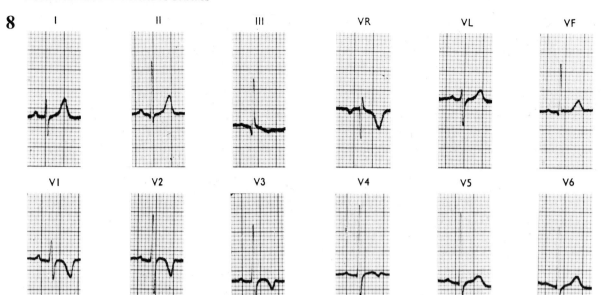

8  **Normal electrocardiogram, early childhood.** The range of normality in childhood is much wider than in later life and space precludes its full illustration. At no time of life is it more important to avoid electrocardiographic diagnosis of abnormality in isolation from clinical data. The tracing illustrates one fairly constant finding—inversion of T waves in the anterior chest leads. Note that the QRS mean axis is about $+90°$, which is normal at this age.

9  **Notched T waves in childhood.** Bifid T waves are a normal finding in childhood. They are usually best seen in the antero-septal chest leads—in this example, V3 and V4—though they can be seen in other leads. It is important not to mistake them for additional P waves. Note the easily seen U waves in this trace. There is also incomplete right bundle branch block and anticlockwise rotation.

10  **Normal electrocardiogram, new-born infant.** At this period of life right axis deviation and right ventricular dominance are the rule. The apparent P pulmonale in V2 is due to the superimposition of P on T.

**9**

| I | II | III | VR | VL | VF |
|---|---|---|---|---|---|

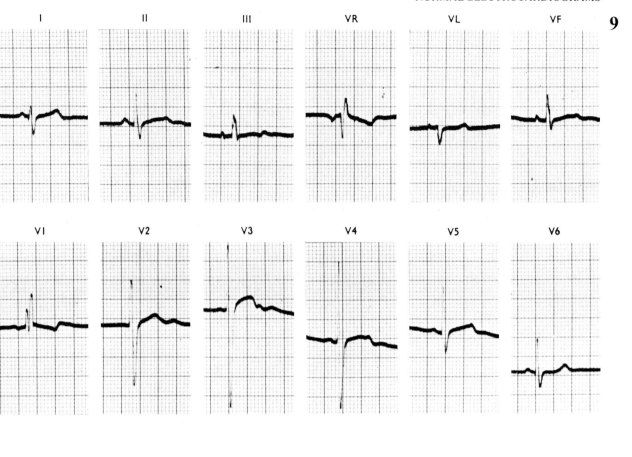

| V I | V2 | V3 | V4 | V5 | V6 |
|---|---|---|---|---|---|

**10**

| I | II | III | VR | VL | VF |
|---|---|---|---|---|---|

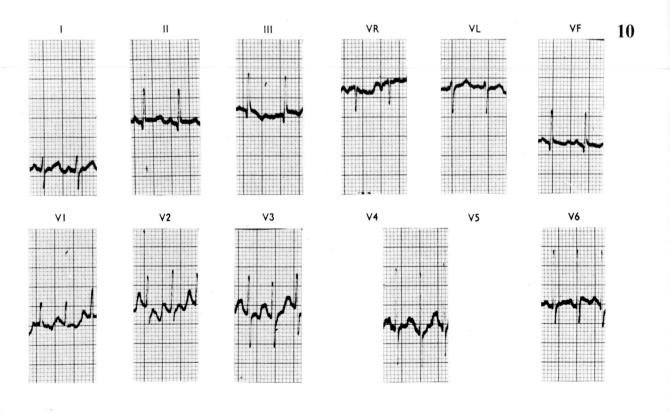

| V I | V2 | V3 | V4 | V5 | V6 |
|---|---|---|---|---|---|

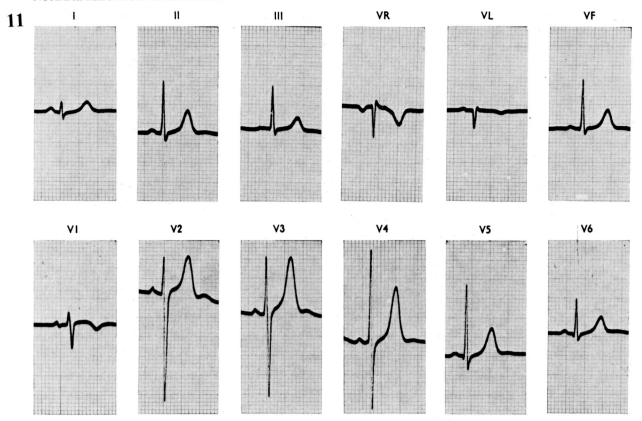

**11 Normal electrocardiogram, exuberant voltages of later childhood and adolescence.** Although after early childhood adult standards of normality may be applied, there are two principal points of difference to keep in mind—the tendency towards a rightward directed QRS axis; and voltages, particularly in the chest leads, which later in life would be regarded as exceeding the limits allowable. At this period of life the diagnosis of left or right ventricular hypertrophy should be made with great caution, and of course, never without reference to clinical findings.

**12 Persistence of T inversion over the right ventricle into adult life.** T waves are normally inverted in leads V1–3 or 4 in childhood but gradually become upright except in V1 by adolescence. In some subjects T inversion in the right ventricular leads persists longer as in this 18-year-old girl.

**13 Sickling pattern.** ST elevation of 1–2mm is present. It is more marked in some leads than others. The ST segment remains concave upwards and the T wave stays upright. This pattern is a normal variant; it is commoner in some races than others.

The appearances resemble those of acute pericarditis (**414**), in which, however, the ST elevation is usually more marked, and of course, progresses to T wave inversion. Similar appearances are seen transiently in the earliest hours after acute myocardial infarction (see **380**, **382**) or Prinzmetal angina (**377**, **378**) but the distribution of changes and the presence of reciprocal ST depression are of assistance in avoiding error. Exercise abolishes the sickling pattern (**14**).

**12**

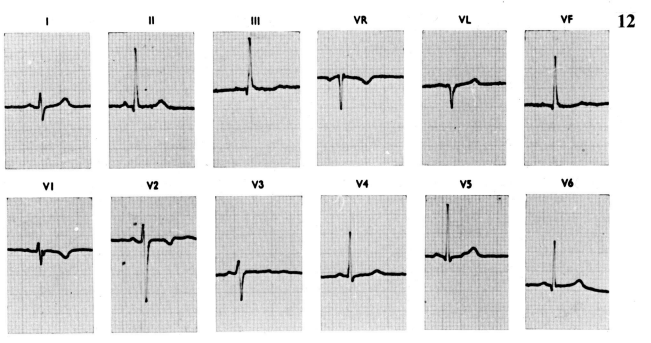

**13**

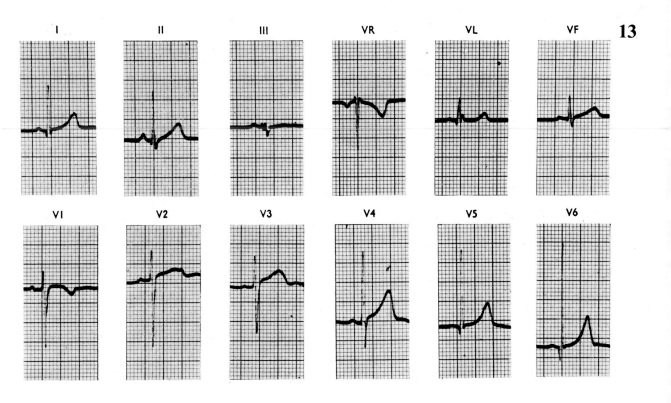

**14**

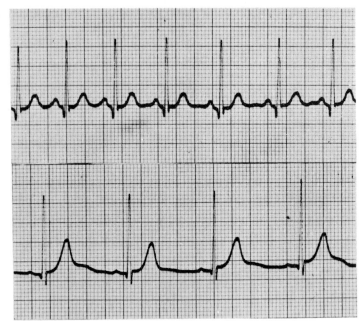

**14 Sickling pattern, effect of exercise.** Upper line, exercise. Lower line, on return to rest.

**15**

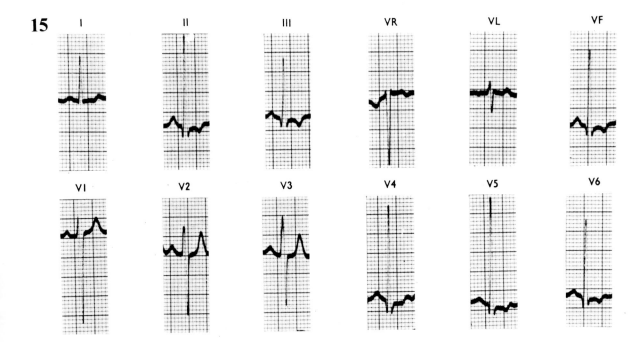

I    II    III    VR    VL    VF

VI    V2    V3    V4    V5    V6

**15 The 'suspended' heart.** The finding on a chest x-ray of the so-called 'suspended' heart (see **468**) is accompanied by electrocardiographic changes which may easily be misinterpreted as those of disease. These subjects tend to be tall and the heart is usually vertical. They present in adolescence or early adult life and frequently have the rather exuberant QRS voltages of this period. There is T wave inversion in II, III and VF, and because of the heart's position, often in V5 and V6 as well. The QRS axis is usually within the normal range at about $+75°$.

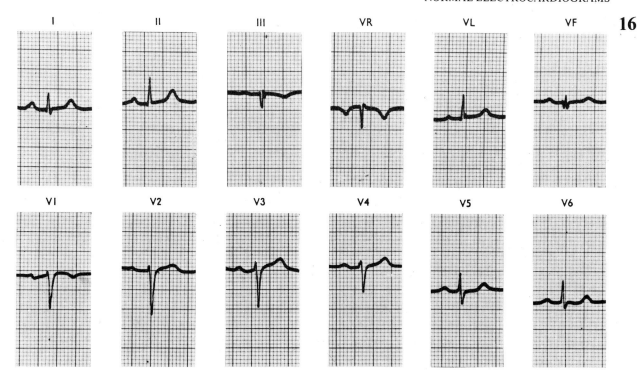

I    II    III    VR    VL    VF

VI    V2    V3    V4    V5    V6

**16  Obesity.** Generalised low-voltage curves; these are also seen in pericardial effusion (**417**), constrictive pericarditis (**416**), myxoedema (**424**) and congestive cardiomyopathies (**443–445**).

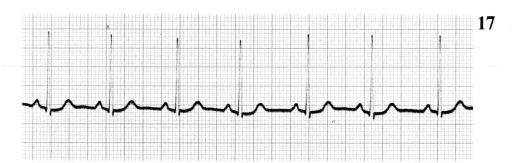

**17  Sinus rhythm.** P waves are normal and unchanging in shape, the PR interval falls within the normal limits, and every P wave is followed by a narrow QRS of normal contour. The heart rate depends on age among many other factors, and will lie between 60 and 100 beats/minute in adults, 75 and 125 beats/minute in young children, and 110 and 150 beats/minute in neonates. Even in a short strip, minor beat-to-beat variations in rate may be seen.

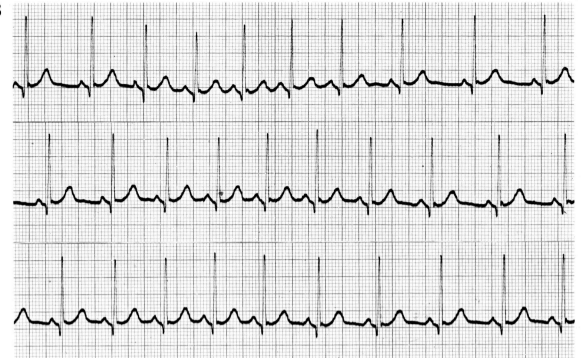

**18   Sinus arrhythmia.** The heart rate accelerates on inspiration and slows on expiration, the effect being exaggerated on deep breathing and disappearing on exercise. All beats originate in the sino-atrial node. The PR interval remains unchanged. The cause is rhythmic variations of vagal tone induced by respiration acting on the sino-atrial node.

The three rows of the illustration are one continuous strip.

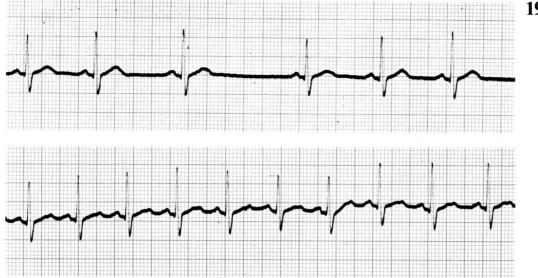

**19  Sinus arrhythmia abolished by exercise.** Upper
line, rest. Lower line, exercise.

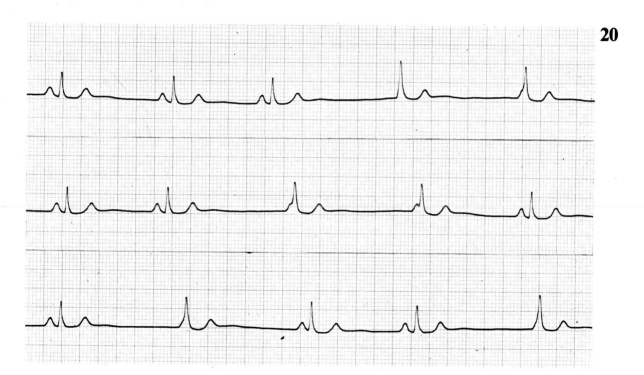

**20  Sinus arrhythmia with junctional escape.** The
heart rate accelerates as normal during inspiration
but the vagal slowing during expiration is so
marked that actual arrest of sino-atrial node
activity occurs. Activation of the heart is taken over
by the atrioventricular junction—'junctional
escape'.

In this example, junctional escape occurs after the
third complex on the top line. Reappearance of
sino-atrial node activity produces a P wave which
can be seen deforming the second junctional beat at
the end of the line. Junctional escape recurs in the
centre of the middle line and again at the beginning
and end of the bottom line. Junctional escape is
readily abolished by exercise. Note the slightly
different shape of the junctional beats (see **113**).

**21**

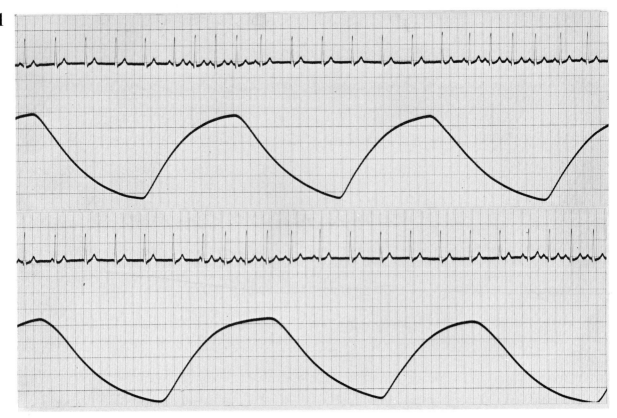

**21  Sinus arrhythmia unrelated to respiration.** In this uncommon situation, regular alternating acceleration and deceleration of sino-atrial nodal discharge is uninfluenced by respiration, as can be seen by studying the respiratory trace below the electrocardiogram (peaks, inspiration; troughs, expiration). In addition, in this instance, slowing is extreme and amounts to sinus arrest, so that, as in the previous illustration, junctional escape occurs. With exercise, this arrhythmia disappears.

**22**

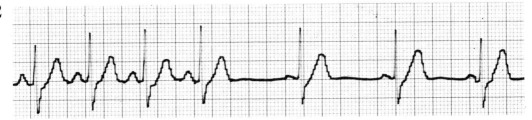

**22  Shifting pacemaker in the sinus node.** Different parts of the sino-atrial node have differing rates of impulse formation. Naturally, the fastest dominates the rest but occasionally, it will fail to discharge, and another pacemaker will emerge. Because the impulse enters the atria by a different route, the P wave may alter in shape, as in this example. Note too, the change in PR interval—shorter with the slower of the pacemakers.

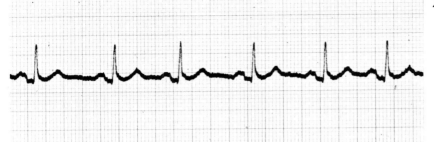

**23  Atrial T wave.** Atrial repolarisation is rarely visible but may be manifest in a slight depression of the isoelectric line between P and QRS.

**24**

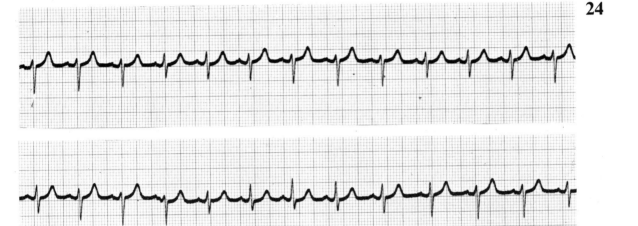

**24  Respiratory variation in QRS contour.** It is not uncommon for respiration to alter the position of the heart in relation to one or more of the leads sufficiently to cause a major alteration in contour of the QRS complex. This is most likely to happen with one of the limb leads. It may lead to confusion until the reason is suspected and confirmation obtained by deeper breathing. The example illustrated shows quiet respiration (above) and deep breathing (below). Further examples are illustrated in **25** and **26**.

III

aVF

I I

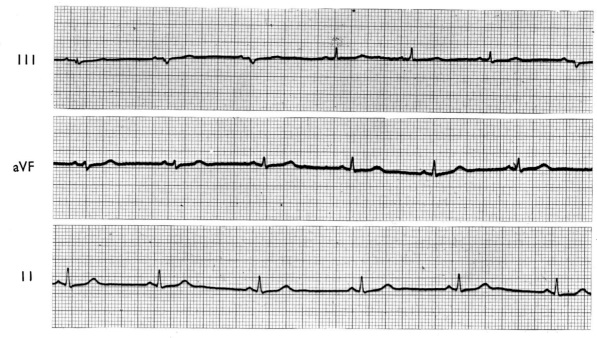

**25    Effect of respiration on Q waves in lead III.** This is a particular example of the respiratory variation in QRS contour described in **24**. Since old inferior infarction is often difficult to diagnose (**401, 402**), Q waves in inferior leads must be viewed with suspicion. Inspiration will often abolish them in lead III, indicating their benign character.

In the illustration, the subject has taken a deep breath after the third complex.

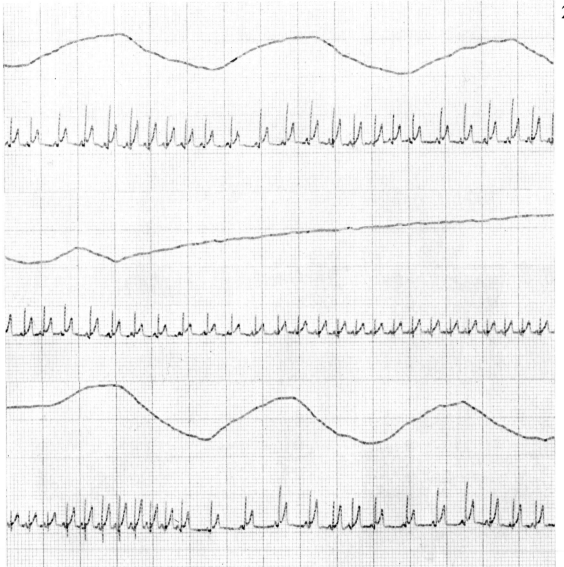

**26  Valsalva's manoeuvre.** A normal response is detectable by a slowing of the heart when the period of strain ends. This example illustrates a complete Valsalva's manoeuvre. The three rows are one continuous strip. Respiratory movements are shown by the single line above the electrocardiogram. The upper row shows normal respiration; note the pronounced sinus arrhythmia and the respiratory variation in the QRS contour (**24**). The middle row shows the period of strain; respiration stops and there is reflex tachycardia towards the end. The diminution in QRS size parallels the increasing effort to hold the strain and is, of course, artefactual. On the lowest row, strain is released and breathing recommenced. Tachycardia is abruptly replaced by the characteristic reflex bradycardia.

27

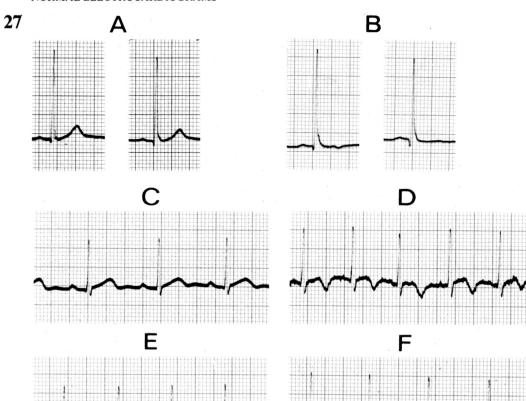

**27 Normally labile T waves.** Transient T wave flattening and even inversion may occur in normal subjects in response to a variety of physiological stimuli and may be mistaken for myocardial ischaemia or other pathological causes of T wave changes (see **357**) if the possibility is not kept in mind. A shows leads V4 and V6 in a normal young man before food and B the same leads after a meal. The lower four traces show the effect of hyperventilation in another healthy young man: C, the basal record; D, during voluntary over-breathing (note the muscular tremor and baseline shift and the nervous tachycardia); E and F, recovery. See **12, 15, 131,** and **162** for the effect of other physiological influences on T waves.

**28 Dextrocardia inadvertently recorded with conventionally placed limb and chest leads.** The results are: Lead I is upside down and leads VR and VL are interchanged (arm leads transposed), leads II and III are interchanged (leg leads transposed), lead VF is unaffected, and progressive diminution in the size of the QRS complexes, associated with T wave inversion, from V1 to V6 (chest leads farther and farther from the ventricular mass). The trace may be mistaken for myocardial ischaemia with lateral infarction if the mistake is not realised. The real clue is the inverted P wave in I and VL, indicating that the sino-atrial node is not on the right-hand side of the heart. Inadvertent transposition of the arm leads in a normal subject mimics this tracing in many respects, but is readily differentiated by the normal contour of the chest leads (see **31**).

Analysis of this tracing is rendered easier by reference to **29**.

**29 Dextrocardia recorded with all limb leads reversed and chest leads placed on the right.** The same patient as **28**. Normal tracing.

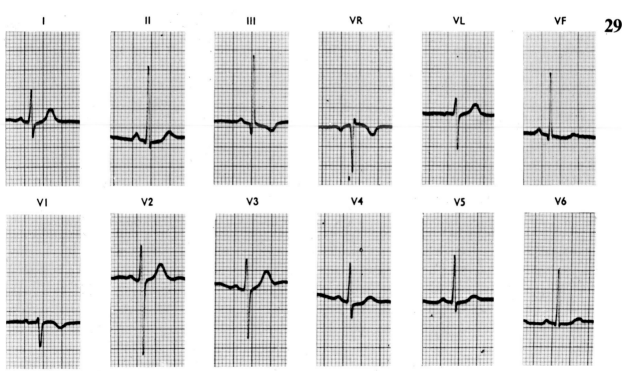

**30**

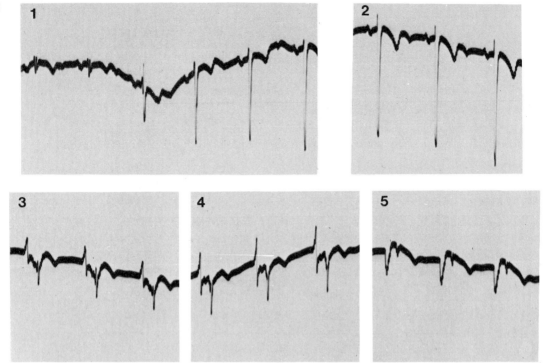

**30 Normal intracardiac electrocardiograms.** Inside the right heart and great veins the electrocardiogram shows considerable variation in morphology, depending on the site of recording. The differences are of physiological interest.

1. Inside the pulmonary artery (first two complexes only—the rest of the trace shows withdrawal to the right ventricle). In the pulmonary artery the complex is of low voltage, and all waves are inverted. These findings reflect the isolation of the recording electrode from the heart itself, and the fact that the myocardial forces point away from it.

2. Inside the right ventricle. The QRS and T wave are large, but predominantly negative once again, for the same reason as above. The P wave remains small, and depending on the exact site of recording, usually positive, at least in part. Note the (negative) U wave.

3. Low right atrium. Inside the great veins and right atrium the P wave becomes the dominant wave of the electrocardiogram, the QRS and T wave being inconspicuous again (note they are still negative). In the mid and low right atrium the P wave is upright, for the recording electrode is below the sino-atrial node.

4. High right atrium and low superior vena cava. In this position the P wave is biphasic, the electrode being close to the sino-atrial node.

5. High superior vena cava. Here, the P wave is negative as the electrode is above the sino-atrial node. Note the diminutive QRST.

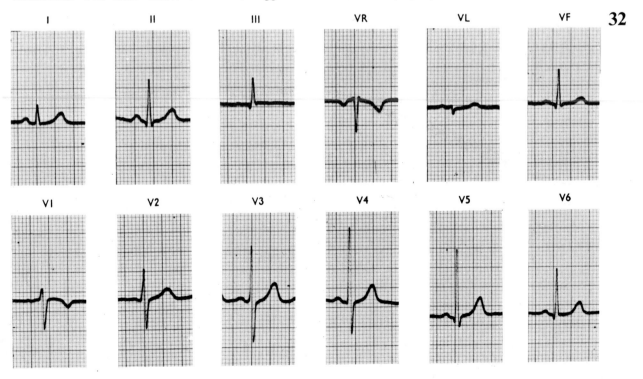

**31, 32  Recording fault, arm leads reversed in error.**
The results of this mistake are that lead I is upside down, leads II and III are transposed, as are leads VR and VL. Lead VF and the chest leads are unaffected. The limb leads, therefore, suggest dextrocardia, but the normal chest leads provide the answer. Compare with the correct tracing shown in **32**. This error is often seen but is readily recognised if the possibility is kept in mind; see also dextrocardia (**28, 29**).

32

**33**

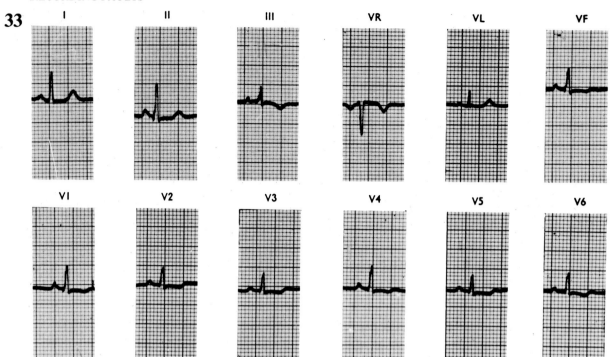

**33, 34 Recording fault, failure to switch lead selector to V position from the VF position when recording chest leads.** Lead VF is recorded seven times. This mistake is surprisingly common and usually unrecognised. The correct tracing is shown in **34**.

**34**

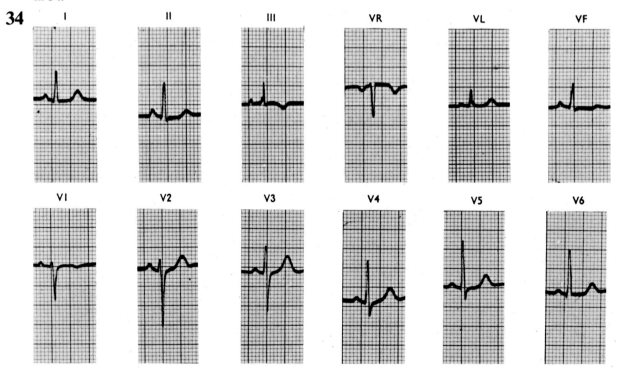

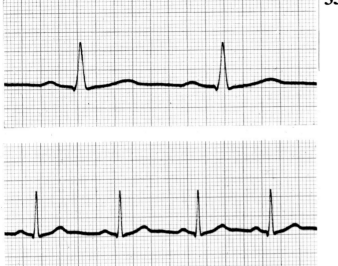

**35  Recording fault, inadvertent recording at double
speed (50mm/sec).** Wide QRST complexes, a broad
P wave, and a prolonged PR interval are the result.
The clue is the apparent sinus bradycardia. Once
again this obvious mistake is often unrecognised.
The correct trace is shown below.

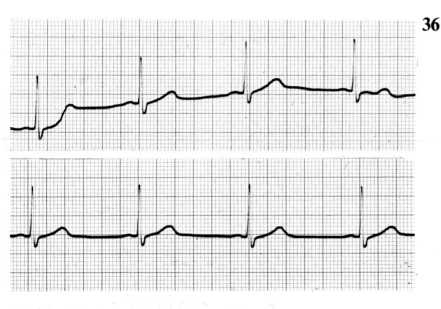

**36  Recording fault, variable baseline.** This makes
assessment of the ST segment difficult. In this
example, ST depression is apparently present. The
stable trace below is normal.

**37**

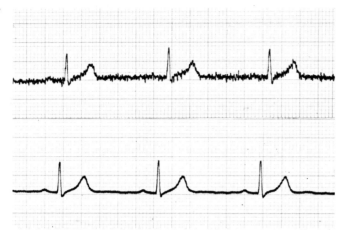

**37    Recording fault, muscle tremor.** If the patient is not properly relaxed electrical disturbance of the baseline occurs (upper line). The proper trace is shown below. Note how difficult it is to see P waves; atrial fibrillation may be mis-diagnosed.

**38**

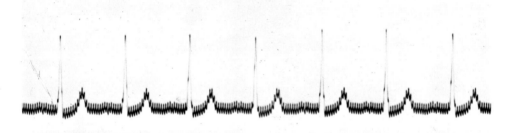

**38    Recording fault, 50-cycle AC interference.** This obscures P waves and minor ST segment shifts.

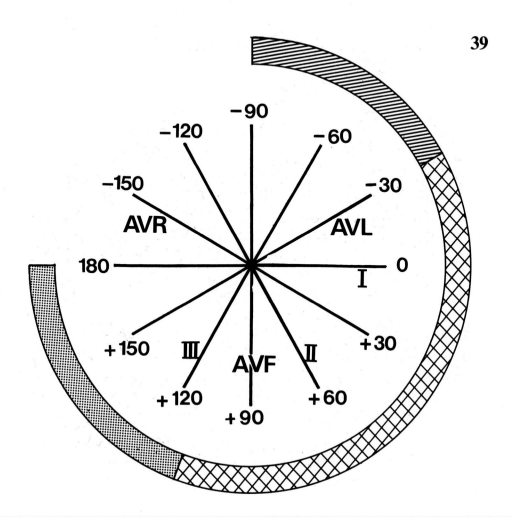

**39 Diagram for the calculation of mean frontal axis.** The axis may be determined for the P wave, the T wave, the initial and the terminal 0.04 second of the QRS complex, and the entire QRS complex, but only the last of these is in common use and the others will not be specifically referred to.

The accurate calculation of the mean QRS axis in the frontal plane necessitates planimetry. Fortunately, it is possible to arrive at a rough approximation at a glance, as long as the axis reference diagram is kept in mind, with results accurate enough for clinical purposes. If, in any of the six limb leads, the QRS complex is equiphasic, the axis lies roughly at right angles to the plane of that lead as represented in the axis diagram. Thus, for instance, equiphasic complexes in lead II mean an axis either of $-30°$ ($+60$ minus 90), or of $+150°$ ($+60$ plus 90). A glance at the other leads indicates at once which of these two possibilities is correct. In the example given, if the axis is $-30°$, the QRS will be essentially positive in lead I and negative in lead III, whereas if the axis is $+150°$, the reverse will be true. This method may also be used when no complex is equiphasic, simply by remembering the value of the plane assigned to each lead; it will be found that the axis must then lie between two adjacent planes and can be guessed at to within 15°. The examples of various QRS axes which follow are intended to illustrate this method of axis calculation.

The limits of normal are from $-30°$ to $+110°$, right axis deviation being from $+110°$ to $+180°$ and left axis deviation, from $-30°$ to $-90°$. Axes in the region from $+180°$ to $-90°$ are rare and may be either right or left. These zones are indicated on the circular strip surrounding the diagram. The axis normally shifts progressively leftwards with age.

**40**

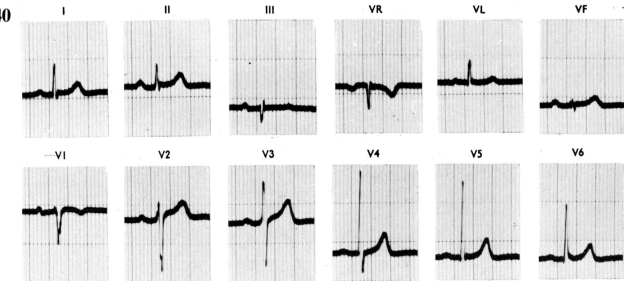

**40 Normal QRS axis of zero.** The QRS complex is equiphasic in VF and positive in leads I and VL. See **39**.

**41**

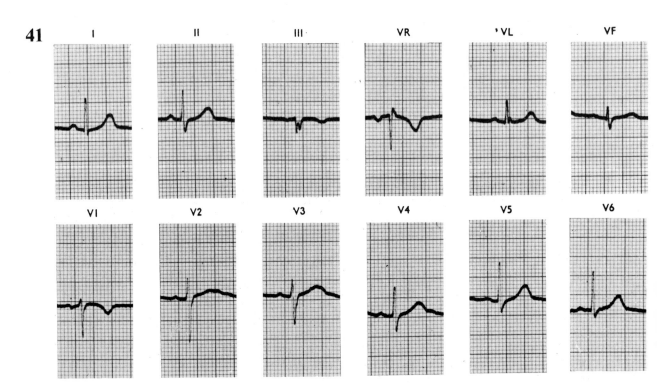

**41 Normal axis of −15°.** Allowing for width, the QRS complex is nearly equiphasic in VF and II. In the former, it veers to the negative and in the latter, to the positive side of the plane of the axis. Thus, the axis must lie between the two—a little less than zero (which would be at right-angles to VF) and a little more than −30° (which would be at right-angles to II). Minus 15° is a reasonable approximation. Note the confirmation afforded by the positive deflection in lead I. See **39**.

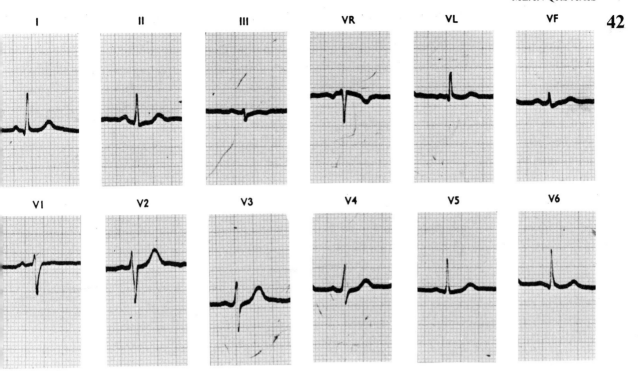

**42**  **Normal axis of +30°.** The QRS complex is very nearly equiphasic in lead III and positive in leads I and VL. As the QRS in III is actually slightly negative, a value of +25° may be more accurate. See **39**.

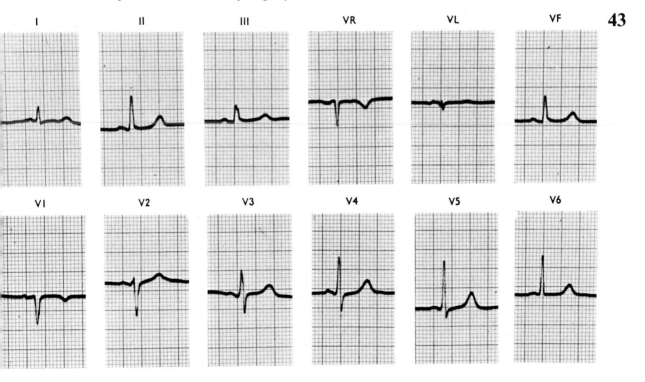

**43**  **Normal axis of +60°.** The QRS complex is very nearly equiphasic in lead VL and positive in leads I and II. See **39**.

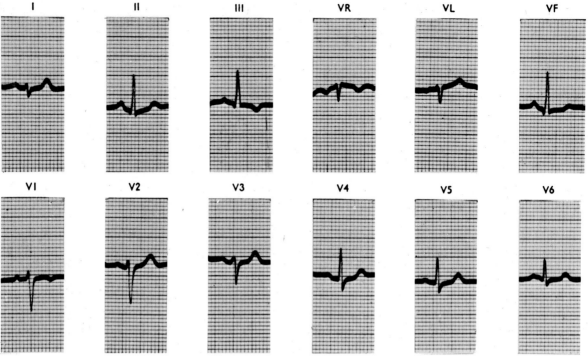

44 **Normal axis of** +95°. The QRS complex is nearly equiphasic in lead I and positive in leads II and III. Actually, it is a little negative in I but nowhere near equiphasic in VR. Thus, the axis is a trifle more than +90° but much less than +120° (which is what it would be if QRS was equiphasic in VR); 95° is a reasonable approximation. See **39**.

45 **Right axis deviation.** The QRS complex is nearly equiphasic in VR and strongly negative in leads I and VL. This makes the axis +120°, or perhaps a little more since the QRS is actually just positive in VR: +130°. To be as much as +150° (the next reference plane rightwards) there would have to be equiphasic QRS complexes in lead II which is not the case. See **39**.

Note the presence of atrial fibrillation.

46 **Right axis deviation.** The QRS complex is equiphasic in lead II, negative in lead I, and positive in lead III. The axis is thus +150° (**39**). Note the presence of P pulmonale in II and deep S waves across the chest leads. There is a tiny R wave in VL and the QS pattern in I is probably misleading in suggesting infarction; a tiny initial R wave has probably been damped out. This trace was taken from a case of cor pulmonale (see **313**).

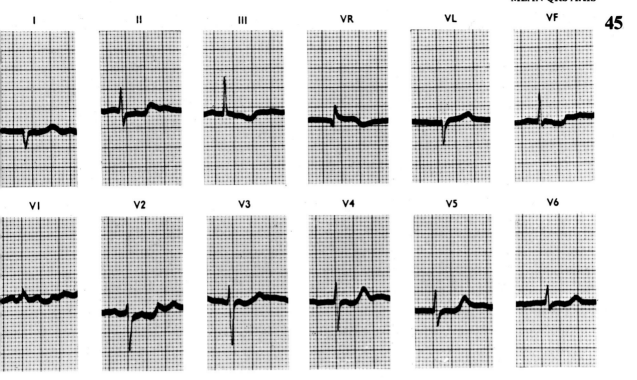

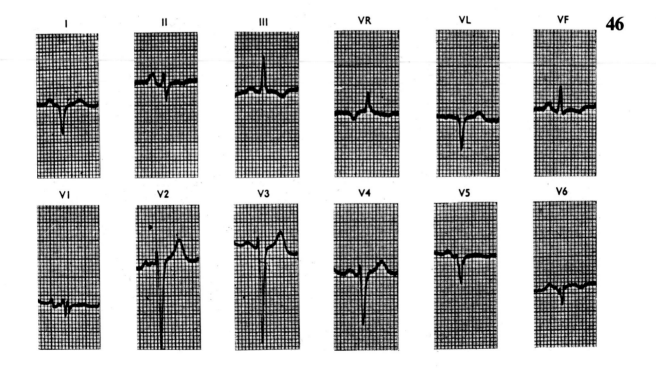

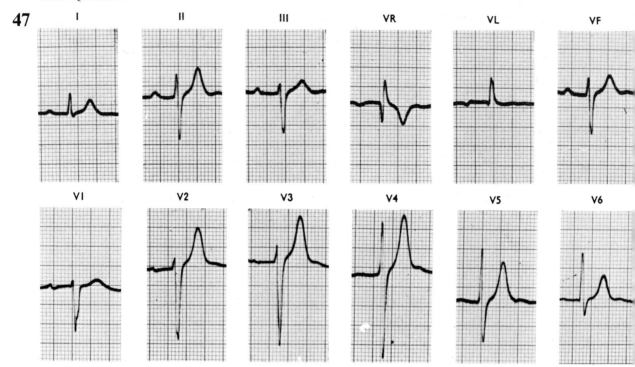

| I | II | III | VR | VL | VF |
|---|---|---|---|---|---|

| VI | V2 | V3 | V4 | V5 | V6 |
|---|---|---|---|---|---|

**47 Left axis deviation.** The QRS complex is equiphasic in lead VR, positive in lead VL and negative in lead III. The axis is thus −60°.

Note the prolonged PR interval. See **39** and **320–341**.

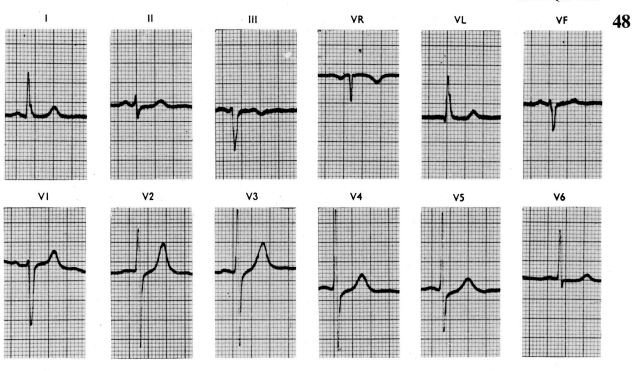

**48   Left axis deviation.** The QRS complex is nearly equiphasic in lead II, positive in lead I and negative in lead III. Actually, it is slightly negative in lead II, thus carrying the axis just beyond the limit of normality, probably −40°. See **39**.

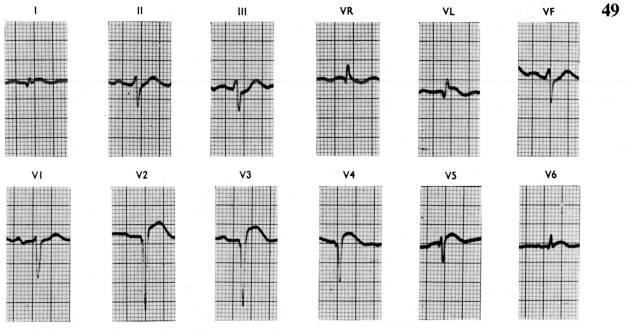

**49   Left axis deviation.** The QRS complex is equiphasic in lead I and negative in leads II and III. The axis is thus −90°. See **39**.

Note the presence of an extensive full-thickness infarction.

**50**

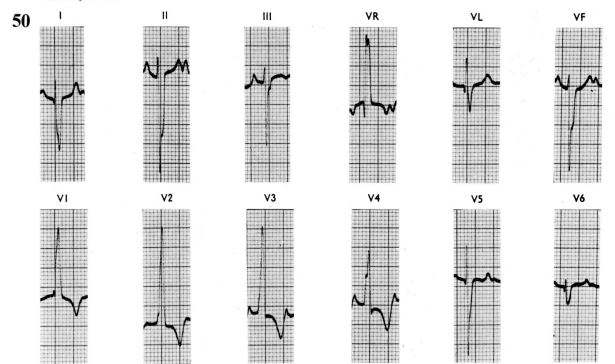

**50 Axis in the range −90° to −180°.** The QRS complex is nearly equiphasic in VL (actually slightly negative), negative in I, II and III, and positive in VR. The axis is thus about −130°. See **39**. The presence of right ventricular hypertrophy and incomplete right bundle branch block make it likely that this is extreme right, rather than left, axis deviation. Note the presence of P pulmonale (in lead II).

**51**

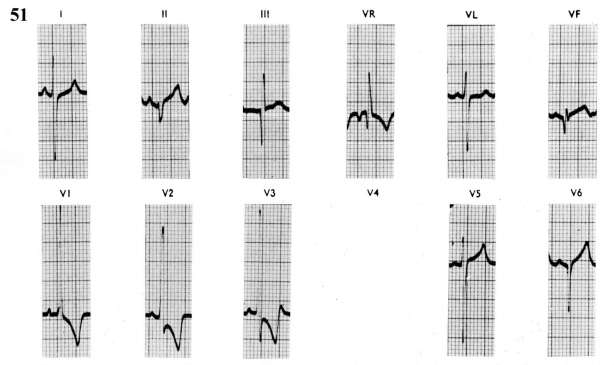

**51 Axis in the range −90° to −180°.** The QRS complex is equiphasic in lead III, and negative in leads I and II. The axis is thus −150°. See **39**. The right ventricular hypertrophy indicates that this is extreme right axis deviation. There is early P pulmonale. N.B. V2 recorded at half sensitivity.

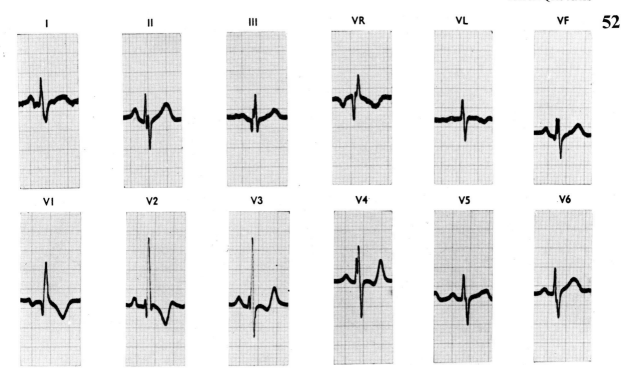

**52, 53 Indeterminate axis.** The calculation of the mean frontal QRS axis is only possible because usually, the vector loop of the ventricular forces is elongated and therefore has a definite direction. In some instances however, the loop is round and wide and in these patients the mean axis cannot be calculated because the forces have no obvious resultant. Two examples are shown, both showing the pattern of incomplete right bundle branch block. In the limb leads all complexes are equiphasic.

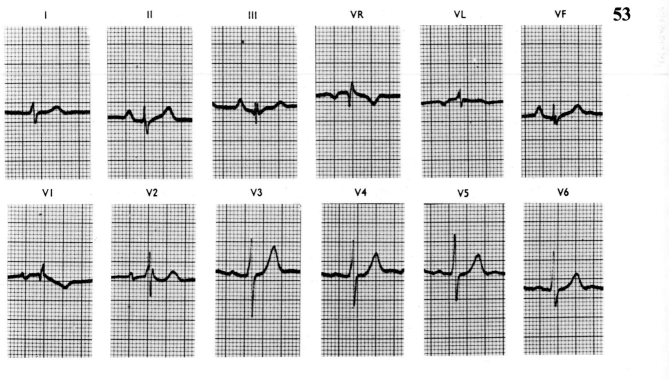

**54**

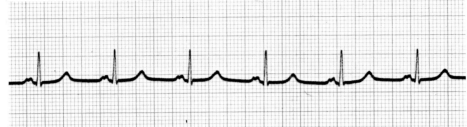

**54 Early P mitrale.** The P wave is bifid but its duration is less than 0.12 second.

**55**

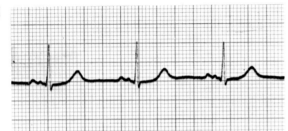

**55 P mitrale.** The P wave is bifid and has a duration of 0.12 second or more. The first peak represents right atrial, and the second, left atrial activation.

**56**

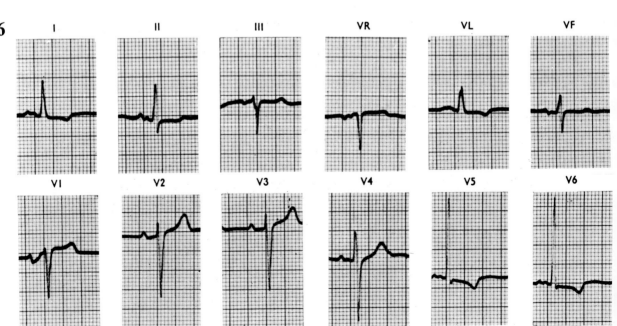

**56 P mitrale, 12-lead electrocardiogram.** P mitrale is seen better in some leads than in others. In VI the second (left atrial) component is negative.

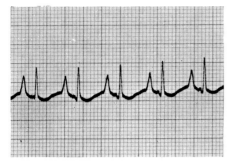

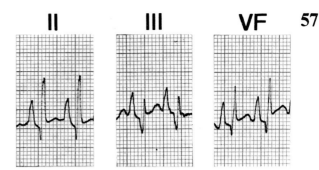

**57   P pulmonale.** The P wave is tall and peaked, being at least 2.5mm in height. The right-hand trace shows a more marked example; leads II, III and VF from a baby with severe right atrial hypertrophy. Here, P waves attain a height of 6mm, rivalling the QRS complexes in these leads. See also **58** and **311–315**.

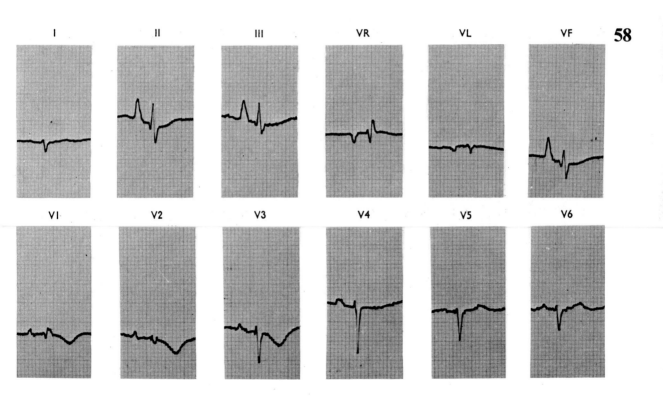

**58**

**58   P pulmonale, 12-lead electrocardiogram.** Note that P pulmonale is seen better in some leads than others, notably II, III and VF. In other instances it is also well seen in V1 and V2. Note the right axis deviation and the rS pattern of right ventricular hypertrophy (see **311, 312**) in the chest leads.

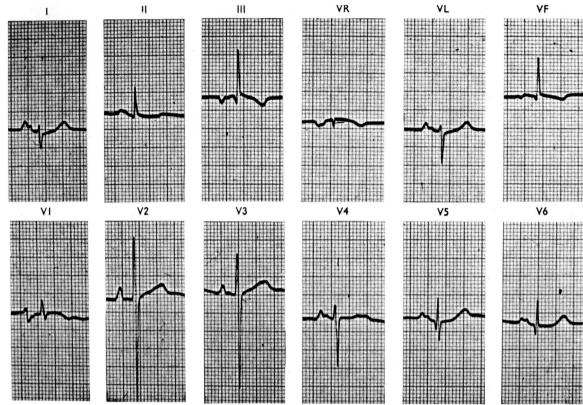

**59**   **Combined P mitrale and pulmonale.** The first peak of the P wave is tall, but there is a second peak and the duration is 0.12 second or more. The usual source is a case of mitral disease with pulmonary hypertension. Note the biventricular hypertrophy and right axis deviation. (See **317**.)

See also **453**.

# SINO-ATRIAL ARRHYTHMIAS

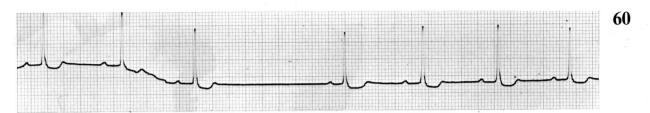

**60   Sino-atrial block.** Sporadic failure of discharge of the sino-atrial node. The atria are not activated and the P wave is absent. Unless an escape beat occurs there is a pause equal to twice the basic interval between sinus beats.

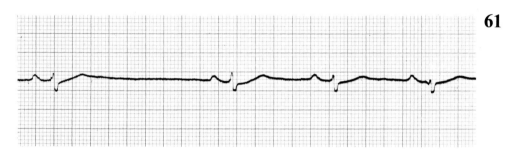

**61   Partial sino-atrial block, Wenckebach periods.** Like heart block proper, sino-atrial block may be partial. Since the actual discharge from the sino-atrial node (as distinct from its effects) cannot be seen, the presence of partial block has to be inferred from subsequent events. This record (unfortunately incomplete) begins with a sinus beat followed by a pause due to a dropped beat. The next three beats show a progressive reduction in interval between events (here, P waves) that is characteristic of Wenckebach periods (**241**). Confirmatory evidence would be a longer P–P interval after the dropped beat than before it, and a P–P interval enclosing the dropped beat less than twice the P–P interval preceding it. If, as seems probable, the three-beat cycle on this trace was followed by a dropped beat similar to the one recorded, then this confirmation exists.

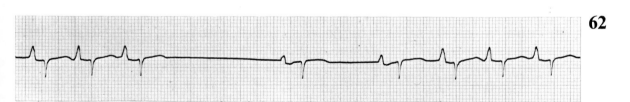

**62   Sinus arrest.** Failure of discharge of the sino-atrial node leads to cessation of the heart beat for a short period unrelated to the basic interbeat interval as in sino-atrial block, though the distinction is not always easy to make. In this situation escape rhythms are very likely to occur but need not do so if the pause is a brief one.

**63**

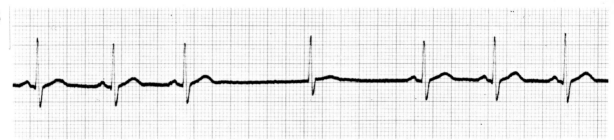

**63 Sinus arrest with atrioventricular junctional escape beat.** Following temporary cessation of sino-atrial node activity a focus in the atrioventricular junction activates the heart for one beat before sinus activity resumes. See also **20**.

**64**

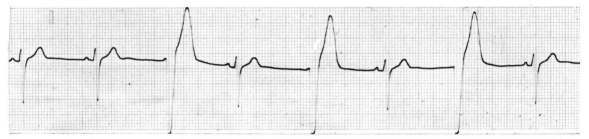

**64 Sino-atrial block with ventricular escape beats.** The situation is similar to **63** but here, the focus which takes over is situated in the ventricles. The cessation of sinus nodal activity in this instance is sino-atrial block because the gap is approximately twice the basic interval between sinus beats.

**65**

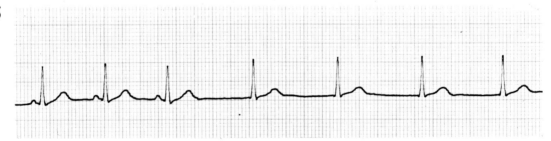

**65 Sinus arrest with atrioventricular junctional escape rhythm.** Cessation of sino-atrial nodal activity leads to control of the heart being assumed by an atrioventricular junctional escape rhythm at a slower rate. See also **20**.

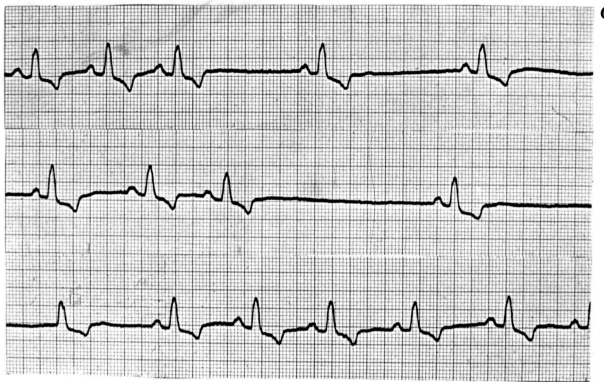

**66   Carotid sinus hypersensitivity.** Pressure on the
carotid sinus produces episodes of sino-atrial block
or sinus arrest, often prolonged. This occurs mostly
in the elderly. The three lines are a single strip cut
up. There is bundle branch block present.

**67**

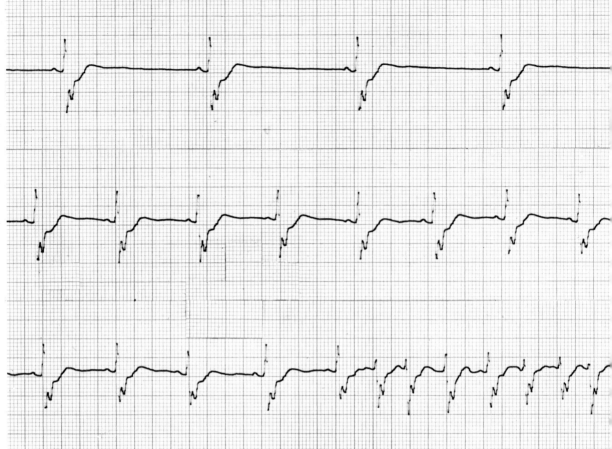

**68**

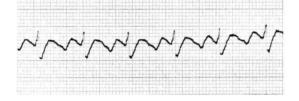

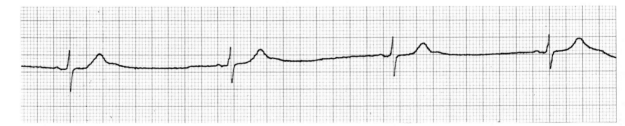

**67, 68 The sick sinus syndrome.** This is characterised by periods of marked sinus brady-cardia, atrioventricular junctional bradycardia, or sinus arrest, alternating with episodes of tachy-arrhythmias such as atrial or atrioventricular junctional tachycardia, atrial fibrillation, or atrial flutter. Figure **67** shows a continuous strip in three rows. It begins with sinus bradycardia, returns to sinus rhythm at normal rates, and on the last line, changes to rapid atrial fibrillation. Aberrant conduction of the QRS complex is present throughout. Figure **68** shows two traces taken at different times from the same patient. Above, the rhythm is atrial flutter with 2:1 block; below, extreme sinus bradycardia is present.

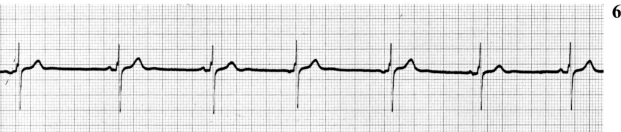

**69 Wandering pacemaker between the sinus node and atrioventricular junction.** When the sinus node and atrioventricular junction have nearly identical rates of discharge, control of the ventricle may pass from one to the other in a random fashion as either speeds up or slows down. The trace illustrated begins with a junctional complex followed by two sinus beats. The fourth complex is also junctional, though its preceding P wave (see **74**) differs slightly in shape from that seen in complex 1. Complex 5 resembles complex 1. Complex 6 has a P wave that is biphasic, and unlike any of the others. The last beat is sinus. Despite the slight irregularity of rate, none of these junctional beats is sufficiently premature to be labelled as an extrasystole. See also **20** and **22**.

**70**

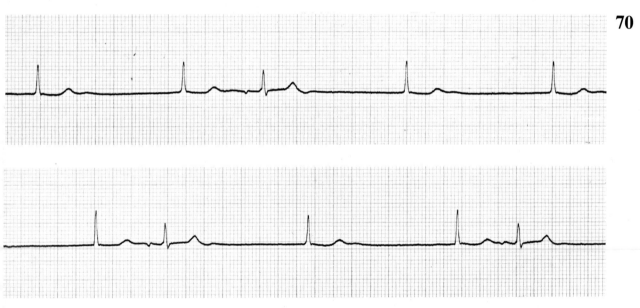

**70 Escape capture bigeminy.** This term is applied to the situation illustrated: an irregular sinus bradycardia at a very slow rate with atrioventricular junctional escape beats. The result is that a P wave appears sandwiched between two QRS complexes, mimicking reciprocal beats (see **79**). In fact, although the P waves in this trace are biphasic and might be mistaken for retrograde P waves, they appear too late for this, and the interval between the preceding junctional beat and the P waves can be seen to alter.

**71**

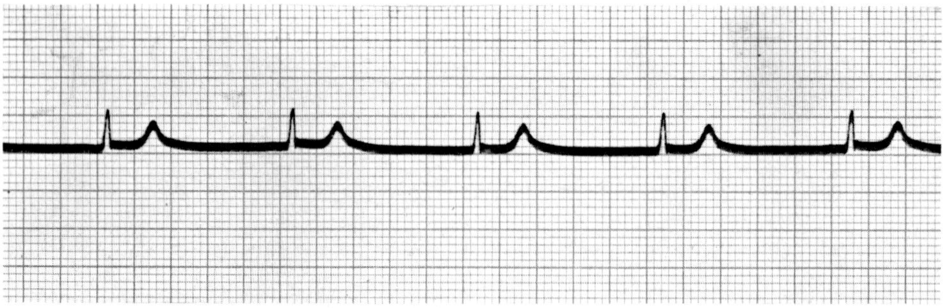

**71 Atrioventricular junctional rhythm.** No P waves are visible. Either they are buried in the QRST complex, antegrade and retrograde conduction times being identical, or atrial standstill is present. To exclude atrial fibrillation with junctional rhythm (see **220**) it is necessary to examine the baseline in several leads carefully for 'f' waves, for they can be inconspicuous (**216**).

**72**

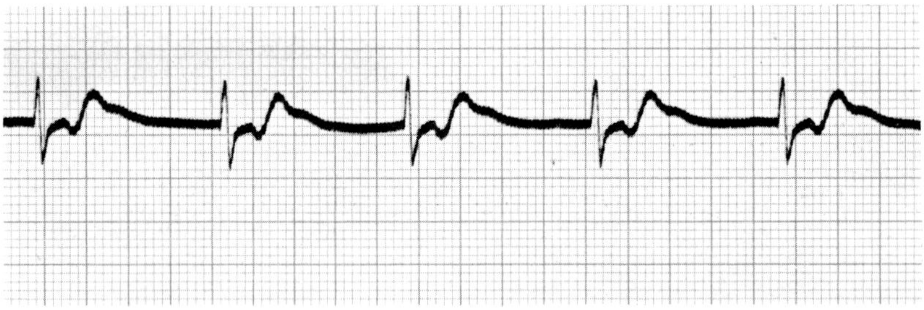

**72 Atrioventricular junctional rhythm.** In this instance there is delayed retrograde conduction to the atria, so inverted P waves follow the QRS complexes and distort the ST segments.

**73**

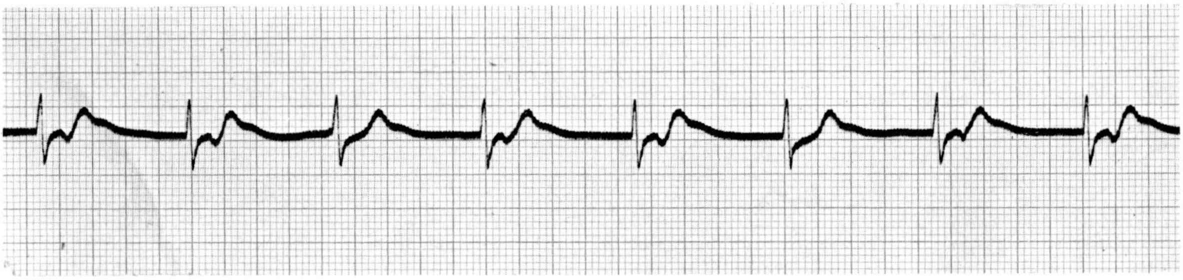

**73 Atrioventricular junctional rhythm with 2:1 retrograde block.** In this example, retrograde atrial activation occurs after alternate beats only in two places.

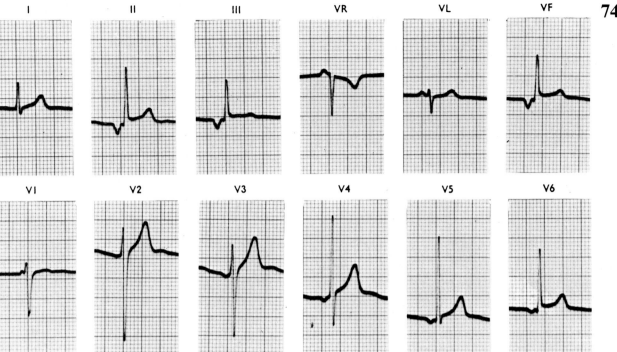

**74 Coronary sinus rhythm.** This name was originally applied to junctional rhythm with inverted P waves immediately preceding the QRS complexes, the reasoning being that the pacemaker was likely to be situated in the proximal part of the atrioventricular node near the mouth of the coronary sinus to account for early atrial activation, but the exact origin of such rhythms arising in the atrioventricular junction cannot be determined from the surface electrocardiogram. See **119**. The pattern is produced by marked delay in antegrade compared with retrograde conduction and the PR interval may be short or normal. The inverted P waves are best seen in II, III, and VF.

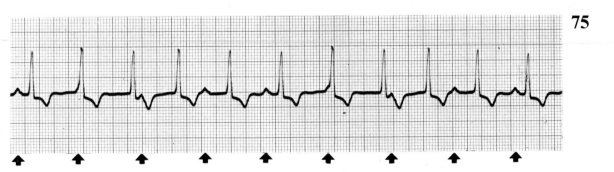

**75  Atrioventricular junctional rhythm: atrioventricular dissociation.** The ventricles are paced by the atrioventricular junction. The atria are beating independently at a slower rate and, therefore, retrograde block is present. Note the increased height of the QRS complex when a P wave coincides with it. P waves are arrowed.

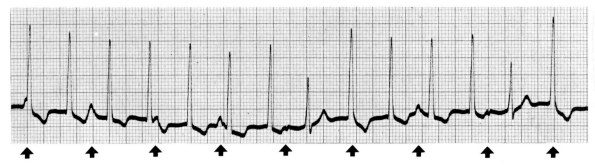

**76 Atrioventricular junctional rhythm with retrograde block and capture beats.** Atrioventricular dissociation is present, with the ventricles controlled by the atrioventricular junction and beating faster than the atria. P waves are arrowed to assist analysis. The fifth and eighth P waves find the atrioventricular junction non-refractory and a normal sinus beat follows—i.e. a capture beat. Although retrograde block is present (for no inverted and out-of-time P waves can be seen), this does not mean that there is no attempt at retrograde conduction and indeed there is indirect evidence for this in the long PR interval of the capture beats, implying impaired conduction in the atrioventricular junction due to partial refractoriness. This state of partial refractoriness accounts for the timing of P waves that are, or are not, successful in capturing the ventricles—e.g. the second P wave might expect to do so if the PR interval were shorter. Note the difference in the shape of the junctional and sinus beats though both are clearly supraventricular in origin (**113**), and the increased height of the QRS complexes when P coincides with them.

**77 Atrioventricular dissociation with paired capture beats.** The illustration shows a continuous strip in three rows. The ventricles are controlled by a junctional rhythm at a rate faster than the discharge of the sinus node. P waves are arrowed. At frequent intervals the P wave falls onto the ST segment and after a long PR interval a capture beat of slightly different contour is produced. The next beat on every occasion is another sinus (capture) beat with a normal PR interval, and thereafter junctional rhythm resumes. The second capture beat is only possible because of the delay imposed by the long PR interval of the first capture beat (for without this the faster junctional rhythm would anticipate it) and this is because each junctional beat is accompanied by concealed retrograde conduction into the atrioventricular junction above the junctional pacemaker itself—hence the long PR interval, due to partial refractoriness, or, looked at another way, the prematurity of the P waves which capture. Note too that the PR interval of the second capture beat varies directly with the prematurity of the first P wave to capture—another manifestation of residual, partial junctional refractoriness.

**78 Atrioventricular dissociation and capture beats with partial heart block.** In this example of atrioventricular dissociation with capture beats, forward conduction through the atrioventricular junction, when it occurs, is complicated by Wenckebach block. All P waves are arrowed to assist analysis. The complex marked 1 is premature and is a capture beat from the preceding P wave. Note the long PR interval—explained in **76**. The next beat (2), though preceded by a P wave, is junctional, and not conducted, for it follows beat 1 by the basic inter-beat interval of the junctional rhythm, and the apparently normal PR interval is, paradoxically, too short for antegrade conduction in this situation. The next beat again (3) is much earlier and no intervening P wave is seen. This reveals the true state of affairs; beat 3 is a capture beat with a much longer PR interval than the first— i.e. it relates to the P wave immediately before beat 2. Thereafter junctional rhythm resumes.

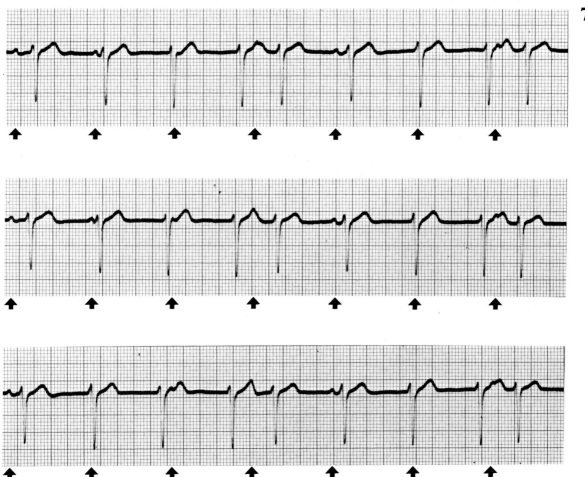

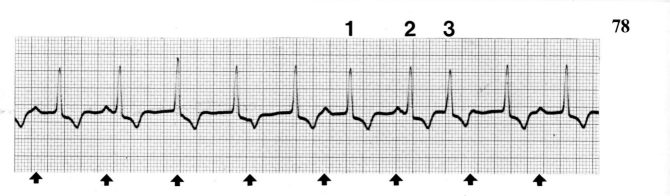

**79**

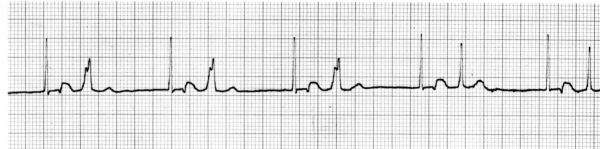

**79  Reciprocal beats.** This phenomenon depends on the presence of two paths of conduction within the atrioventricular junction which may be separately activated so that an impulse may traverse the junction in one direction and immediately return in the other by a different route. The trace illustrates the only common situation in which this occurs. The basic rhythm is junctional, and each QRS is followed by a clearly retrograde P wave. This in turn re-traverses the junction to capture the ventricles in a series of reciprocal beats. The first three reciprocal beats show aberrant conduction; the last two do not. The difference may be explained by the marginally longer PR interval of the latter. See also **121**.

**80**

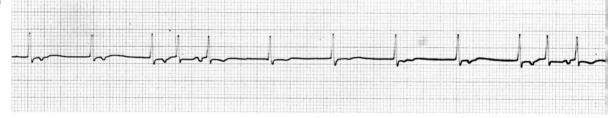

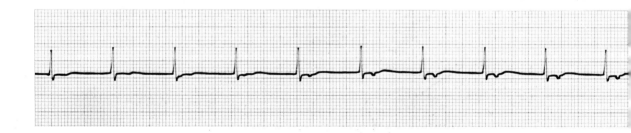

**80  Reciprocal beats with partial retrograde block.** The illustration is a continuous strip in two rows. It begins with junctional rhythm with retrograde conduction to the atria as evidenced by the inverted P waves deforming the ST segments. The third *RP* interval is a little longer than the preceding ones and is late enough to find the ventricle responsive when it re-enters the atrioventricular node by the alternative pathway (see **79**). This reciprocal beat is in its turn conducted retrogradely through the junction and now the RP interval is longer. The next beat, though a trifle premature, may well belong to the basic junctional rhythm for it seems to follow the preceding P wave too closely to be related to it in view of the time relations of the reciprocal beat. For two beats thereafter, retrograde conduction ceases altogether but reappears towards the end of the top line, when the whole cycle is repeated. Once again (lower line) retrograde conduction is lost for several beats after the episode of retrograde Wenckebach block.

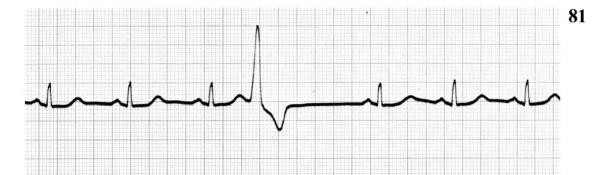

**81 Ventricular extrasystole.** The QRS shape is bizarre and the T wave abnormal; no preceding P wave is present. Usually, though not invariably, the QRST will have the contour of left rather than right bundle branch block in the appropriate lead (see **92**). The sino-atrial node discharges at the usual time but the impulse finds the ventricle refractory; the P wave is not usually visible, being obscured by the T wave of the extrasystole. A pause follows until the next sinus beat is due—the so-called 'compensatory' pause. The interval between the two beats enclosing the extrasystole is, therefore, equal to twice the interbeat interval of the basic sinus rhythm and the compensatory pause is said to be 'full'.

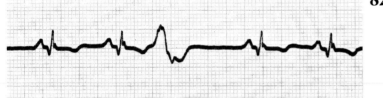

**82 Ventricular extrasystole.** In this instance, the blocked P wave which occurs during the ventricular extrasystole can be seen deforming the ST segment.

**83**

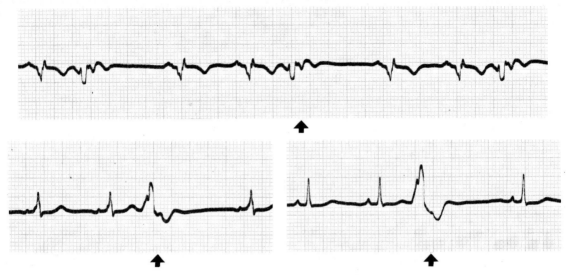

**83 Ventricular extrasystole, retrograde conduction.** The retrograde activation of the atria by a ventricular extrasystole is not uncommon but it is not always possible to demonstrate, for it tends to occur roughly at the time that the next normal P wave is due in any case. It may be suspected when there is a deformity in the ST segment of the extrasystole which is definitely premature in relation to the next expected P wave and has a different shape from it (usually inverted). The illustration shows three leads from one electro-cardiogram. In each, the arrow points to such a deformity in one of the extrasystoles which fulfils these criteria. The inverted blip in the upper strip is the most convincing. Note that it is not easy to decide whether the inverted wave or the positive deflection which follows it is the abnormal P wave, and this is where the timing becomes all-important. Recapture of the ventricles may occur (i.e. a reciprocal beat, see **79**) and will provide additional evidence—in fact, many apparently interpolated extrasystoles may be examples of this mechanism.

**84**

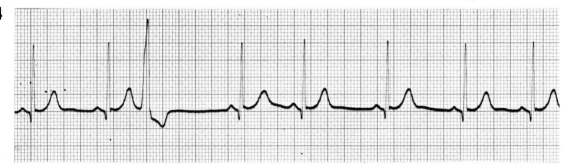

**84 Ventricular extrasystole; effect of sinus arrhythmia on compensatory pause.** For obvious reasons (**81**) a change in the basic rate alters the length of the post-extrasystolic pause. This is most commonly seen with sinus arrhythmia as the heart slows and speeds up. Also see **122** and **101**. In this trace the pause following the ventricular extrasystole is, thus, incomplete because the next beat is early.

Note the slight alteration in T wave height in the post-extrasystolic beat (see **85, 86**).

**85**

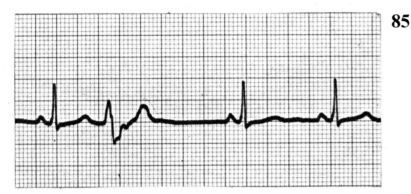

**85 T wave changes in the first post-extrasystolic beat.** The first complex after the extrasystole shows a flat T wave compared to surrounding beats. Sometimes the T wave is taller. Opinions differ as to whether this indicates myocardial disease. See also **84, 86, 117, 122**.

**86**

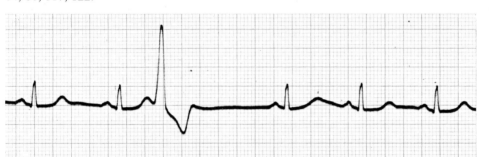

**86 T wave changes in the first post-extrasystolic beat.** In this example, there is prolongation of the QT interval, the T wave is a little taller, and the U wave is much more prominent.

**87**

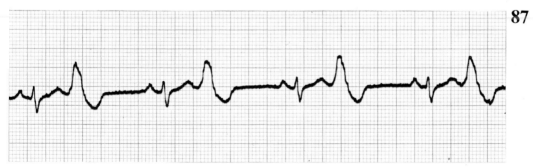

**87 Coupling with unifocal ventricular extra-systoles.** Every alternate beat is a ventricular extrasystole having the same contour and following the previous sinus beat by the same interval or 'coupling time', indicating a single point of origin. Such a rhythm is often stable over a very long period.

　　N.B. Coupling time is measured from the beginning of the QRS of the preceding beat to the beginning of the extrasystole.

**88**

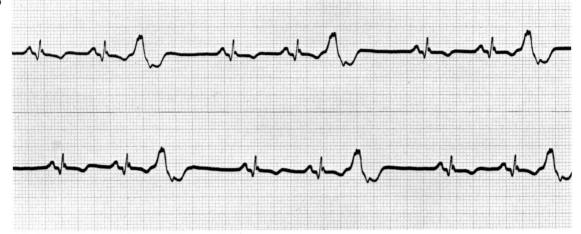

**88 Unifocal ventricular extrasystoles occurring regularly after every second sinus beat.** As defined in **87**, these extrasystoles are unifocal. The two lines are a single strip cut up.

**89**

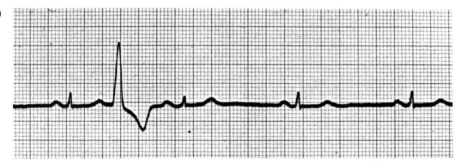

**89 Interpolated ventricular extrasystole.** A ventricular extrasystole falls between two sinus beats without interrupting the basic sinus rhythm. This is most likely to occur when the extrasystole occurs early in diastole and the basic heart rate is slow. Note the prolongation of the PR interval of the post-extrasystolic beat due to concealed conduction retrogradely into the atrioventricular junction which renders it partially refractory to the next beat (see **76** and **120**).

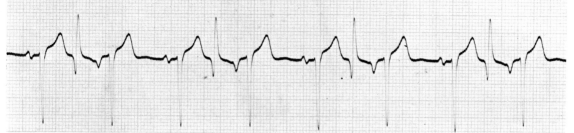

**90 Regularly occurring interpolated ventricular extrasystoles.** Note the prolongation of the PR interval of the post-extrasystolic beats, the P wave deforming the T wave of the extrasystole.

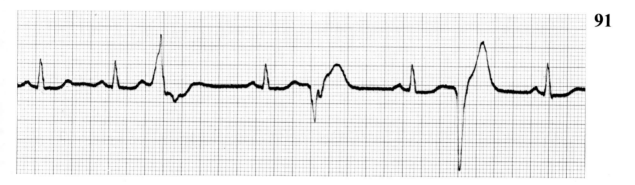

**91**

**91 Multifocal ventricular extrasystoles.** The three ventricular extrasystoles on this trace all have different shapes and all have different coupling times, thus confirming their different sites of origin. The latter point is important since unifocal extrasystoles occasionally vary in contour (see **94**).

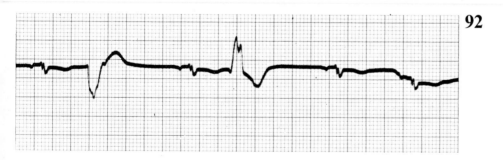

**92**

**92 Multifocal ventricular extrasystoles, ventricle of origin.** This is best determined in a lead in which characteristic patterns are produced in bundle branch block, e.g. V1, as in the illustration. Extrasystoles arising in the right ventricle show the pattern of left bundle branch block (first extrasystole) and those arising in the left ventricle, the pattern of right bundle branch block (second extrasystole).

**93**

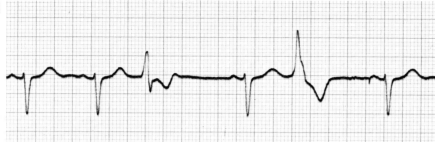

**93 Unifocal ventricular extrasystoles with varying contour.** There are two extrasystoles on this trace and at first sight they appear to arise from different foci. There is, however, an alternative explanation. To be certain that two extrasystoles arise from different foci, one of the criteria is that they should have different coupling times. Here, the coupling times are identical, thus raising the possibility that both arise from the same focus but pursue different conduction paths within the ventricle. *Multiform* extrasystoles of this kind are often seen in digitalis toxicity. See also **95, 226, 228**.

**94**

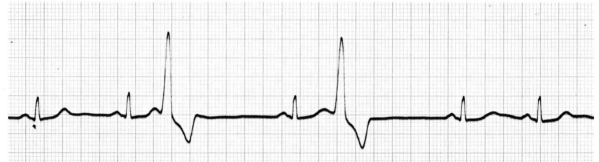

**94 Multifocal ventricular extrasystoles of similar contour.** The two ventricular extrasystoles on this trace appear very similar in shape but they have slightly different coupling times and are, therefore, multifocal, though from adjacent sites.

**95**

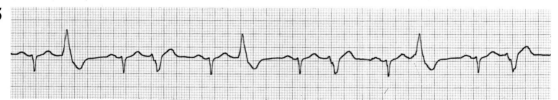

**95 Coupling with alternation of ventricular extrasystoles.** Every other beat is a ventricular extrasystole, and alternate extrasystoles show a different contour, pointing in opposite directions. Although this suggests two foci, probably in different ventricles, all the extrasystoles have the same time relationship to the preceding beat and this is probably another example of unifocal, multiform extrasystoles (see **93**). Another example of this arrhythmia is illustrated under atrial fibrillation (**226**).

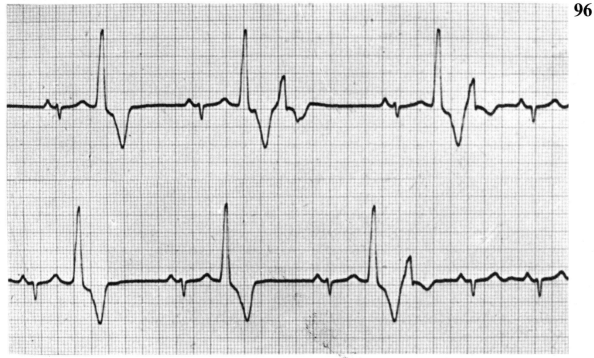

**96   Linked ventricular extrasystoles.** There are two extrasystolic ventricular foci in this trace. The discharge from one is linked to the other. The two lines are a single strip cut up.

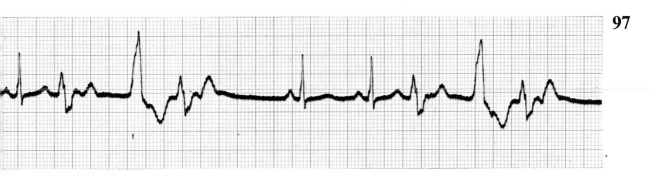

**97   Linked ventricular extrasystoles.** Another, more complex example, in which a sequence of three extrasystoles recurs.

**98**

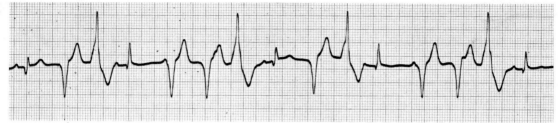

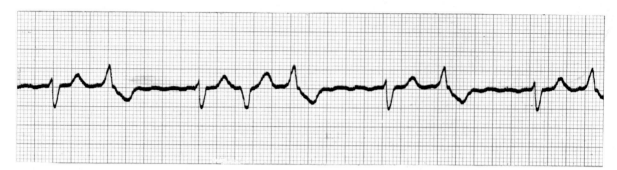

**98 Bidirectional ventricular extrasystoles.** Although coupled and linked ventricular extrasystoles of any kind are commonly due to digitalis intoxication, the occurrence of brief runs or pairs of extrasystoles in which successive beats point in opposite directions suggests digitalis toxicity more strongly. Two examples are illustrated, one in sinus rhythm and the other in atrial fibrillation.

**99**

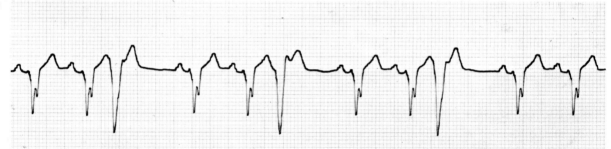

**99 Very premature ventricular extrasystoles.** The timing of ventricular extrasystoles is of some importance. If they are very premature, the QRS of the extrasystole may fall close to the peak of the T wave of the preceding beat—the so-called 'R on T' phenomenon. At this point in the cardiac cycle the risk of inducing ventricular tachycardia and fibrillation by small electrical potentials is very high (see **183**, and also **210** and **235**).

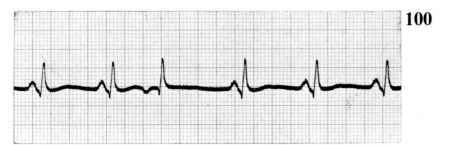

**100**

**100 Atrial extrasystole.** The third beat is premature; it has the same QRS shape as surrounding beats. It is preceded by a P wave which is of a different shape to the normal P waves because it arises well away from the sino-atrial node. There is slight prolongation of the PR interval of the extrasystole because its premature appearance finds the atrioventricular junction still partially refractory. The extrasystole discharges the sino-atrial node prematurely, so the compensatory pause which follows is 'incomplete', i.e. the interval between the two sinus beats enclosing the extrasystole is less than twice the basic interbeat interval of the sinus rhythm. See **81**.

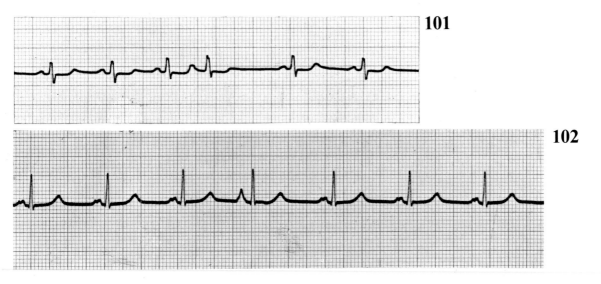

**101**

**102**

**101, 102 Atrial extrasystole beat with long compensatory pause.** Not all atrial extrasystoles are followed by an incomplete compensatory pause. There are three reasons: a changing heart rate (**101**) which may even produce a longer than full compensatory pause; an extrasystole occurring relatively late in diastole (**102**, fourth beat) which fails to reach the sino-atrial node before its next discharge takes place, so that, although the sinus node cannot capture the now-refractory atria, the fundamental rhythm of the heart is undisturbed, as happens with ventricular extrasystoles; or depression of the automaticity of the sinus node following its premature discharge.

**103**

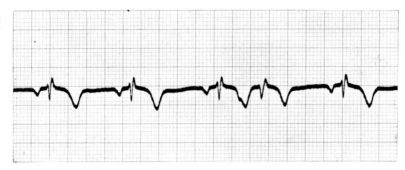

**103  Atrial extrasystole.** The illustration shows marked prolongation of the PR interval of the extrasystole (the P wave can be seen deforming the descending limb of the T wave of the beat before). This occurs when the atrial extrasystole is fairly early in diastole so that the refractoriness of the atrioventricular junction is relatively high. (Extrasystoles arising low in the atrium may have short PR intervals and are indistinguishable from junctional extrasystoles, see **119**.)

**104**

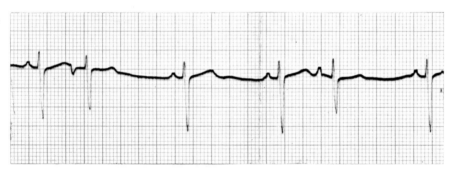

**104  Multifocal atrial extrasystoles.** The second and fifth beats are both atrial extrasystoles but differ in P wave shape, PR interval, and timing relationship to the preceding complex. Clearly, they arise from different foci. Note the different QRS shape these beats have; this is discussed in **106, 107**.

**105**

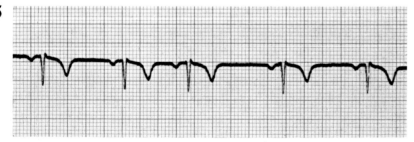

**105  Atrial extrasystole.** In this example, the atrial extrasystole has a P wave which is identical with the P waves of surrounding beats and a PR interval which is only marginally longer. These features indicate that the extrasystolic focus is situated very close to the sino-atrial node itself. True sino-atrial nodal extrasystoles are very rare: they have P waves and PR intervals which are identical with those of surrounding beats and the next beat follows after an interval identical to that of the interbeat interval of the fundamental sinus rhythm.

**106**

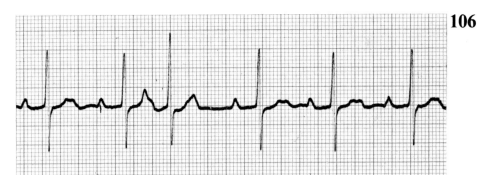

**107**

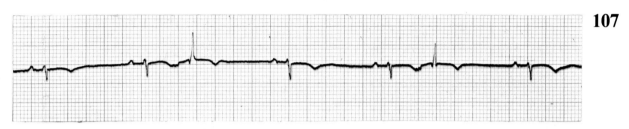

**106, 107 Variation in the contour of the QRS complex of atrial extrasystoles.** Although arising above the atrioventricular junction, atrial ectopic beats do not necessarily have the same QRS contour as surrounding beats, even if the duration of QRS is not prolonged. Presumably this is due to a slight alteration in ventricular activation caused by incomplete recovery from the refractory state. Figure **106** shows such an extrasystole (third beat).

Depending on the lead, this alteration may be dramatic—**107** shows two extrasystoles arising from the same focus (third and sixth beats) which show an entirely different contour, yet they are clearly atrial extrasystoles. Note that all three extrasystoles show a prolonged PR interval and have P waves deforming the T waves of the preceding beat. See also **103** and **111**.

**108**

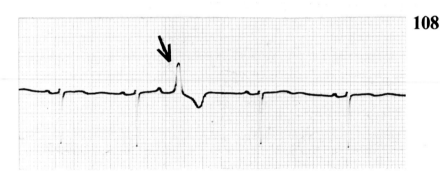

**108 Atrial extrasystole with aberrant conduction.** The marked beat is premature. It is an atrial extrasystole, being preceded by a P wave which deforms the T wave of the beat before, and being followed by a pause which is less than fully compensatory, but the QRS is wide and bizarre in shape due to aberrant conduction.

**109**

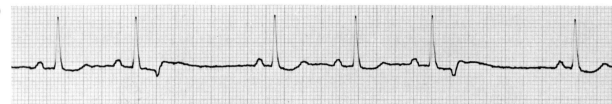

**109 Blocked atrial extrasystoles.** The second and fifth beats of this record show a deformity in the ST segment caused by the inverted P waves of atrial extrasystoles which, on account of their prematurity, find the atrioventricular junction refractory, and are thus blocked.

**110**

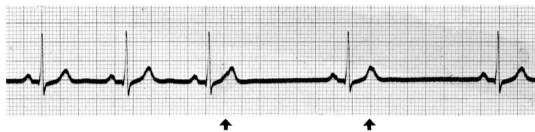

**110 Blocked atrial extrasystoles mimicking sino-atrial block.** In this trace a sudden drop in rate raises the suspicion of sino-atrial block, but the rate is not exactly halved as it should be, and close examination of the T waves of the third and fourth complexes reveals that they are deformed by P waves (arrowed). These are atrial extrasystoles which are blocked because they are so premature.

**111**

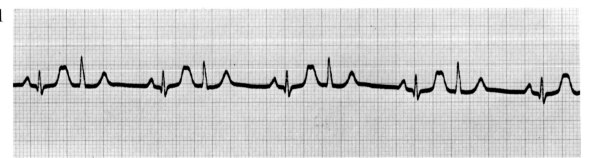

**111 Coupling with atrial extrasystoles.** The P wave of each extrasystole deforms the T wave of the preceding T wave giving it a bifid apex. As usual, the PR interval of the extrasystole is prolonged and in addition, it shows a different QRS shape (see **106, 107**).

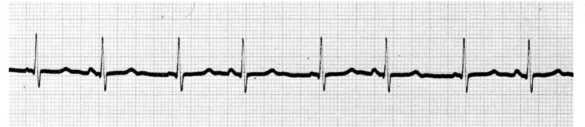

**112   Coupled supraventricular beats.** In this trace, complexes which are all clearly supraventricular are occurring in pairs. The PR interval of the first beat of each pair is below the limit of normality while the PR interval of the second is normal. The possible interpretations are: sinus rhythm with the Lown–Ganong–Levine syndrome (see **171**) and coupled atrial extrasystoles, junctional rhythm with coupled atrial extrasystoles, or sinus rhythm with junctional escape beats (i.e. the sinus beats are the second of each pair).

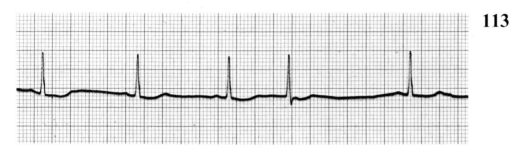

**113   Atrioventricular junctional extrasystoles.** The fourth beat is premature. It has a narrow QRS complex or normal duration and is clearly supraventricular in origin. Note that it differs slightly in shape from surrounding sinus beats, as is often the case in beats arising in the atrioventricular junction, presumably because the pathway of ventricular activation is slightly altered by the abnormal site of origin of activation within the atrioventricular junction itself (see also **76, 116**). In this instance no P wave accompanying the junctional QRS can be seen for certain though it may be deforming the T wave. P waves with junctional extrasystoles are dealt with in **114, 115**.

**114**

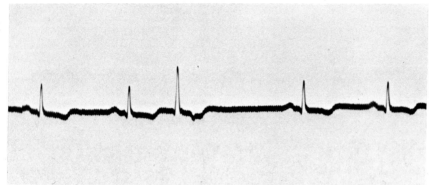

**115**

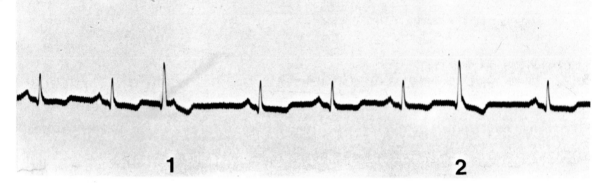

1                                         2

**114, 115 Atrioventricular junctional extrasystoles and P waves.** Junctional extrasystoles may or may not be conducted retrogradely to the atrium. If they are (**114**) an inverted P wave is seen deforming the ST segment, as in junctional rhythm (**72**). In such cases, the post-extrasystolic pause may or may not be fully compensatory, obeying the same rules as with atrial extrasystoles (see **100**–**102**). If retrograde block is present (**115**) the next normal P wave will either be seen in the ST segment of the extrasystole (1) or will coincide with its QRS (2), the post-extrasystolic pause being full, as with a ventricular extrasystole. Note that in **115** the different P wave position is due to two things—a change in heart rate and an alteration in the timing of the extrasystoles with respect to preceding beats. Junctional extrasystoles preceded by inverted P waves (as in coronary sinus rhythm—see **74**) cannot readily be distinguished from low atrial extrasystoles. See **103** and **119**.

**116**

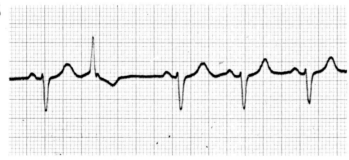

**116 Junctional extrasystole, markedly different QRS contour.** The difference in the contour of a junctional extrasystole as compared to surrounding sinus beats may be marked, as with atrial extrasystoles (see **107**); lesser changes in contour are common (**113, 114, 115, 118, 120, 121**). And see **70, 122, 230, 261**.

**117**

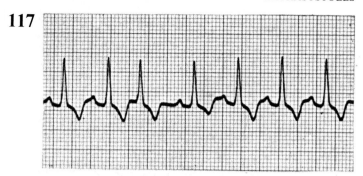

**117 Junctional extrasystole, post-extrasystolic T wave change.** The alteration in the T wave of the first post-extrasystolic beat which was described with ventricular extrasystoles (**85, 86**) may also be seen after junctional (and atrial) extrasystoles. Here, a junctional extrasystole (third complex) is followed by a complex showing less deep T wave inversion. See also **122**.

**118**

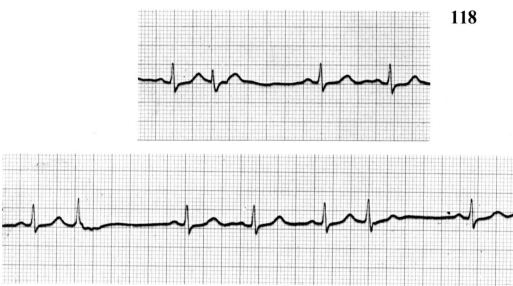

**118 Multifocal junctional extrasystoles.** The two rows of this trace are one strip cut up. Three junctional extrasystoles are seen; all show different contours and follow preceding beats by different intervals. Retrograde P waves can be seen after the first two but not the last. It is likely that these extrasystoles arise from slightly different sites within the atrioventricular junction.

**119**

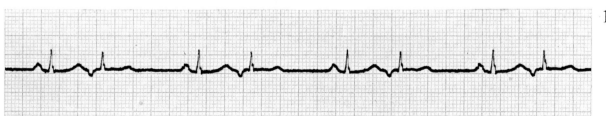

**119 Coupled junctional extrasystoles.** This trace shows coupling with supraventricular extrasystoles preceded by inverted P waves. Taken with the short PR interval, these complexes are reminiscent of coronary sinus rhythm (**74**) and may be junctional. Atrial extrasystoles are an alternative explanation. (See **111**, and also **103**).

**120**

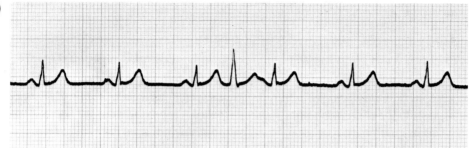

**120 Interpolated junctional extrasystole.** The fourth complex is interpolated between two sinus beats. It has a wider complex of different shape to the rest but still falls within the limits for a supraventricular complex. Note the prolonged PR interval of the first post-extrasystolic beat caused by concealed retrograde conduction of the extrasystole into the proximal part of the atrioventricular junction. (See also **89**.)

**121**

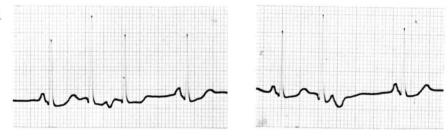

**121 Reciprocal beat following a junctional extrasystole.** Two short strips are illustrated. Both contain a junctional extrasystole differing in shape from surrounding beats. On the left, the extrasystole is followed by an inverted, premature P wave of retrograde atrial activation, and this in turn is followed by a reciprocal beat (see **79**). Note that although this beat resembles other sinus beats it is not preceded by a normal P wave. At first sight this sequence resembles an interpolated extrasystole, and the latter *are* usually followed by a prolonged PR interval, but the prematurity of the retrograde P wave, and its shape, indicate the correct answer. On the right, another junctional extrasystole from the same lead is shown for comparison. In this instance retrograde block is present and the ST segment of the extrasystole is deformed by the next normal P wave.

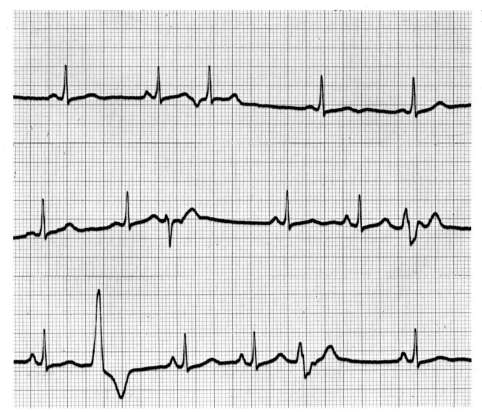

**122 Multiple and multifocal ventricular and supraventricular extrasystoles.** This short record illustrates well the three types of extrasystoles; it is a single strip in three rows. There are five extrasystoles.

1. Top line. Atrial extrasystole; no change in QRS shape, inverted P wave in preceding ST segment; compensatory pause incomplete.
2. Middle line. Junctional extrasystole; change in shape of QRS which is, however, supraventricular; inverted P wave follows QRS (deforming ST segment); compensatory pause incomplete.
3. Middle line. Ventricular extrasystole; bizarre QRS shape, full compensatory pause.
4. Lowest line. Ventricular extrasystole from a different focus from 3.
5. Lowest line. Ventricular extrasystole from the same focus as 3.

Note that the compensatory pauses are measured by reference to beats immediately surrounding the extrasystole in question; here the changing heart rate makes this imperative (see **84**). Note too the post extrasystolic T wave flattening produced by all the extrasystoles, bearing in mind that the only sinus beats definitely *not* preceded by an extrasystole are the second and fourth on the top line, the first, second and fourth on the middle line, and the third on the lowest line; the rest show T wave flattening. (See **85**, **86** and **117**.)

**123 Parasystole.** This term is used when an independent focus somewhere in the heart (commonly the ventricles) competes for control with the normal rhythm (which may, or may not, be sinus). Rarely, more than one such focus is present. For this situation to occur, the abnormal focus must be protected by 'entrance block', for otherwise it would be discharged by the normal rhythm and parasystole would not be possible. The abnormal beats resemble ordinary extrasystoles, and, dependent on the rates of the competing foci, appear with greater or lesser frequency. The clue to the presence of parasystole is that the apparent extrasystoles, although all having the same morphology and therefore obviously arising from the same focus, do not follow the preceding sinus beat by the same interval, as is readily seen in the example of ventricular parasystole illustrated. Measurement of the inter-beat intervals between parasystolic complexes shows that these are either identical or are a simple multiple of some common denominator. Note that the rate of formation of the impulses is not necessarily absolutely regular (time between each pair shown in seconds). Obviously, the more parasystolic beats that appear, the easier it is to recognise the arrhythmia, for these minor fluctuations in timing summate over long periods. The last cardinal feature of parasystole, fusion beats, occur occasionally as both foci chance to capture the ventricles simultaneously. The result is a beat intermediate in morphology between the other two, preceded, if the basic rhythm is sinus, by a P wave which by its timing *could* be conducted (starred beat). Naturally, it also fits into the timing of the parasystolic rhythm. Occasionally, a parasystolic beat fails to appear when it would seem the timing might be favourable (not on this record); this is due to 'exit block' around the abnormal focus, or perhaps to intermittency of discharge. See also **185, 188**.

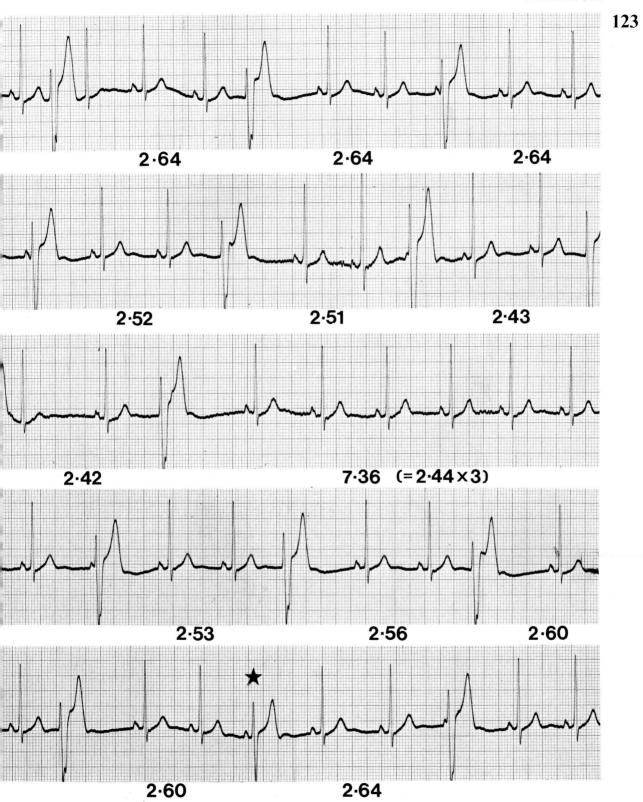

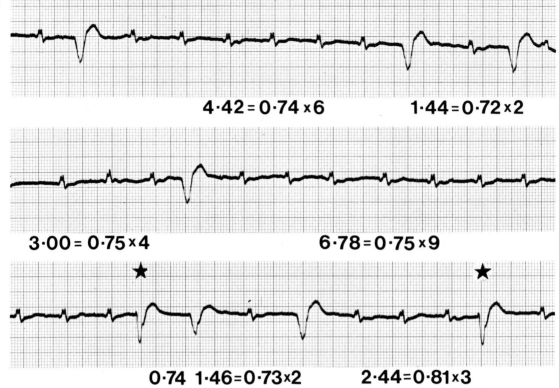

**124 Ventricular parasystole in atrial fibrillation.**
Parasystole is discussed in **123**. In atrial fibrillation, ventricular parasystole is identifiable by the occurrence of wide QRS complexes of abnormal contour which do not follow the preceding beat by a fixed coupling interval and therefore cannot be extrasystoles or escape beats (see **224, 230**). Calculation of the intervals separating these beats reveals a more or less fixed relationship between them. In the example shown, the interval calculation in seconds is shown beneath the trace. Note the longer interval at the end—this indicates a slowing of the parasystolic focus. The alternatives are that this is an extrasystole or is due to aberrant conduction, but these seem unlikely. Note the morphology of the two beats marked with a star— these seem intermediate in shape between the parasystolic beats and the rest, and are fusion beats.

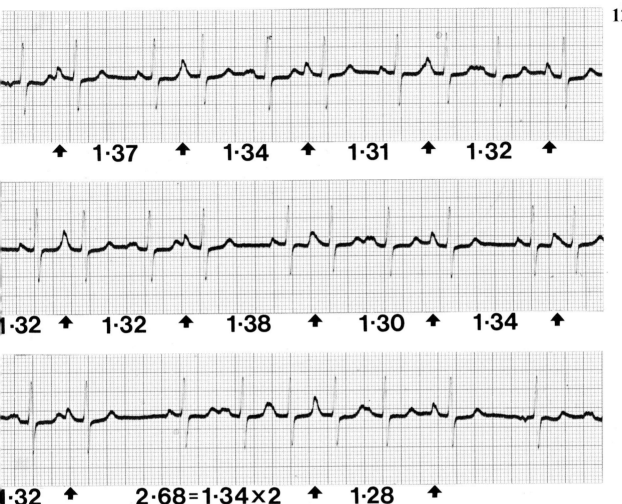

**125  Atrial parasystole.** Parasystolic foci are rarer in the atria than in the ventricles. The trace shows a continuous strip in three rows. There are frequent beats (arrowed) showing tall pointed P waves quite different from the bifid P waves of the basic rhythm. At first sight these appear to be extrasystoles, for they are premature, but their varying relationship to preceding beats raises the possibility of parasystole and measurement between them reveals that they are indeed separated by more or less fixed intervals (figures are in seconds). The basic rhythm is grossly disturbed by so frequent a parasystolic entry, and elsewhere in the longer trace of which this was a part was rather irregular, so the effect of the parasystolic focus on the sinus node is difficult to determine, but usually, the sinus node is discharged.

**126**

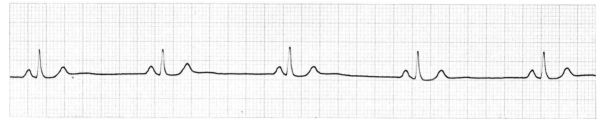

**126  Sinus bradycardia.** The P waves and the QRST complexes are normal, as is the PR interval. The heart rate is below 60/minute. Sinus brady-cardia is abolished by exercise or atropine.

**127**

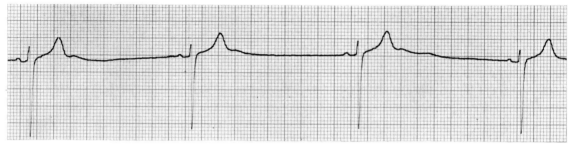

**127  Marked sinus bradycardia.**

**128**

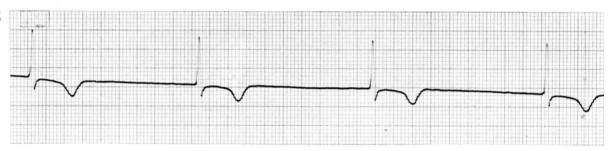

**128  Marked junctional bradycardia.** Sinus arrest is present.

**129**

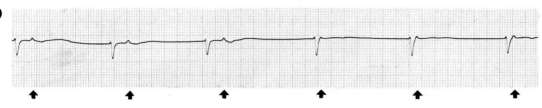

**129  Combined sinus and junctional bradycardia.** Severe sinus bradycardia is present at a regular rate of about 40/minute (P waves arrowed). There is in addition an irregular junctional bradycardia at a similar rate, but there is no relation between the two. The apparent possible connection in the first three beats is seen to be illusory as the trace proceeds.

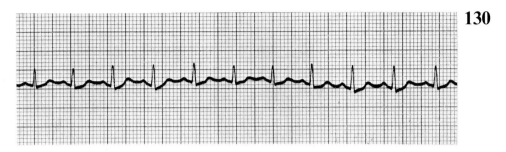

**130**

**130 Sinus tachycardia.** The heart rate at rest exceeds 100 beats/minute and may reach 130–140 beats/minute, as in this example. During exercise, of course, even faster rates occur (180/minute). At very rapid rates, the P wave may merge with the preceding T wave. Sinus tachycardia is distinguished from paroxysmal tachycardia most easily by its fluctuation in rate (but see **152**). Minor beat-to-beat differences can be seen and usually the rate will slow down as the tracing proceeds if nervousness is the cause. Even in this brief example, the rate is slightly slower at the end.

**131**

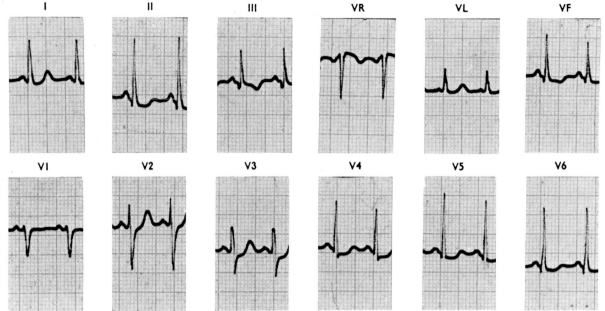

**131, 132 Sinus tachycardia, ST–T changes.** Prolonged sinus tachycardia as in chronic anxiety states may be associated with ST segment depression and T wave inversion. Figure **131** shows such a tracing in a 24-year-old woman; the heart rate varies between 120 and 140/minute. Figure **132** was taken the same night under heavy sedation when the heart rate was 84/minute; the electrocardiogram is now normal. Note the short PR interval (see **171**); there was no history of paroxysmal tachycardia, however.

**132**

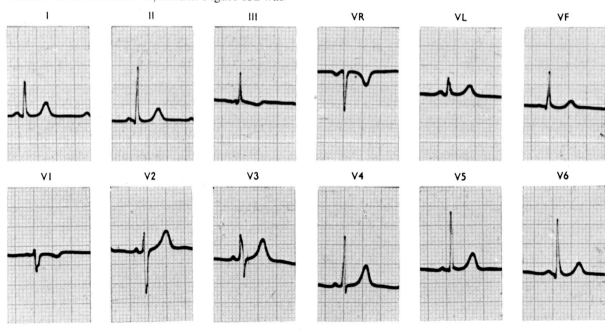

**133**

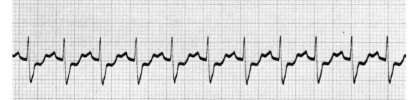

**133 Paroxysmal atrial tachycardia.** The appearances are identical to sinus tachycardia but the rate is usually faster—between 150 and 200/minute. Rates above this may be seen (especially in children) but a 1:1 response is then less likely to occur. The P waves frequently have an abnormal contour but this is only likely to be recognised if an earlier electrocardiogram is available for comparison. Atrial tachycardia is typically absolutely regular but may not be so (see **152**).

**134**

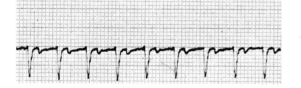
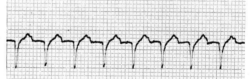

**134 Paroxysmal junctional tachycardia with retrograde conduction to the atria.** P waves can be seen deforming the T wave in both the leads illustrated. See **72**.

**135**

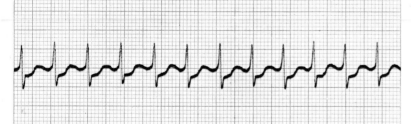

**135 Paroxysmal supraventricular tachycardia.** It is not always possible to identify P waves in an episode of paroxysmal tachycardia which nevertheless clearly arises above the ventricles because the QRS is narrow and thus define it as either atrial or junctional. In the trace illustrated for instance, the T wave has a slight deformity of its downstroke which may or may not be a P wave. The term 'supraventricular' tachycardia is used.

**136**

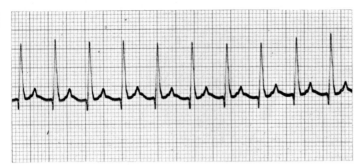

**136 Paroxysmal atrial tachycardia with grade 1 block.** The trace shows supraventricular tachycardia with a P wave closely following the QRS. If this P wave were inverted, junctional tachycardia with retrograde conduction would be the diagnosis, but as the P wave is upright, this is probably atrial tachycardia with grade 1 block.

**137**

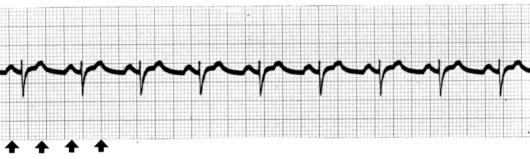

**138**

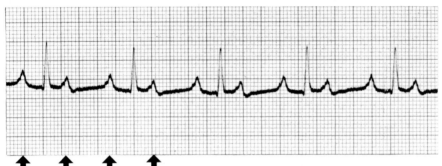

**137, 138 Paroxysmal atrial tachycardia with 2:1 atrioventricular block.** The ventricles respond to every alternate P wave, either with a normal PR interval (**137**) or with a prolonged one (**138**). In both cases one of each pair of P waves must be sought in the T wave (first four arrowed in both traces). The atrial rate in **138** is rather slow for paroxysmal tachycardia but this was taken from a sustained trace.

**139**

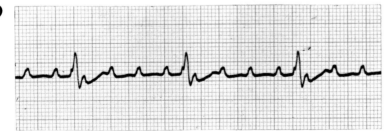

**139 Paroxysmal atrial tachycardia with 4:1 atrioventricular block.** The atrial rate is about 200/minute and the ventricles can be seen responding to every fourth P wave (one P wave immediately follows each QRS). The resulting heart rate is only 50/minute. This degree of block is unusual in atrial tachycardia though not uncommon in atrial flutter. The atrial rate here is too slow for this to be flutter.

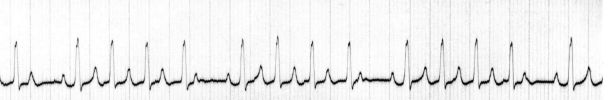

**140 Paroxysmal atrial tachycardia with type 1 grade 2 atrioventricular block.** The illustration shows regularly occurring P waves at about 180/minute with the ventricles responding in Wenckebach periods (5:4 conduction). The second, third, and fourth P waves of each cycle summate with the T wave of the previous beat.

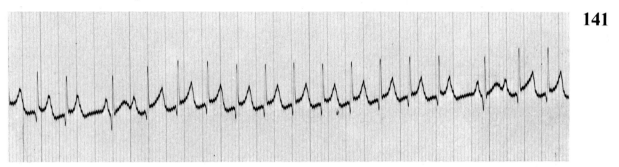

**141 Paroxysmal atrial tachycardia with type 2 grade 2 atrioventricular block.** In the tachycardia illustrated the PR interval of the established arrhythmia is prolonged so that the P wave summates with the T wave of the previous complex. From time to time a beat is dropped and the following complex has a short PR interval because the conducting system has had more time to recover, and this enables the P waves to be identified with certainty. Then the PR interval lengthens again for one beat before the former stable situation is resumed.

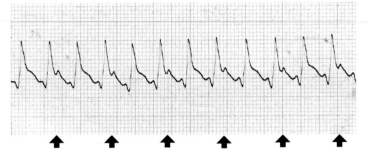

**142 Paroxysmal junctional tachycardia with partial retrograde block.** Every alternate QRS complex in this paroxysmal tachycardia is followed by a P wave which, although upright, bears such a consistent relationship to the QRS that retrograde conduction must be present and the two cannot be independent. The QRS complexes are wide and although junctional tachycardia with aberrant conduction is the more likely diagnosis, ventricular tachycardia, which may occasionally show retrograde atrial activation, is also possible. The P waves are arrowed.

**143**

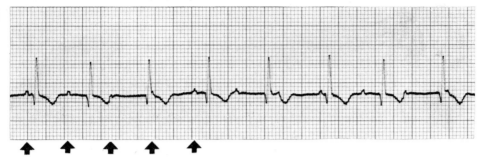

**143 Paroxysmal atrial tachycardia with complete atrioventricular block.** The atrial rate is about 140/minute. Independent junctional rhythm is present at about 95/minute. A series of P waves are arrowed to assist analysis.

**144**

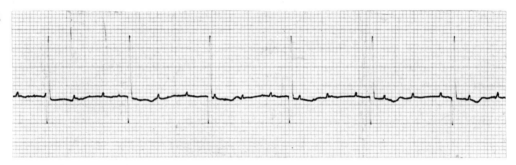

**144 Atrial tachycardia with atrioventricular block, digitalis intoxication.** Atrial tachycardia with block (partial or complete) is one of the arrhythmias which may be induced by digitalis. One helpful point of distinction from atrial tachycardias of other cause is the small size of the P waves. Here, they are diminutive. N.B. on this criterion, the tachycardia in **143** may also have been digitalis induced.

**145**

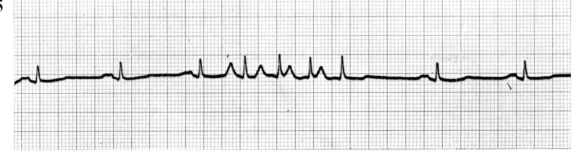

**145 A brief paroxysm of atrial tachycardia.** The trace shows a four beat burst of atrial tachycardia. The P waves of the arrhythmia are tall, and the first summates with the T wave of the preceding complex and is taller than the rest. Each beat of the tachycardia shows a longer PR interval than the one before so that Wenckebach block is present but the paroxysm stops before a beat can be dropped.

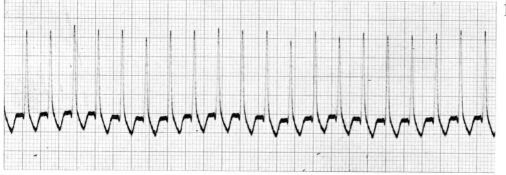

**146 Paroxysmal supraventricular tachycardia in a baby.** The rate is about 230/minute.

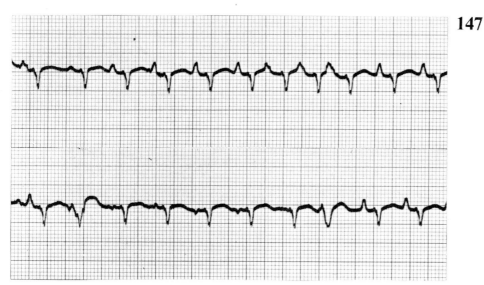

**147 Multifocal atrial tachycardia.** The two lines are a single strip. Atrial tachycardia is present but the rate is constantly changing as different foci in the atria compete for control. Note the varying P wave shapes and PR intervals. Occasionally, aberrant conduction is present (unless these are extrasystoles).

**148**

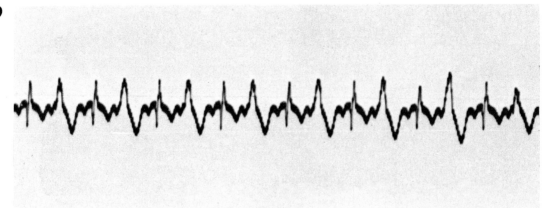

**149**

**148, 149 Paroxysmal supraventricular tachycardia with aberrant conduction.** The differential diagnosis is from ventricular tachycardia. In atrial tachycardias, P waves may be seen immediately before each widened QRS but this will not help in junctional tachycardias. Features favouring a supraventricular origin are a QRS pattern of right bundle branch block and absolute regularity of rate, but these are not completely reliable (**152**).

Figure **149** shows atrial tachycardia with aberrant conduction (probably via an accessory tract in view of the shorter PR interval) in every other beat only. (Also see **212, 234**).

**150**

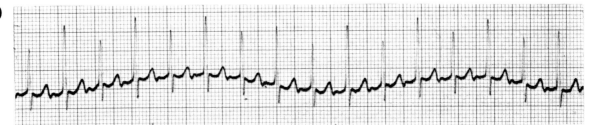

**150 Electrical alteration in paroxysmal tachycardia.** Alternate complexes show a different QRS pattern. Presumably, this is a fatigue phenomenon, every other impulse finding some part of the conduction pathway refractory. In this example, the alternation is slight, affecting the height of the QRS complex only.

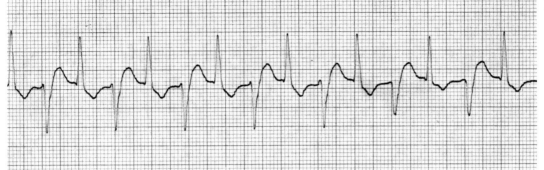

**151 Bidirectional tachycardia.** In some instances, electrical alternation of the QRS (see **150**) can be extreme, resulting in every other complex pointing in opposite directions. The tachycardia is usually junctional in such cases and the cause, digitalis intoxication. The tracing shown was recorded in a patient with atrial fibrillation undergoing digitalisation; the burst of tachycardia occurred without warning. This pattern may be due to alternating block of each of the two divisions of the left bundle branch. (See also **98**.)

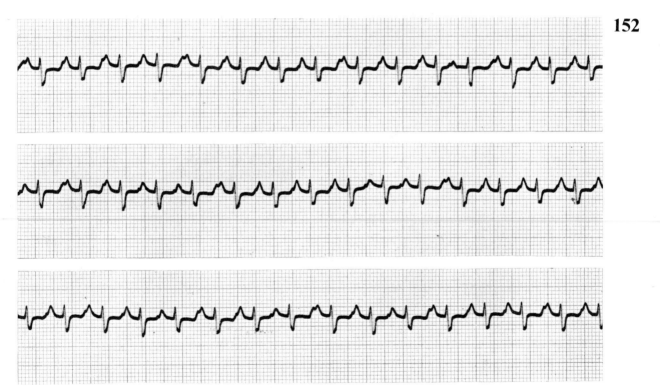

**152 Irregular paroxysmal atrial tachycardia.** In most cases paroxysmal supraventricular tachycardias are perfectly regular, but this is not always so. The tachycardia illustrated shows an irregular atrial rhythm and the irregularity is increased by minor variations in PR interval, reflecting slight changes in refractoriness of the atrioventricular junction with different cycle lengths and prematurity of the P wave.

**153**

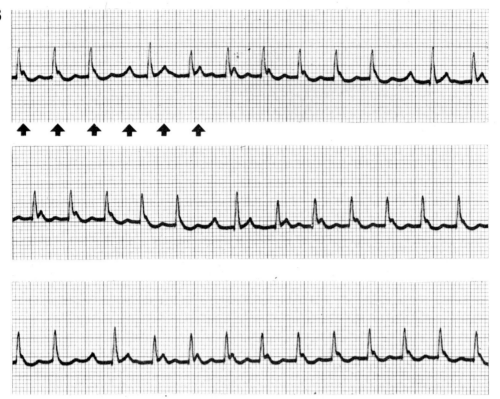

**153 Simultaneous atrial and junctional tachycardia.** The illustration shows a continuous strip in three rows. Throughout the record there is paroxysmal atrial tachycardia at a rate of just over 150/minute. A series of P waves is arrowed to assist analysis. In addition there are repetitive bursts of self-limiting junctional tachycardia. The end of each one is followed by a brief pause after which the next P wave is conducted (PR interval 0.26 second) to produce a QRS of different contour. Then the junctional tachycardia recommences. Its rate is slightly slower than that of the atrial tachycardia so that the P waves seem to 'move' backwards into the QRS complexes (and see **155**). The apparently lengthening PR interval ending in a dropped beat raises the alternative possible explanation of atrial tachycardia complicated by a Wenckebach type of conduction but this seems less likely because of the length of some of the cycles, the fixed rate of the ventricles, and the different shape of the conducted beat. However, see **245**.

**154**

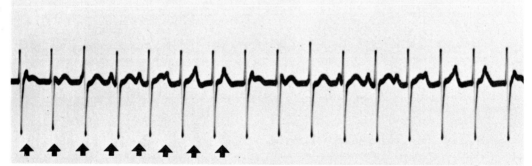

**154 Simultaneous atrial and junctional tachycardias.** Another example of the combination of two simultaneous supraventricular tachyarrhythmias, the atrial being the faster. They are quite autonomous. A series of P waves is arrowed to assist analysis.

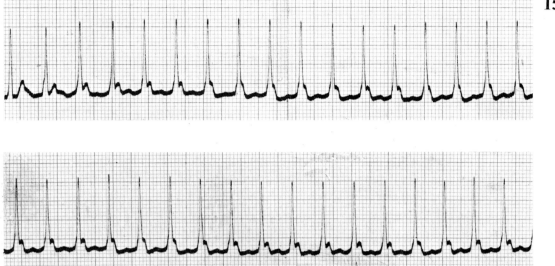

**155 Synchronisation in simultaneous atrial and junctional tachycardia.** When atria and ventricles are dissociated but have similar rates there is a tendency for one focus to adjust its rate to keep time with the other. This may be a transient or a persistent phenomenon. Combined tachycardias such as that illustrated in **155** afford a good opportunity for this to occur though it is also seen in slower rhythms. The trace is a continuous strip cut up. Note how the P waves appear to 'move' away from and back to the QRS complexes in what appears to be otherwise two dissociated tachycardias, although in fact it is the QRS complexes that accelerate at the start of the record to 'join' the P waves. N.B. the same explanation may explain the appearances in **153**.

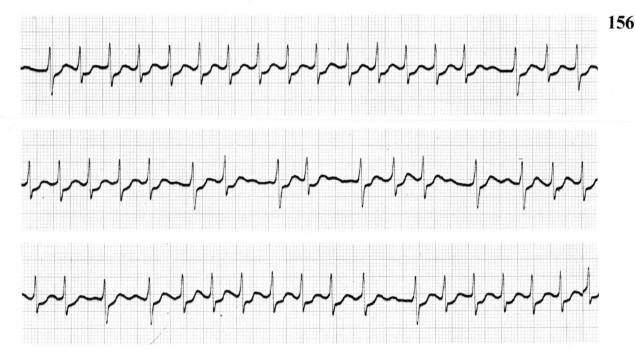

**156 Repetitive supraventricular tachycardia.** Paroxysms of supraventricular (junctional?) tachycardia follow each other with only one or two sinus beats intervening. See also repetitive ventricular tachycardia (**181**). The three rows are one continuous strip.

**157**

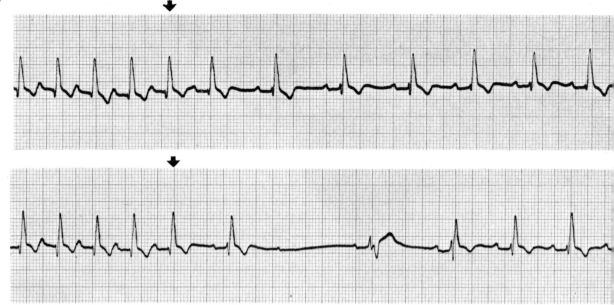

**157 Paroxysmal supraventricular tachycardia, effect of carotid sinus massage.** Two examples are shown, both from the same patient. Carotid stimulation begins to act at the point marked by the arrow. On the upper line, one beat is a little delayed and then the tachycardia is aborted. Note that, as a result, P waves may now be suspected in retrospect, deforming the T waves during the tachycardia. On the lower line, sinus rhythm returns at once, but the next P wave is not followed by a QRS because of transient atrioventricular block; the next beat is probably a fusion beat, part sinus, part junctional escape. Thereafter, sinus rhythm is resumed. Aberrant conduction is present throughout.

**158**

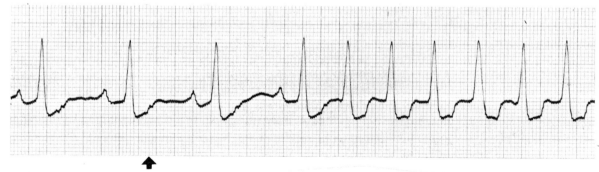

**158 Reciprocating tachycardia.** In many cases, paroxysmal supraventricular tachycardia appears to be due to a circus movement of the excitation wave around two conducting pathways having different refractoriness—for instance, the atrioventricular junction and the bundle of Kent in patients with the Wolff–Parkinson–White syndrome. Because one of the pathways may be refractory at the time, the impulse travels down the other route, stimulates the ventricles and at the same time is enabled to return to the atria via the first, now non-refractory path. By now, the second route has recovered and the cycle recommences. The trace shown begins with four beats with a long PR interval. A blip in the ST segment (arrowed in one complex) indicates atrial re-entry which however, is not reconducted forwards through the atrioventricular junction. After the fourth beat a re-entry tachycardia begins. The re-entry blip can still be seen but the normal P waves have vanished.

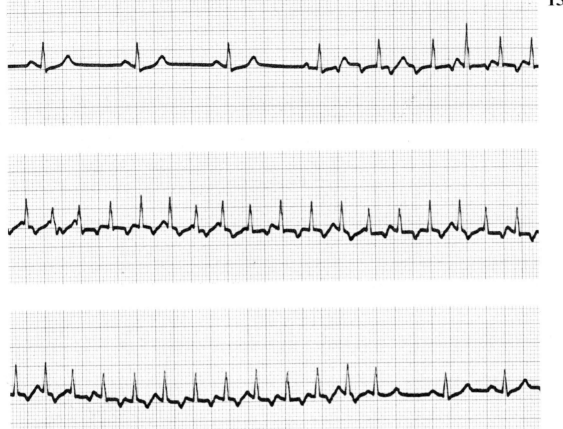

**159  Reciprocating tachycardia.** Another example showing the onset of atrial retrograde activation particularly well because of the presence of 2:1 block at the start of the arrhythmia. Later 1:1 conduction develops (with a varying PR interval). The ventricular rhythm is slightly irregular as is sometimes seen in supraventricular tachycardias (see **152**). Eventually the paroxysm ends with a complex which is not followed by an inverted P wave, indicating that the retrograde pathway has stopped conducting spontaneously. Other methods of termination are discussed in **160** and **161**. The three rows are a single strip cut up.

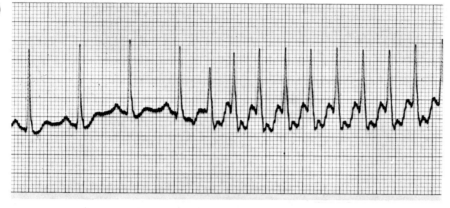

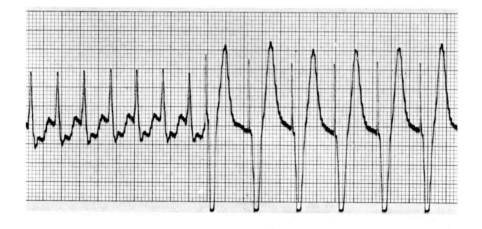

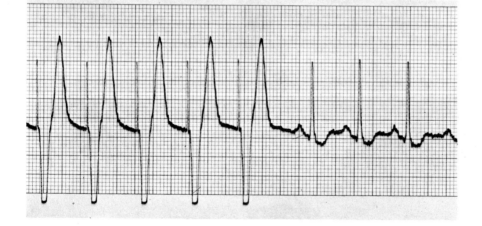

**160 Control of reciprocating tachycardia by pacing.** Reciprocating tachycardia is explained in **159**. It can be stopped by rendering one of the two pathways refractory at the crucial moment. This can happen spontaneously with a suitably timed extrasystole if this is retrogradely conducted into the atrioventricular junction (and for years a catheter-induced extrasystole has been known to be a useful way of terminating many tachycardias complicating cardiac catheterisation—see **161**) but a paced beat (i.e. an iatrogenic extrasystole) will do as well.

The illustration shows a continuous strip in three rows. After the fourth sinus beat atrial re-entry is visible as an inverted P wave deforming the T wave,

and a reciprocating tachycardia is set up. In the centre line, the arrhythmia is interrupted by ventricular pacing and control of the heart is instantly achieved. The pacemaker is slowed a little (though this is not necessary for success) and on the lowest line it is turned off abruptly. Sinus rhythm resumes. Note that in this instance a series of paced beats is used but, in theory, one is enough. This record was taken from a patient in whom paroxysmal tachycardia could not be controlled by drugs. The pacemaker used was the induction coil variety (see **729**) and the patient was able to switch it on and off at will, applying the external coil to the praecordium whenever necessary.

**161**

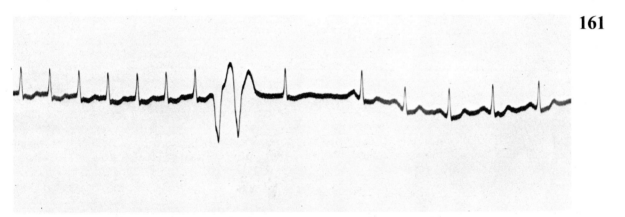

**161 Termination of reciprocating tachycardia with ventricular extrasystoles.** This is explained in **160**. The trace shows a supraventricular tachycardia terminated by two ventricular extrasystoles. A junctional beat follows; then sinus rhythm resumes.

**162**

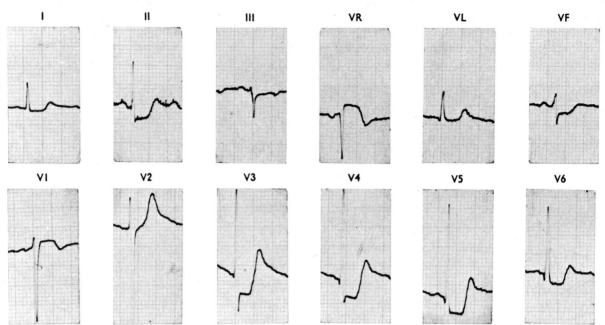

**162, 163 ST–T changes following paroxysmal tachycardia.** Transient widespread ST–T abnormalities may be seen after an attack of paroxysmal tachycardia and, while in a diseased heart the significance of such changes may be disputed, they may unjustly throw suspicion on a healthy heart.

Figures **162**, **163** show the electrocardiogram of a young woman of 20 who, despite the voltages suggesting left ventricular hypertrophy, had a clinically normal heart. Figure **162** was taken shortly after paroxysmal tachycardia and **163** some weeks later.

**163**

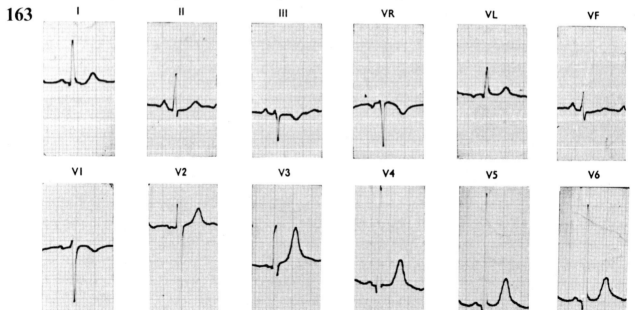

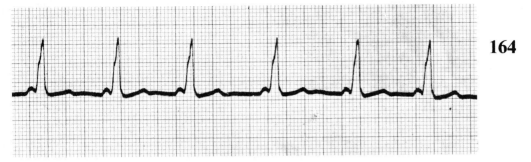

**164**

**164 Wolff–Parkinson–White syndrome.** The PR interval is less than 0.12 second and the QRS complex is widened by a slur or 'shoulder' on its upstroke—the delta wave. The overall duration of P combined with QRS is normal. The PR interval is short because the excitatory impulse bypasses the atrioventricular junction via an accessory conducting pathway—usually, the bundle of Kent. Thus, the interventricular septum is directly activated before the rest of the ventricular mass and this produces the delta wave. If the contribution of this 'pre-excitation' is small, the rest of the QRS and the T wave will be unaffected (but see **165, 166**).

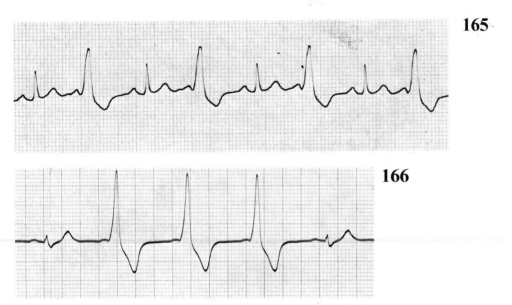

**165**

**166**

**165, 166 Intermittent Wolff–Parkinson–White syndrome.** The abnormal pattern is often intermittent or transient. Figure **165** shows the W.P.W. syndrome in alternate beats. In this instance the delta wave is not well defined, for the later portion of the QRS is abnormal as well as the early portion. Furthermore, the T wave of these complexes is inverted. The W.P.W. complexes are thus completely different to the normal ones. These additional changes reflect the degree to which the pre-excitatory impulse has been able to activate the ventricles preferentially—i.e. the contribution it has made to the fusion beat that is the W.P.W. complex. Thus, the diagnosis of myocardial ischaemia or other causes of abnormal T waves, of infarction, of ventricular hypertrophy, and of aberrant conduction of the QRS is extremely difficult, if not impossible, once the W.P.W. syndrome has been identified. N.B. the possibility that the appearances in **165** are due to coupling with ventricular ectopics late enough to land just after the next P wave may be entertained, but these are rare, and the mimicry would not survive an alteration in heart rate. In fact, the alternation in this trace was stable and sustained. See also **169**.

Figure **166** shows the transient appearance of three W.P.W. complexes in an otherwise normal electrocardiogram—another manifestation of intermittent W.P.W. syndrome. Once again, there is total alteration in the contour of the complex.

**167**

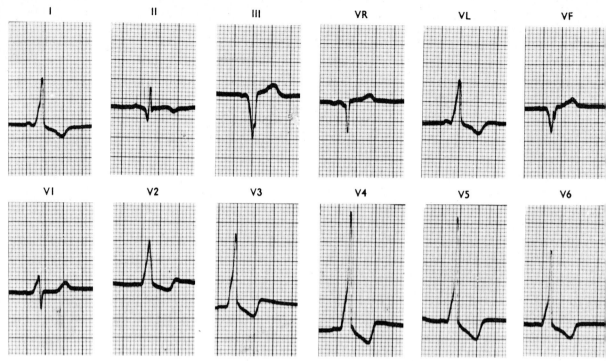

**167, 168 Wolff–Parkinson–White syndrome, 12-lead electrocardiogram.** There are two different patterns—type A, in which the bundle of Kent links the left atrium and left ventricle, and type B, in which the connection is on the right. Type A shows upright delta waves in all chest leads (**167**) and type B, negative delta waves in right praecordial leads (**168**—VI only in this instance).

Note how easily the appearances may be mistaken for ventricular hypertrophy, bundle branch block, or, in leads showing broad negative delta waves, for myocardial infarction. The PR interval is the clue. Note the left axis deviation, especially in **168**. See also **165**, **169** and **170**.

**168**

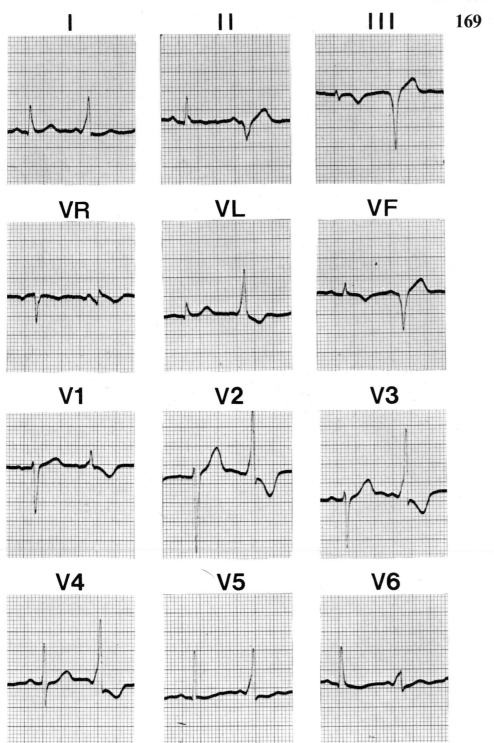

**169 Alternating Wolff–Parkinson–White syndrome, 12-lead electrocardiogram.** The profound and often misleading effect which the development of the W.P.W. syndrome may have on the electrocardiogram (**168**) is graphically illustrated in this record, taken from a patient with sustained alternating W.P.W. complexes (see **165**). Each of the twelve leads shows, first, a normal complex and, second, the W.P.W. one (type A pattern —**167**). Note the complete change of axis (from +30° to −60°) and the mimicry of an inferior infarction. Bundle branch block might also be misdiagnosed by the unwary. And see **170**.

**170**

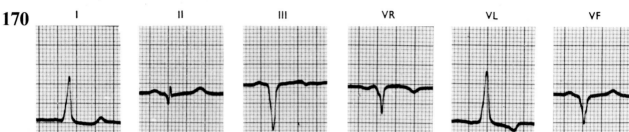

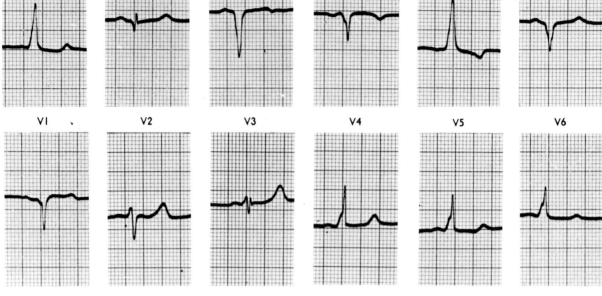

**170 Wolff–Parkinson–White syndrome with normal PR interval.** This rare variant is due to the presence of 'Mahaim fibres', a tract connecting the atrioventricular node directly to the interventricular septum. Thus, pre-excitation is produced and delta waves are seen, but the atrioventricular node itself is not bypassed and the PR interval remains normal. Misdiagnosis of infarction or bundle branch block (**167–169**) is even more likely to occur.

**171**

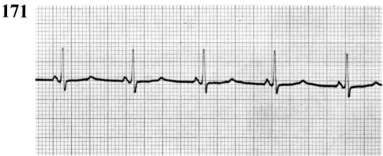

**171 Lown–Ganong–Levine syndrome.** A variant of the Wolff–Parkinson–White syndrome. The PR interval is short (under 0.12 second) but no delta waves are present. This is due to the presence of a James' tract, another accessory conducting pathway which connects the atrium to the lower part of the atrioventricular node itself. Thus, the normal slowing of the excitation wave in the node is avoided and the PR interval is shortened. As in the Wolff–Parkinson–White syndrome reciprocating paroxysmal tachycardias are favoured by the dual conducting pathways (**158, 159**).

**172**

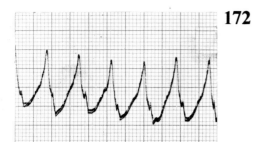

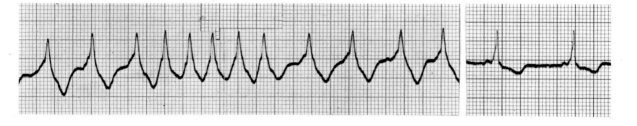

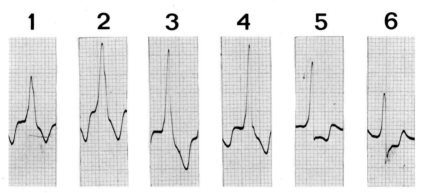

1  2  3  4  5  6

**172 Tachyarrhythmias in the Wolff–Parkinson–White syndrome.** During the paroxysmal tachycardias of the reciprocating type (**158, 159**) which are so characteristic of the W.P.W. syndrome, the characteristic QRS format is usually lost, but occasionally it persists. The upper line of **172** illustrates a brief example of junctional tachycardia in which this is the case. Paroxysmal tachycardia is not the only arrhythmia which may occur, atrial fibrillation (centre line, left) also being quite common. Note the short strip on the right in the centre line which shows the same lead during sinus rhythm and confirms the presence of the W.P.W. syndrome. The lowest line shows the chest leads (V1–6) of the same patient during another episode of atrial fibrillation. All three examples underline the difficulty of making the correct diagnosis, for in the absence of identifiable P waves and thus of a PR interval recognition of the delta wave becomes all important and this may not be easy (**165**). The result is that ventricular tachycardia may be suspected, especially when atrial fibrillation is the arrhythmia. However, although ventricular tachycardia may be irregular it rarely shows the abrupt burst of speed that can be seen in the middle of the left-hand strip in the centre line. See also **234** for a similar problem.

**173**

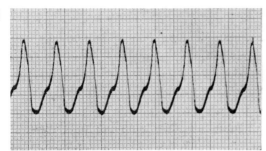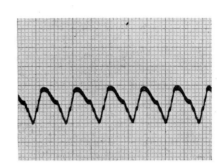

**173 Ventricular tachycardia.** The main differential diagnosis is from supraventricular tachycardia with aberrant conduction (**148**) and the distinction may be very difficult. In general, ventricular tachycardia is much more likely to show the pattern of left bundle branch block. Irregularity of rate (see later) is also helpful but not diagnostic, as these two examples show. Other points are discussed in **174–179**. See also **172, 212, 234**.

**174**

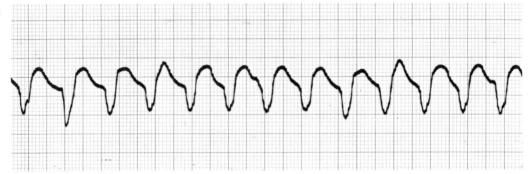

**174 Ventricular tachycardia.** Diagnostic points in this trace are the slight irregularity of the rate and the variability of the QRS contour. Both these features are unusual in supraventricular tachycardias with aberrant conduction.

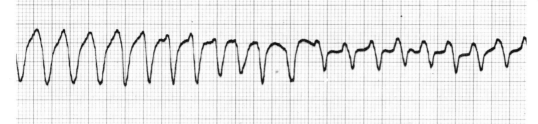

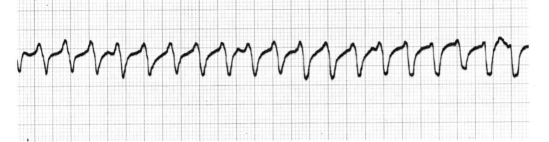

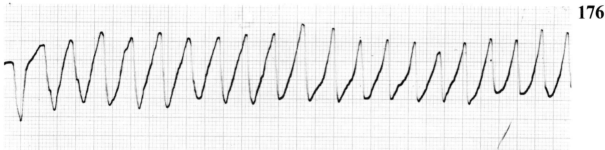

**175, 176 Ventricular tachycardia, changing QRS pattern.** This is a feature strongly suggestive of ventricular tachycardia. Two examples are illustrated. Figure **175** is a continuous strip in two rows. The imperceptible alteration in direction from a complex pointing downwards to one pointing upwards seen in **176** is typical.

**177 Ventricular tachycardia with independent atrial activity.** If, as is usually the case, there is no retrograde conduction to the atria in an episode of ventricular tachycardia, the independent P waves may sometimes be seen continuing to appear at a slower rate. In this trace P waves can be identified in two places (arrowed). The same appearances may be seen in junctional tachycardia with aberrant conduction if retrograde block is present so this is not a diagnostic point.

**177**

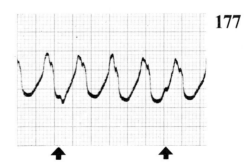

**178**

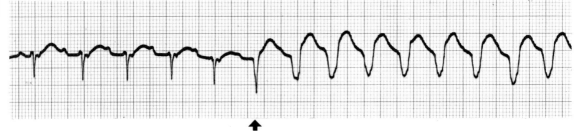

**178 Ventricular tachycardia and fusion beats.**
Fusion beats are a strong pointer towards a tachycardia being ventricular rather than supraventricular for they indicate that the heart is controlled intermittently from two sources at once. They may occur during the tachycardia or as it begins or ends. The trace shows a series of sinus beats with a lengthening PR interval passing into ventricular tachycardia, the first beat of which (arrowed) is in time with both rhythms and intermediate in contour—a fusion beat.

**179**

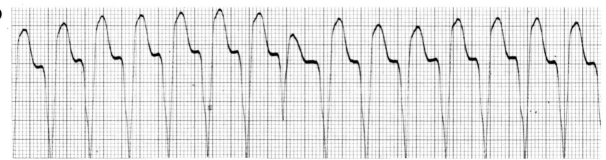

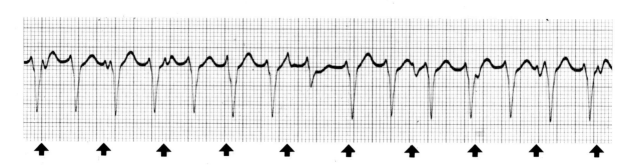

**179 Ventricular tachycardia with independent atrial activity and capture beats.** When independent atrial activity due to retrograde block is present during a tachycardia with broad QRS complexes, the occurrence of capture beats (like fusion beats—see **178**) favours the diagnosis of ventricular tachycardia rather than junctional tachycardia with aberrant conduction because they imply that the atrioventricular junction is free to conduct in an antegrade direction. The upper line shows such a tachycardia which is interrupted by a complex of different contour. In another lead (lower line) P waves can be seen (arrowed). Once again a different beat is seen. It follows one of the P waves by a suitable interval and is a capture beat related to this P wave. In addition, it is in time with the other beats and has a shape resembling them in part, so it has a fusion beat as well (as in the complex on the upper line).

**180**

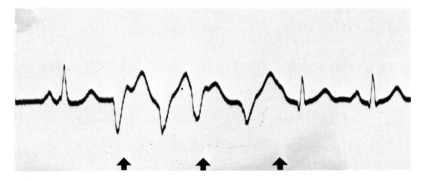

**180 Ventricular tachycardia.** Three or more ventricular extrasystoles in a row are defined as ventricular tachycardia. The trace shows four consecutive multiform ventricular extrasystoles. P waves continue undisturbed (arrows) and the last of them is conducted with a long PR interval (see **89**) to restart sinus rhythm.

**181**

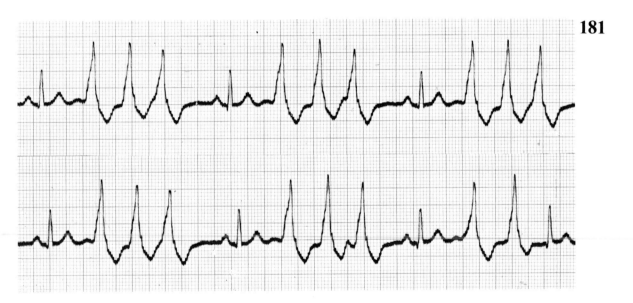

**181 Repetitive paroxysmal ventricular tachycardia.** Short bursts of ventricular tachycardia follow each other in quick succession. Paroxysms may last a few beats only and are sometimes represented by a single extrasystole. It is unusual to record an electrocardiogram free of tachycardia. The history often extends over many years (in the case illustrated it was fifteen years). Repetitive atrial and junctional tachycardias also occur (see **156**) and the tachycardia in **159** came from another patient with this syndrome. The two lines are a single strip cut up.

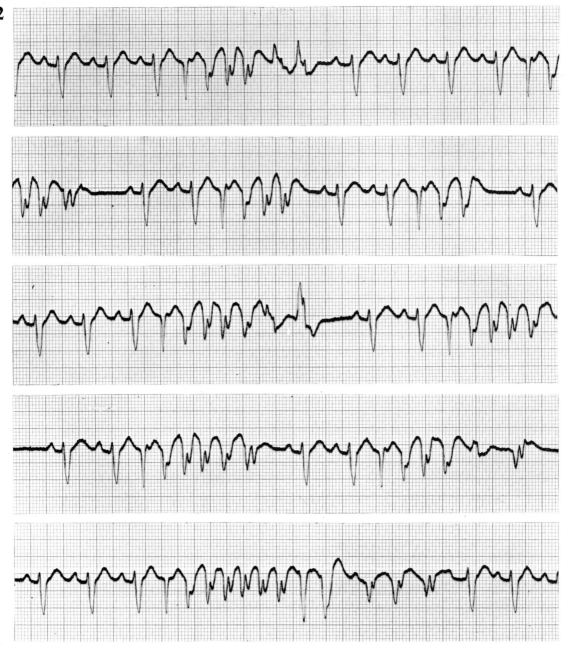

**182   Repetitive tachycardia.** Another example of this arrhythmia in which most paroxysms begin with an identical series of complexes—first, a narrow complex which is probably a junctional extrasystole; then, several beats showing aberration which manifests the same sequence of patterns. The multiform character and direction of later beats in longer paroxysms suggest that this is a repetitive ventricular tachycardia. Throughout a very long trace the duration of paroxysms varied from three to twenty beats, and sinus rhythm never returned for more than a second or so. N.B. the sinus beats show aberrant conduction. The five rows are a single strip cut up.

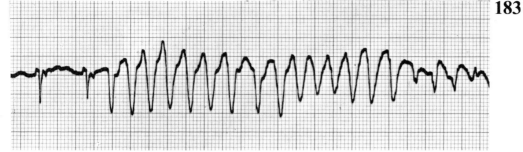

**183   Ventricular tachycardia and fibrillation following a ventricular extrasystole.** Ventricular extrasystoles coinciding with the apex of the T wave of preceding beats are likely to produce ventricular tachycardia (see **99**). The illustration shows an extrasystole occurring very soon after the second sinus beat. It triggers a burst of ventricular tachycardia which by the end of the trace appears to be degenerating into ventricular fibrillation. (See also **210, 235.**)

**184–186 Accelerated idioventricular rhythm.** The heart is controlled by a ventricular focus at a rate (between 50 and 100 roughly) that is too slow to be labelled ventricular tachycardia. The arrhythmia is seen most often after myocardial infarction and, as illustrated in these three examples, tends to occur intermittently in short paroxysms of varying length interspersed with sinus rhythm. The onset of such a paroxysm may be by acceleration of the abnormal focus relative to sinus rhythm (**184**, end of line), by a parasystolic mechanism (**185**—intervals in seconds), or by some kind of escape (e.g. following

an extrasystole as in **186**, upper line). Atrial dissociation is usual during a paroxysm (note the P waves 'moving' into the QRS complexes in **186**) but atrial standstill may occur (**184**, **185**). The paroxysm ends in one of various ways—abruptly, by acceleration of the sinus node (**184**, centre), parasystolically (**185**), or following the interruption of an extrasystole (**186**, lower line).

N.B. **185**, **186** are each single strips cut up. The arrowed beats in **184** and the arrowed beat at the end of the second line in **185** are fusion beats.

**184**

**185**

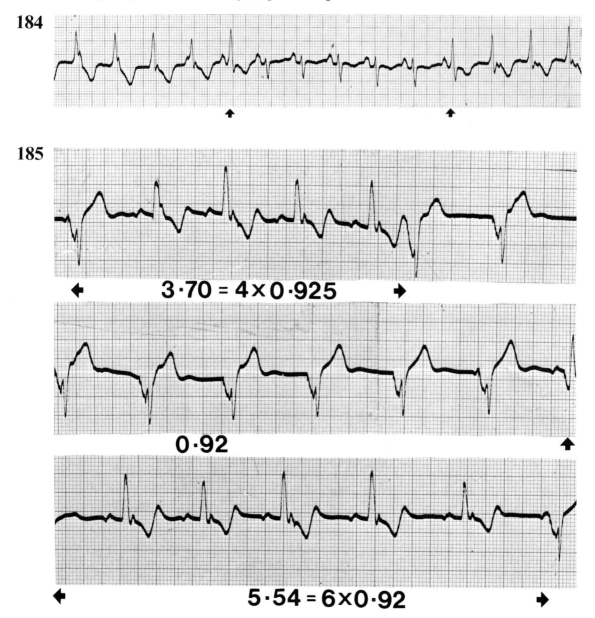

**186**

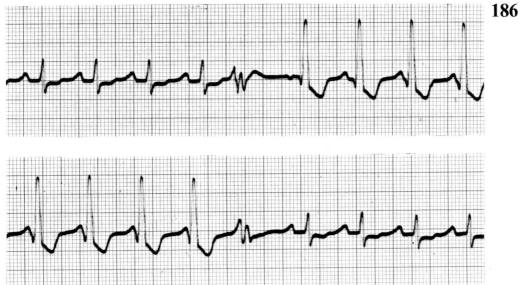

**187**

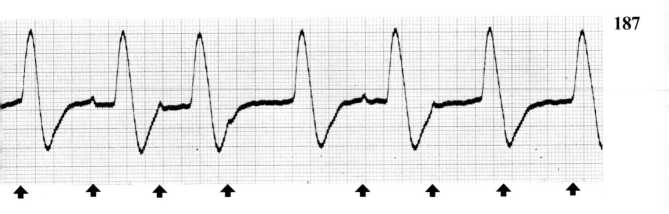

**187 Irregular accelerated idioventricular rhythm.**
The abnormal focus need not be regular, as in this
example. Note the independent P waves, arrowed
where visible.

**188**

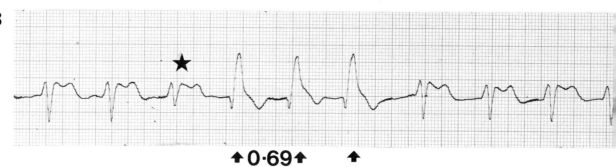

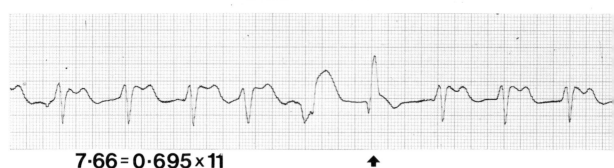

**↑0·69↑**     **↑**

**7·66 = 0·695 × 11**      **↑**

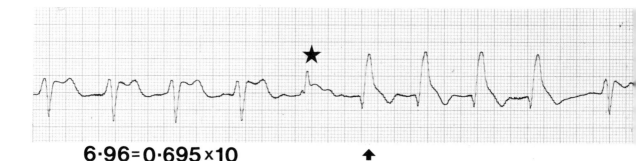

**6·96 = 0·695 × 10**     **↑**

**188 Accelerated idioventricular rhythm, two foci.** More than one focus may control the heart. In this example, which is one continuous strip, two distinct types of complexes occurring at different rates are present. The non-dominant focus is parasystolic (185). Note the presence of fusion beats (starred). The fifth complex on the second line may be an escape beat or even a third focus. P waves are seen only occasionally. Time intervals are in seconds.

**189**

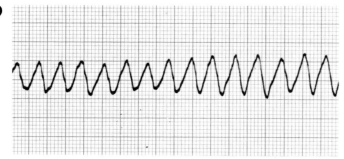

**189 Ventricular flutter.** This term is applied to ventricular tachycardia when the distinction between QRS and T completely vanishes so that a 'saw-tooth' appearance is produced which is reminiscent of atrial flutter. Note the irregularity of rhythm and shape typical of ventricular tachycardia. Ventricular fibrillation usually follows without delay.

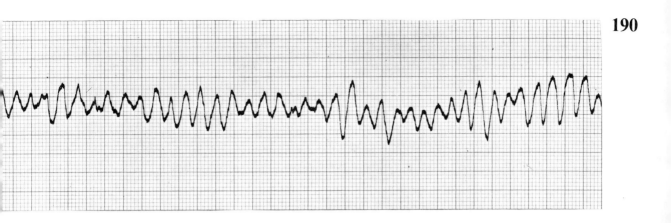

**190   Ventricular fibrillation.** Co-ordinated activity of the ventricles ceases. The electrocardiogram shows irregular waves of no defined shape. In this trace there are short periods suggestive of ventricular flutter. Appearances such as this are favourable for the success of DC shock.

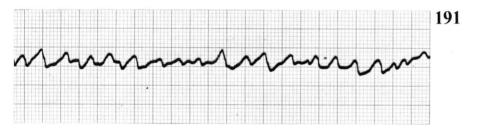

**191   Fine ventricular fibrillation.** This illustration shows ventricular fibrillation with very variable low voltage waves. With such appearances, DC shock is less likely to be successful.

**192**

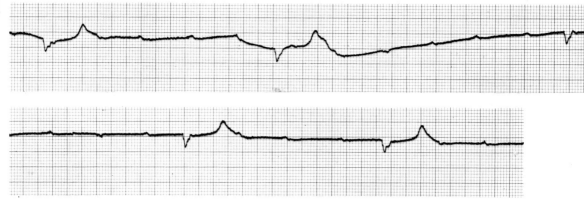

**192–194  Agonal rhythms.** Extreme bradycardia produces effective cardiac arrest. Three examples are shown. In **192** there is an irregular idioventricular focus with continuing atrial activity, **193** shows a similar situation with atrial fibrillation, while **194** illustrates an extreme sinus bradycardia with an irregular, dissociated junctional rhythm. All were recorded immediately before death. Each trace is a single strip cut up.

**193**

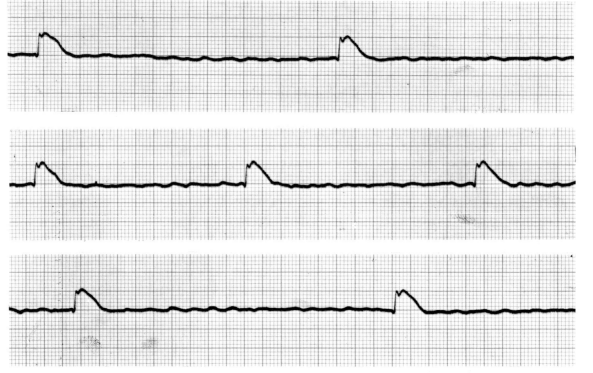

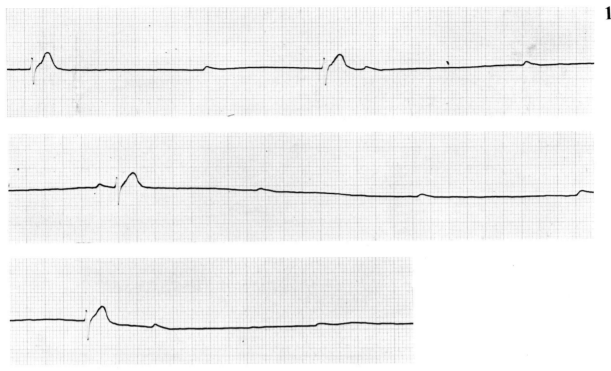

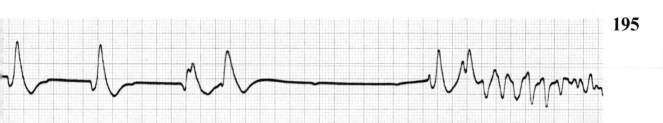

**195 Cardiac arrest.** In this illustration, slow idioventricular activity gives way to asystole and then to ventricular fibrillation.

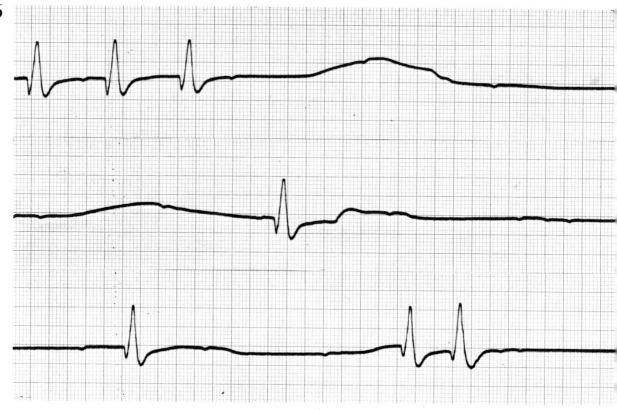

**196 Cardiac arrest.** The illustration shows a continuous strip in three rows. After three idioventricular beats abrupt asystole occurs. The baseline is broken by tiny deflections representing slow atrial activity. Occasional further idioventricular complexes occur at irregular intervals before total asystole.

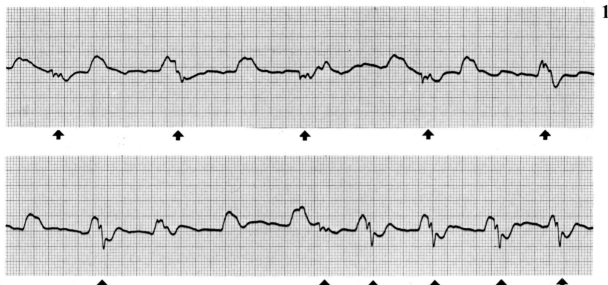

**197  Cardiac massage.** External cardiac massage causes a deviation from the isoelectric line due to physical displacement of the heart within the chest. In the example illustrated, the coarse upward deflections are due to massage artefact. Two kinds of QRS complexes can be seen (all arrowed). In the upper row, there are slow regular complexes of bizarre contour which represent post-mortem electrical activity, **198**. On the lower line, narrower complexes are present and these are closely related to the massage. These are mechanically induced ventricular extrasystoles.

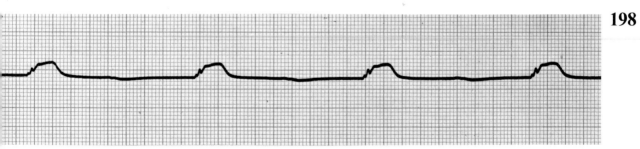

**198  Post-mortem electrical activity.** Often, after effective cardiac contractions have ceased, coarse wide bizarre QRS complexes continue to appear. They may be regular or irregular and they may persist for a surprisingly long time after death. Such electrical activity is not associated with any mechanical pumping action of the ventricles and represents the persistent discharge of a dying, increasingly anoxic focus within the muscle.

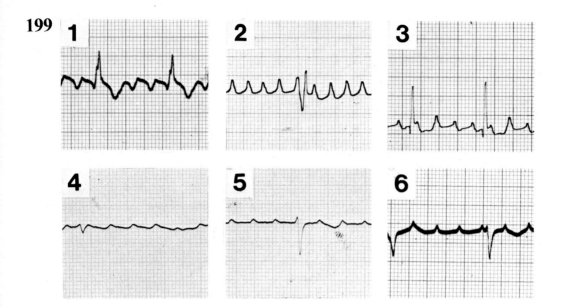

**199** **Atrial flutter, morphology of flutter waves.**
Classically, flutter waves (or 'F' waves) produce the
so-called 'saw-tooth' appearance of the baseline
because their rapid rate hardly permits return to the
isoelectric line, but this depends upon the vector of
the F wave and the lead observed. Furthermore,
flutter waves themselves vary considerably in
contour. The illustration shows six examples of
flutter ranging from the classical appearance (1) to
apparent P waves separated from an isoelectric line
(6). In all, the rate (between 240 and 360/minute)
indicates the correct diagnosis. Atrial tachycardia is
always slower. This point is further illustrated in
**213, 214**.

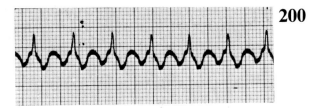

**200**

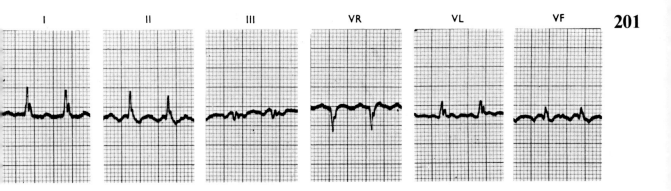

**201**

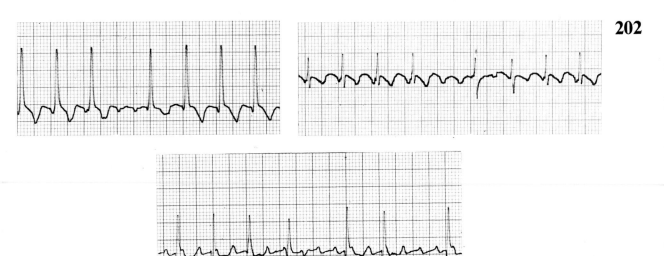

**202**

**200–202 Atrial flutter with 2:1 atrioventricular block.** This diagnosis is often missed because alternate F waves coincide with T waves and are not recognised (**200**) and because not all leads show flutter waves equally well (see **213, 214**). The latter point is reinforced in **201** which shows the limb leads of another patient in flutter with 2:1 block. The clue is the ventricular rate at about 150/minute which should always bring the possibility of flutter to mind. Fortunately, the degree of block often changes spontaneously from 2:1 to a higher ratio (usually 4:1) and the diagnosis becomes obvious. Figure **202** shows three separate examples of this. Of course the same effect may be achieved by carotid sinus massage (see **211**).

**203**

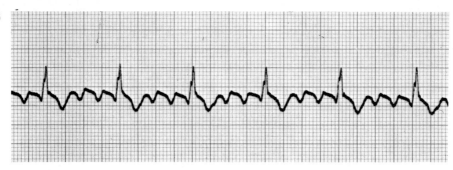

**203 Atrial flutter with 4:1 atrioventricular block.**
When identifying the F waves it is important to
remember those coinciding with the QRS
complexes and T waves. See also **207**.

**204**

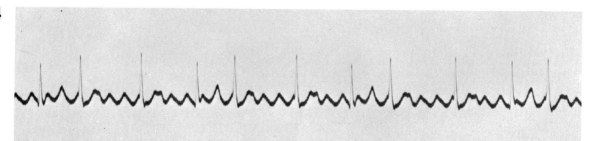

**204 Atrial flutter, 2:1 and 4:1 atrioventricular
block producing paired beats.** When atrial flutter
manifests block varying between 2:1 and 4:1, which
are the only two common ratios, the result is a
tendency to a bigeminal rhythm. In this trace, each
cycle of 2:1 block is separated by two cycles of 4:1
block so that the paired complexes are followed by a
single beat. At the wrist, extrasystoles may be
simulated. Note how summation of an F wave with
a QRS complex increases the height of the latter.
There is also F and T summation in the 2:1 cycle.
Note that the 4:1 cycles of each pair show different
F–QRS conduction relationships; nevertheless,
there are eight F waves to two QRS complexes (or,
including the 2:1 cycle, 10 F waves to three QRS
complexes).

**205**

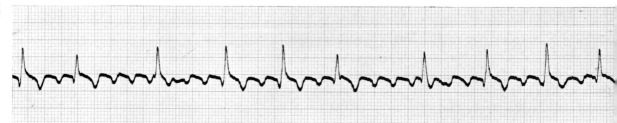

**205 Atrial flutter with irregular atrioventricular
block.** No consistent relationship exists between F
waves and the irregularly spaced QRS complexes.
The pulse at the wrist will be indistinguishable from
that of atrial fibrillation, but rapid regular 'a' waves
may be visible in the jugular venous pulse.

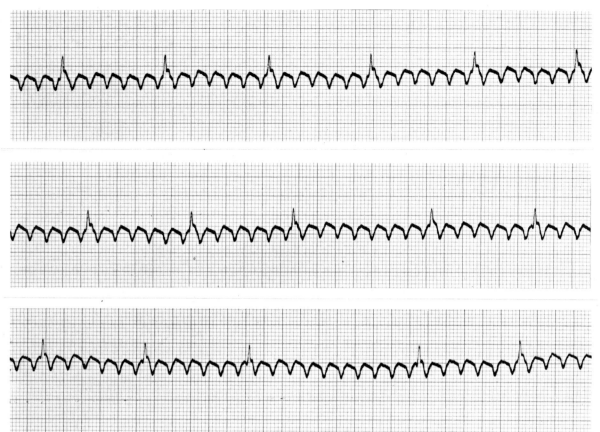

**206 Atrial flutter with higher ratios of partial atrioventricular block.** The three strips illustrated were taken from the same subject. The top line shows 6:1 block; the centre line 6:1 and 8:1 block; and the lowest line contains one cycle of 10:1 block.

Despite these high ratios, complete block is not present as can be seen by examining the consistent relationship of the QRS to the F wave immediately before it (see **209**). Ratios of conduction greater than 4:1 are uncommon.

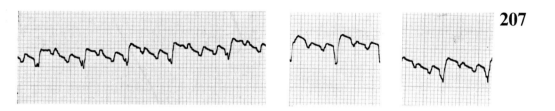

**207**

**207 Atrial flutter with 3:1 atrioventricular block.** This is an uncommon ratio of conduction. Three separate leads are illustrated, all from the same electrocardiogram. Note that one of the F waves coincides with the QRS complex. In the long strip on the left the ratio changes to 4:1.

**208**

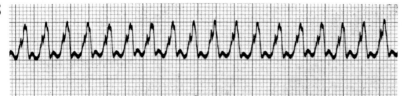

**208   Atrial flutter with 1:1 response.** A 1:1 response to atrial flutter is unusual in adults but may be seen in children. In this example the flutter waves are poorly developed but can be clearly seen between the QRS complexes. The latter show aberrant conduction.

**209**

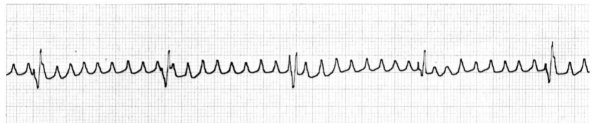

**209   Atrial flutter with complete atrioventricular block.** The flutter waves bear no constant relationship to the QRS complexes which are slow and regular. Note how their morphology is altered by the flutter waves when the two summate.

**210**

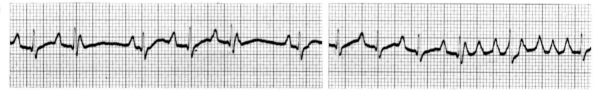

**210   Atrial flutter, onset.** Like atrial fibrillation (see **235**), atrial flutter may be initiated by an atrial extrasystole, particularly when it occurs early and falls in the vulnerable phase of atrial recovery—a situation analogous to ventricular extrasystoles and ventricular tachycardia and fibrillation (**99, 183**). The left-hand trace shows premature P waves deforming the QRS complex of beats 2 and 5. Because they *are* so premature they find the atrioventricular junction refractory and are not conducted (**109**), another consequence being that the prolonged PR interval of the basic rhythm is shortened in the post-extrasystolic beat because of the longer time available for junctional recovery. The same event occurs after the fourth beat in the right-hand trace and on this occasion atrial flutter is initiated.

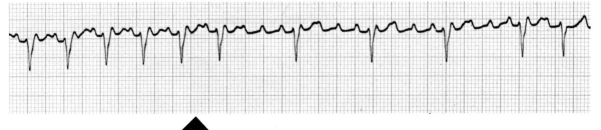

**211  Atrial flutter, effect of carotid sinus massage.**
Carotid sinus stimulation increases the degree of
atrioventricular block in atrial flutter and is thus
useful in diagnosis in difficult cases (see **202**). In the
illustration, the arrow points to the onset of carotid
massage. Note that the effect is typically short-lived.

**212**

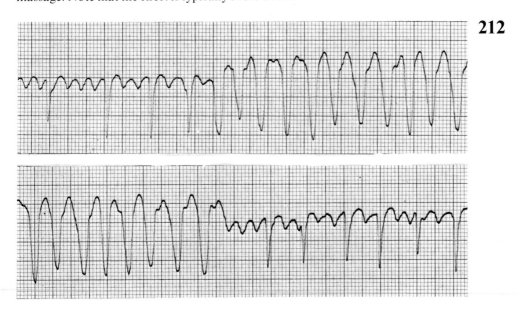

**212  Atrial flutter with aberrant conduction.** The
illustration shows a continuous strip in two rows.
Atrial flutter with irregular block is present. Half
way across the upper row the ventricular response
increases and the rate rises, causing the development of aberrant conduction (see **342**). When the
ventricular rate slows again (lower line) aberrant
conduction disappears. The appearances mimic
ventricular tachycardia (**173**). See also **234**.

**213**

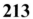

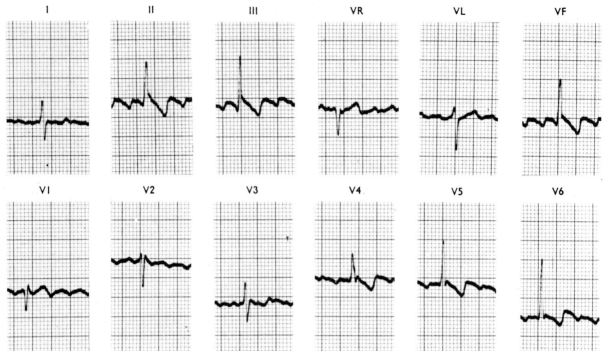

**213, 214    Atrial flutter, 12-lead electrocardiogram.**
Flutter waves are better seen in some leads than in others. Usually, they are well formed in II, III and VF, and are also easily recognised in V1 and V2 (**213**), but sometimes they are obvious in the latter leads only (**214**).

**214**

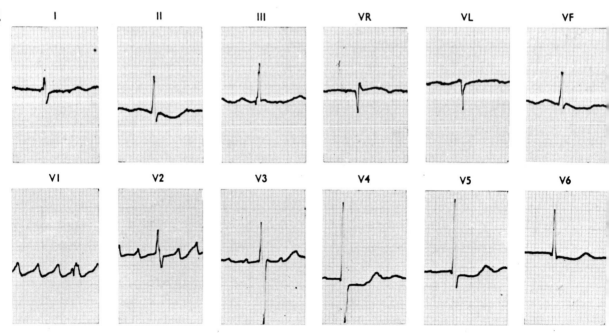

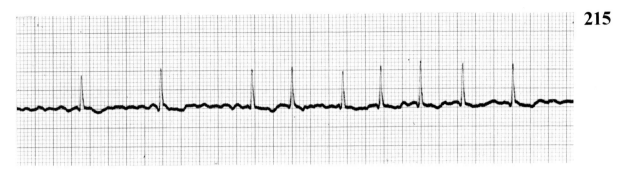

**215   Atrial fibrillation.** The incoordinated activity of the atria is visible as small irregular fluctuations of the isoelectric line at rates up to 600/minute—the 'f' waves. The ventricular response is always irregular, unless complete heart block or atrioventricular dissociation with junctional rhythm is present. (See **219**, **220**.)

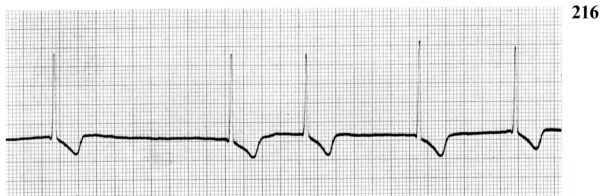

**216   Atrial fibrillation, slow ventricular response owing to heavy digitalisation.** Note the absence of f waves in this particular trace; they are not always visible.

**217**

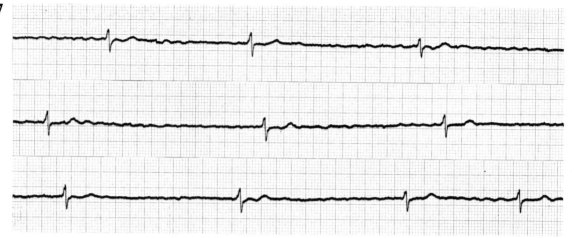

**217 Atrial fibrillation, ultra slow ventricular response.** The trace is a single strip cut up. Extremely slow, irregular ventricular rates like this are usually the result of the combination of digitalis and a beta blocking drug.

**218**

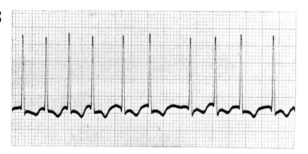
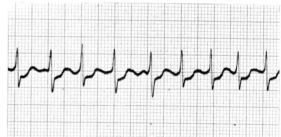

**218 Atrial fibrillation, rapid ventricular response.** In atrial fibrillation the ventricular rate may be very rapid—often between 150 and 180/minute. This is especially so in thyrotoxicosis. The illustration shows two examples. The irregularity of the ventricular response is less evident in the right-hand one: this, and occasional distortions of the baseline which mimic P waves, encourage a search for alternative diagnoses, and indeed supraventricular tachycardias may sometimes be irregular (**152**), but appearances such as this are usually atrial fibrillation.

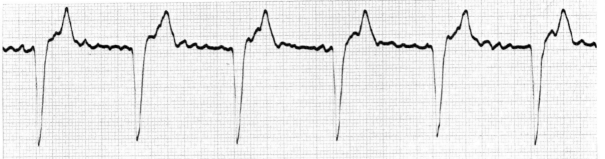

**219 Atrial fibrillation, complete heart block.** Irregular f waves can be readily identified. QRS complexes are wide, indicating their origin below the atrioventricular junction. The ventricular rate is slow and the rhythm regular.

**220**

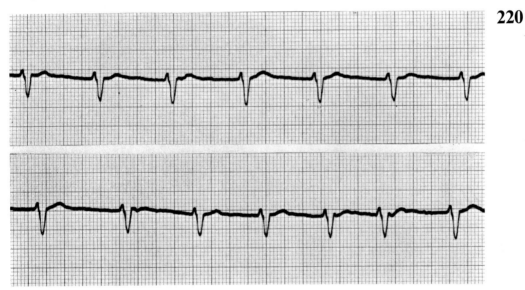

**220 Atrial fibrillation, digitalis intoxication causing atrioventricular dissociation and junctional rhythm.** The upper line shows a regular ventricular rate of 75/minute but no P waves are visible and in fact, there are tiny f waves here and there. The lower strip was taken from the same patient later; f waves are easier to see and the ventricles are irregular—junctional rhythm has stopped. (See also **228.**)

**221**

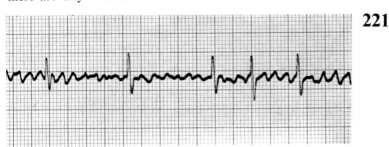

**221 Flutter—fibrillation.** Also called impure flutter. From time to time, the f waves become coarse and almost regular but are faster than classical flutter waves. The ventricular response is always irregular and the appearance has no special significance.

**222**

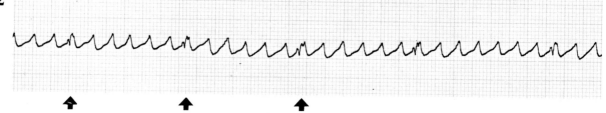

**223**

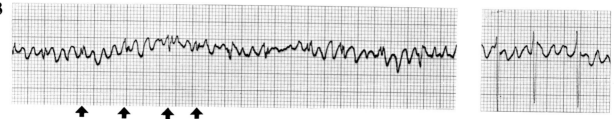

**222, 223 Lead V1 in atrial fibrillation and atrial flutter.** Lead V1 is often used for monitoring purposes. If the QRS complexes are of low voltage as they sometimes are, they may be dwarfed by F waves in atrial flutter (**222**) or the coarse f waves in atrial fibrillation (**223** left, compared to a short strip of V2 on the right). Ventricular flutter or fibrillation is mimicked. The arrows point to some of the discernible QRS complexes.

**224**

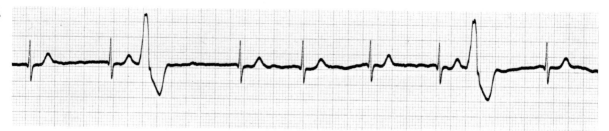

**224 Atrial fibrillation and extrasystoles.** Extrasystoles are not uncommon when atrial fibrillation is present; the problem is recognition. Junctional beats cannot be readily recognised unless they show a QRS contour which is different from that of surrounding beats. Ventricular extrasystoles however are easily identified because of their shape, and two are shown in the illustration opposite. Each follows the preceding beat by the same interval and has the same contour, so they arise from the same focus. Note that this is the one situation where it is impossible to describe an extrasystole as a premature beat for the rhythm is irregular, yet it is usually obvious by eye that the extrasystole is early. If it is not, then the diagnosis should be queried and the possibility of escape beats (**231**) or parasystole (**124**) examined. (See also **98**.) Remember too the possibility of intermittent aberrant conduction, which is also favoured by prematurity (**233**).

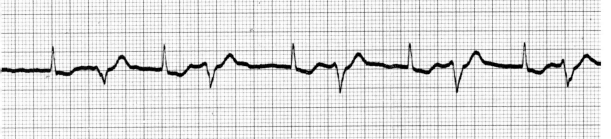

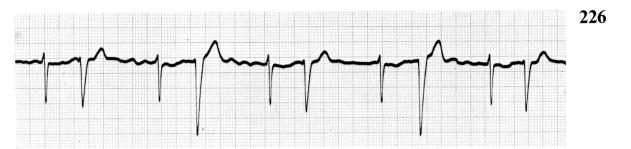

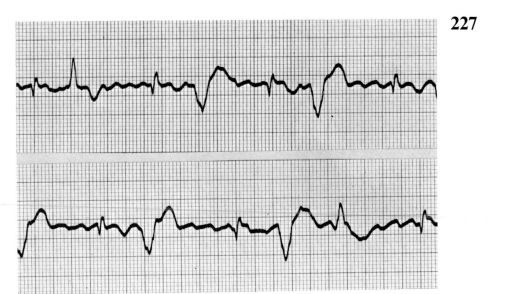

**225–227  Atrial fibrillation and coupled ventricular extrasystoles.** This rhythm is virtually certain to be due to digitalis intoxication. Figure **225** shows extrasystoles with a slightly changing contour which follow the preceding beat by an inconstant interval—i.e. they are multifocal. Figure **226** shows alternation in the contour of the extrasystoles but they all follow the preceding beat by very similar intervals—multiform, unifocal ectopics (see **93**). Figure **227** shows multifocal extrasystoles, and towards the end of the trace, bidirectional linked extrasystoles (see **97**, **98**). Note that although the basic rate is very slow in all three examples, the rhythm remains irregular, so junctional rhythm or complete heart block are not present (**219**, **220**). N.B. **227** is a single strip cut up.

**228**

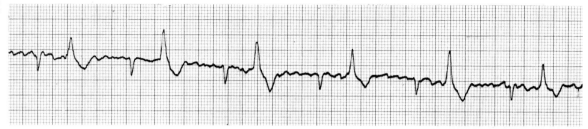

**228 Atrial fibrillation, junctional rhythm and coupled ventricular extrasystoles.** This trace shows even more evidence of digitalis intoxication. In addition to multiform, unifocal coupled extrasystoles, there is junctional rhythm (see **220**).

**229**

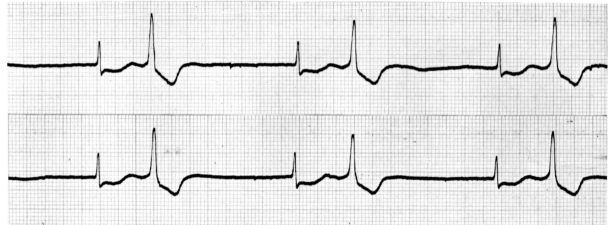

**229 Atrial fibrillation, extreme regular bradycardia and coupled ventricular extrasystoles.** A more severe case of digitalis induced arrhythmia. In addition to coupling, the basic rhythm is regular and the rate so slow that, despite the narrow junctional QRS complex, it is probable that complete heart block is present (see **219** and **263**).

(The two lines are a single strip.)

**230, 231 Escape beats in atrial fibrillation.** Escape beats occur during prolonged diastolic pauses whatever the underlying rhythm. For instance, they are seen in sinus arrest (see **65**), or during the marked bradycardia of sinus arrhythmia (**20**). Clearly, unusually long diastoles in atrial fibrillation with a controlled ventricular rate afford the same opportunity. If the escape beats arise in the atrioventricular junction, it is difficult to recognise them unless their contour differs from the rest. Figure **230** shows an example. The arrowed beats are junctional escape beats, following the preceding complexes by a constant interval. When the escape beats arise in the ventricle the position is easier because of the more obvious difference in QRS contour; **231** shows an example. The three escape beats are readily identified.

The differential diagnosis of ventricular escape beats in atrial fibrillation are extrasystoles (**224**), parasystole (**124**), and aberrant conduction (**233**). N.B. both examples are single strips cut up.

**230**

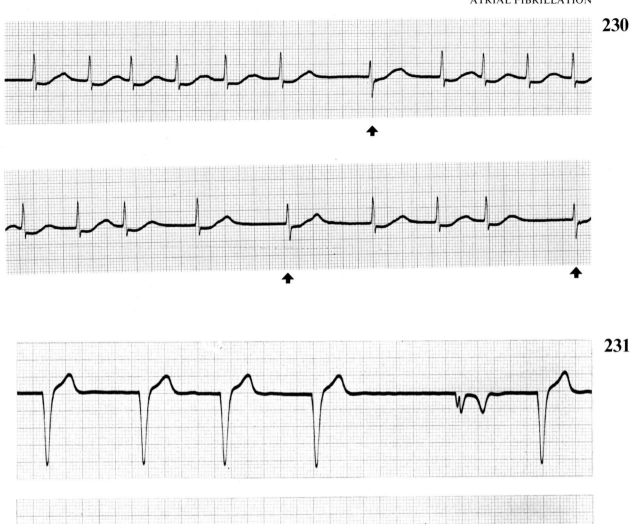

**231**

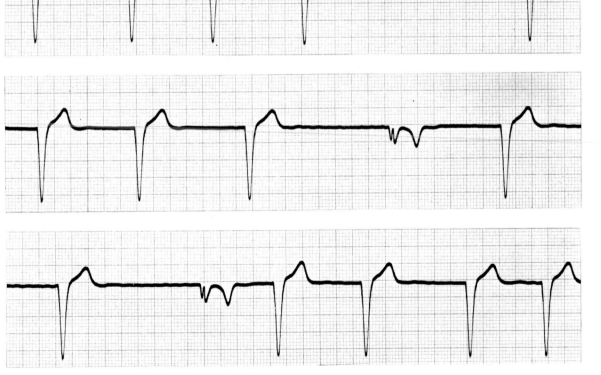

**232**

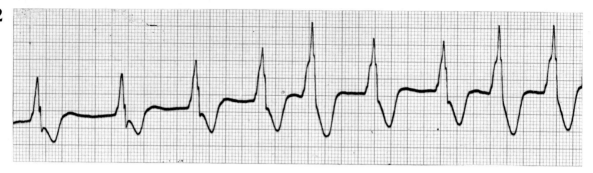

**232  Atrial fibrillation, aberrant conduction.** There
are no P waves, the rate is irregular, and the QRS
complexes are wide and bizarre. When the rate is
much faster (**234**) ventricular tachycardia may be
suspected, but this diagnosis is improbable at this
rate and with this degree of irregularity.

**233**

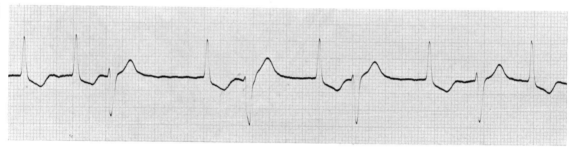

**233  Atrial fibrillation, intermittent aberrant con-
duction.** The basic rhythm (upright QRS complexes)
is irregular and there are no P waves. Four beats are
seen with a somewhat wider, differently shaped
QRS. They do not follow the preceding beat by a
fixed interval, and so cannot be either extrasystoles
or escape beats (see **224, 231**), and they are not
separated by intervals which are mutually multiples
of each other, so this is not parasystole (**124**). Note
the tendency for the aberrant complexes to occur
shortly after a beat which is itself preceded by a
long diastole—this is due to the longer refractory
period which follows such a pause in combination
with a relatively early subsequent beat.

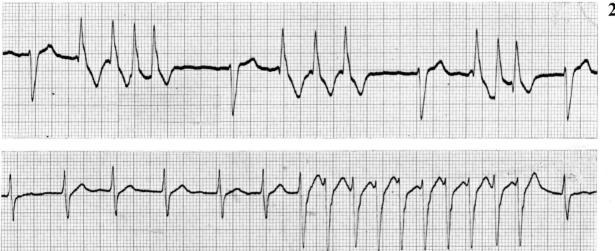

**234 Atrial fibrillation, bursts of aberrant conduction.** In addition to occurring in single, unusually premature beats (233) rate-dependent aberration in atrial fibrillation expresses itself in short bursts due to the marked irregularity of the ventricular response. Two examples are illustrated. The upper one shows several brief runs of aberrant conduction, and the lower one a single, longer episode. Both show the association with an increase in rate (see 342). The obvious differential diagnosis is from ventricular tachycardia. This may cause difficulty, though the irregularity of both rhythms, the rate dependency, and sheer probability favour aberration. As with aberration in supraventricular tachycardia (148) a QRS pattern of right bundle branch block is another helpful, but not a diagnostic, pointer. (See also 212, 232 and 345).

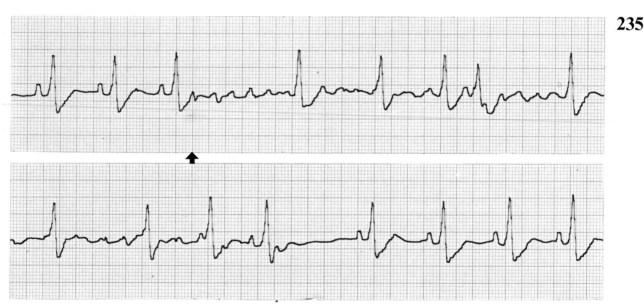

**235 Onset and termination of atrial fibrillation.** The trace is a continuous strip in two rows and documents a brief episode of atrial fibrillation. Three sinus beats are followed by an atrial extrasystole (upright P wave) which, being particularly premature, is not conducted to the ventricles and which triggers the episode of atrial fibrillation (see 210). There is a suggestion of a P wave towards the end of the upper line but successful coordination of atrial activity does not take place until the centre of the lower line. A sinus beat occurs, and once again is followed by a blocked extrasystole, but on this occasion atrial fibrillation is not initiated and sinus rhythm returns. Note the presence of aberrant QRS conduction throughout.

**236**

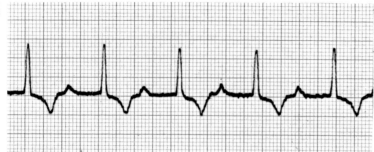

**236 Grade 1 heart block.** The PR interval is prolonged above the upper limit of normal of 0.22 second. In this example it is 0.4 second.

**237**

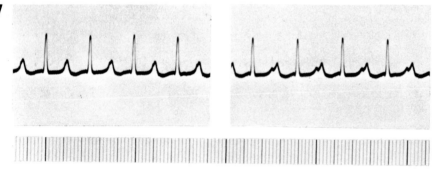

**237 Grade 1 heart block.** If the PR interval is sufficiently long, or if there is tachycardia, the P waves may disappear inside the T wave of the preceding complex. The illustration demonstrates this point. On the left, P waves cannot be seen. When the heart slows (right) the P waves emerge and can be seen following the T waves.

57 56 60 56 56 58 54 **238**

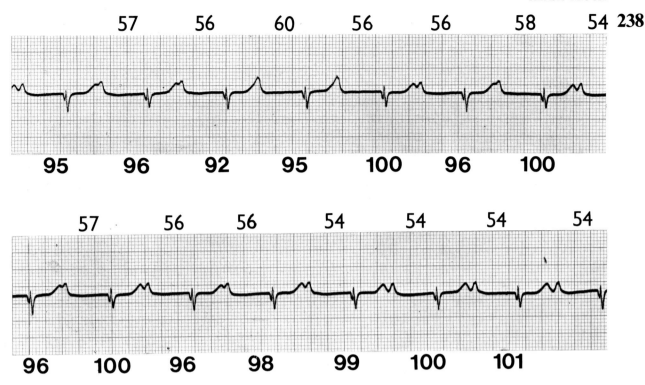

95 96 92 95 100 96 100

57 56 56 54 54 54 54

96 100 96 98 99 100 101

**238, 239 Grade 1 heart block, changing PR interval.** In grade 1 heart block the PR interval may not be constant. The impairment of conduction may alter spontaneously, or in response to a change in atrial rate, for if P waves occur 'earlier' they find the junction rather more refractory. Such changes are likely to be noticeable when the PR interval is long enough to place P near to the preceding T, as in **238** (a continuous strip on two lines). In this trace the figures in heavy type below are the P–P intervals, and the figures above, the PR intervals (the width of the P waves has been assumed where it cannot be seen). At the start of the record the heart speeds up and the PR interval lengthens. Later, it becomes steady, and the PR interval settles down. The changes are slight, but the result is striking and may cause confusion.

Figure **239** shows a similar situation, but here the PR interval appears to be lengthening and shortening in cycles. The figures below are P–P intervals. This is the result of sinus arrhythmia in a child. Again, the earlier the P wave, the longer the PR interval in subsequent beats. The picture is complicated by slight alterations in ventricular rate as it follows the atria and the effect is confusing.

N.B. all figures represent hundredths of a second.

**239**

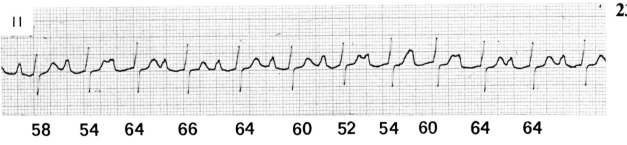

II

58 54 64 66 64 60 52 54 60 64 64

**240**

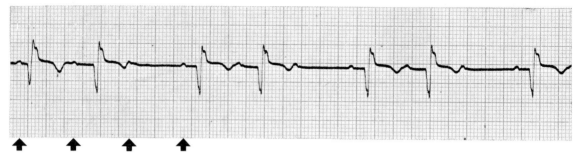

**240  Grade 2 heart block, type 1; Wenckebach periods.** Cycles of beats occur, very often repetitively, in which the PR interval lengthens progressively until conduction fails altogether, the last P wave not being followed by a QRS complex. The resulting short pause when cycles occur one after the other produces a characteristic grouping of beats which should always arouse the suspicion that Wenckebach periods are present. The first PR interval of each cycle is usually normal but may be slightly prolonged. The illustration shows three repeated cycles of 3:2 conduction—i.e. three P waves to two QRS complexes. N.B. the last P wave of each cycle is half hidden in the preceding T wave. Cycle length varies (see **242, 245**) but most show 2:1, 3:2, or 4:3 conduction. See also Wenckebach periods in paroxysmal atrial tachycardia (**140**), in junctional rhythm (**78, 80**), and in sino-atrial block (**61**). N.B. The arrows point to the first four P waves.

**241**

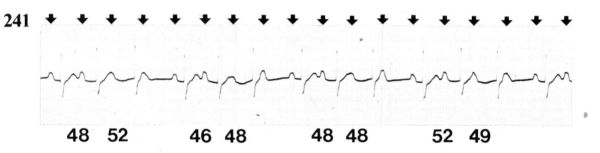

48   52          46   48          48   48          52   49

**241  Grade 2 heart block, Wenckebach periods.** It is characteristic of the conduction defect that each successive PR interval in a cycle increases by an amount which is less than in the previous one, so that classically, the effect is progressively to diminish the interval between QRS complexes making up the cycle—i.e. the ventricular rate speeds up. In practice, changes in sinus rate or in the smooth increments in block interfere with this effect and the ventricular rate may remain constant or even fall. The illustration shows all three. There are four complete cycles of 4:3 block. The figures below are the intervals between the QRS complexes in hundredths of a second. It will be seen that the interval lengthens in the first two cycles, is constant in the third, and shortens in the fourth. It can be seen that the sinus rate alters as the trace proceeds. (P waves arrowed.)

**242  Grade 2 heart block, Wenckebach periods.** Although Wenckebach cycles are frequently constant in length as they follow one another, they may vary. This illustration shows cycles of all lengths from 3:2 to 7:6 (also see **245**). Note again the variability of the timing of the ventricular response referred to in **241** (timings in hundredths of a second). Note too the not uncommon observation that, while at the start of a cycle the rate speeds up as classically described, the last interbeat interval is unexpectedly long (e.g. the first cycle on the top line, the first two cycles on the centre line, and the second cycle on the bottom line). This is because the last increment in the PR interval of the cycle in question is paradoxically greater than the preceding one, rather than less, as is usually the case. The explanation is obscure, The three lines are a single strip cut up.

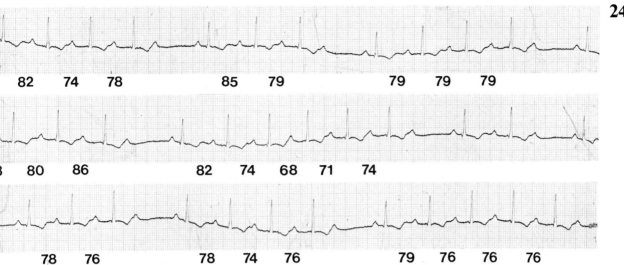

82  74  78        85  79        79  79  79

3  80  86        82  74  68  71  74

78  76        78  74  76        79  76  76  76

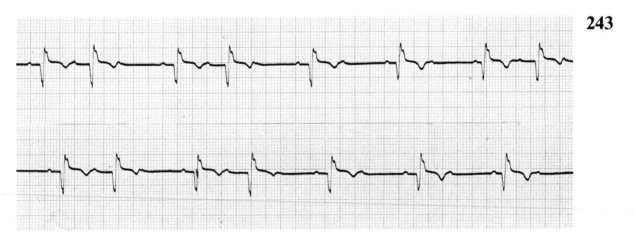

**243**

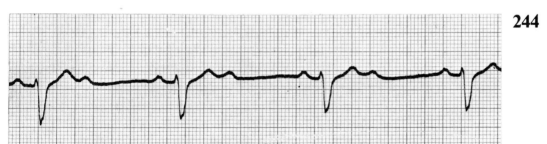

**244**

**243, 244 Grade 2 heart block, type 1; 2:1 conduction.** Partial heart block showing 2:1 conduction may be type 1 (i.e. Wenckebach block with 2:1 cycles) or type 2. Since the two varieties have a different patho-physiology and prognosis, the distinction is worth making. Fortunately, in Wenckebach block the length of the cycles often alters and this may help. For instance 243 shows cycles of 3:2 conduction as well as of 2:1, indicating that the latter is really type 1 block. Another useful point is that the PR interval of the conducted P wave in type 1 block is often prolonged (**244**) whereas it is more often normal in type 2 block—but this is not a reliable guide (see **254**). N.B. **243** is a single strip cut up.

**245**

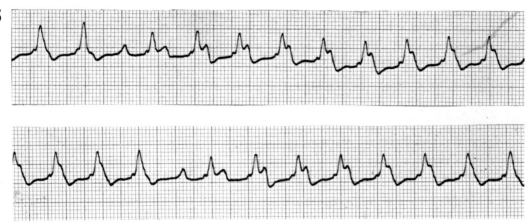

**245 Grade 2 heart block, prolonged Wenckebach periods.** Most Wenckebach cycles are relatively short, whether constant or variable (**242**), and are easily recognised. Prolonged cycles may cause diagnostic difficulty. The illustration shows a single trace in two rows. After the first two QRS complexes a P wave can be seen in a pause. This is followed after a prolonged PR interval by a QRS complex, and subsequent P waves can now be identified immediately following each QRS complex but steadily 'moving backwards' as the trace proceeds to merge with them as the PR interval progressively lengthens still further. The P wave which merges almost exactly with the fourth QRS on the second row is not conducted and the cycle is completed by a dropped beat as on the upper line. The next P wave is now visible and the cycle recommences.

**246**

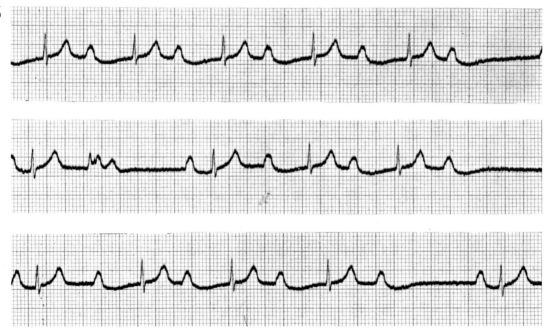

**246 Changing grades of partial heart block.** Heart block is often unstable, changing grade from minute to minute. The illustration shows a continuous trace in three rows. It begins with grade 1 block, the PR interval being fixed, and then passes without warning into Wenckebach periods of varying length.

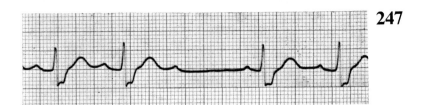

**247**

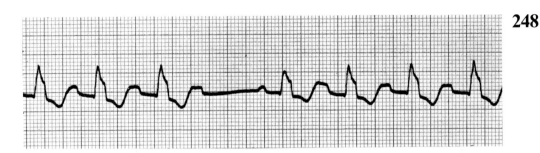

**248**

**247, 248   Grade 2 heart block, type 2; occasional dropped beats.** This is the simplest form of type 2 block. Without warning, and in particular without progressive prolongation of the PR interval beforehand, a P wave is not conducted and a beat is dropped. Classically, the PR interval of conducted beats should be normal but this not a reliable feature as is seen in both the examples illustrated. Both show one dropped beat. Figure **248** is interesting because P waves are practically invisible inside the T wave of the preceding complex and the true nature of the arrhythmia is only discovered when the dropped QRS reveals the next P wave in isolation. Note that in both examples the PR interval of the first beat after the pause is shorter—presumably the conduction paths have had more time to recover. Both traces show QRS aberration.

**249**

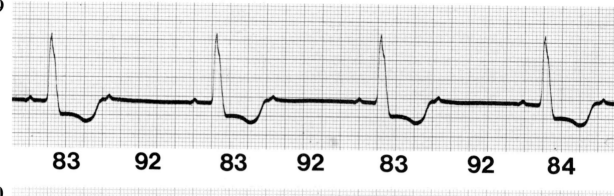

83    92    83    92    83    92    84

**250**

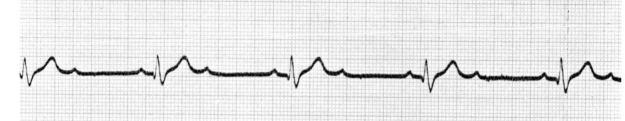

**249, 250 Grade 2 heart block, type 2; 2:1 conduction.** Higher degrees of type 2 heart block are characterised by fixed ratios of conduction. In the commonest, 2:1 block, every alternate P wave is conducted, usually with a normal PR interval. (Prolongation of the PR interval of the conducted beat favours type 1 block—see **244**.) In this degree of block, it is common for the P–P intervals to vary, the P–P interval enclosing the QRS being shorter than the one that does not. This is probably due to alterations in vagal tone induced by the ventricular beat itself. Figure **249** shows this (the figures are P–P intervals in hundredths of a second). The alternative situation is shown in **250**, in which the P–P intervals are fixed. See also **261, 262, 265**.

**251**

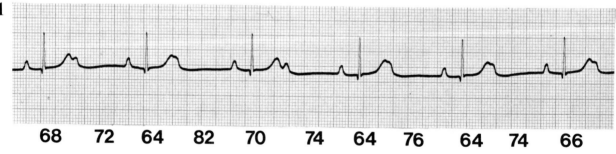

68    72    64    82    70    74    64    76    64    74    66

**251 Grade 2 heart block, 2:1 block.** The alteration in timing of the P wave referred to in **249** is usually a consistent event when it occurs at all, but occasionally the intervals change slightly and this can cause diagnostic difficulty, since the alteration in appearance of the trace suggests complete heart block. The illustration shows such a case. The figures beneath it are the P–P intervals in hundredths of a second.

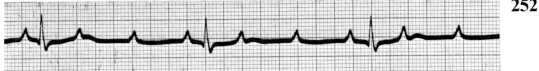

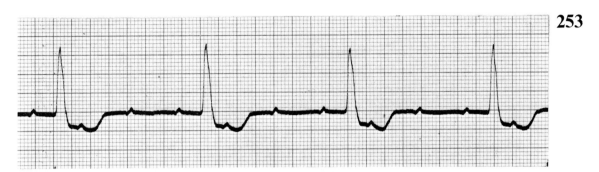

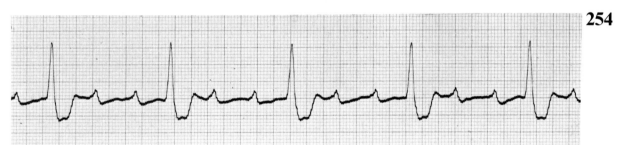

**252–254  Grade 2 heart block, type 2; 3:1 conduction.** The ventricles respond to only every third P wave. The P–P intervals tend to be fixed. The PR interval of the conducted P wave is usually normal (**252**) but may be slightly (**253**) or greatly (**254**) prolonged. In each example it is necessary to identify one of the P waves inside the QRS complex (**254**) or T wave.

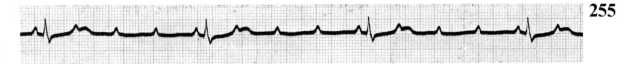

**255  Grade 2 heart block, type 2; 4:1 conduction.** This degree of block is rare. The PR interval of the conducted beat is normal in this example.

**256**

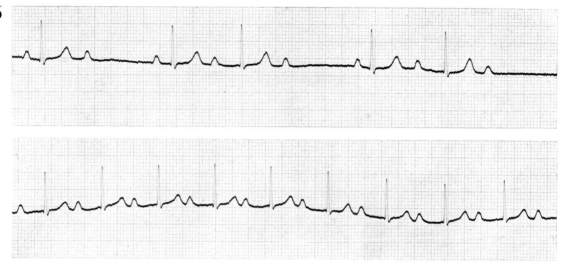

**256, 257   Partial heart block, influence of atrial rate.** The two types of grade 2 heart block behave differently with alterations in atrial rate. In type 1 block, 1:1 atrioventricular conduction can usually be restored with a rise in atrial rate (e.g. with exercise, or atropine); **256** shows this effect. A 3:2 Wenckebach block (above) is converted to grade 1 block with exercise (below).

In contrast, a rise in atrial rate in type 2 block increases the impairment of conduction. Figure **257** shows 2:1 block at rest (upper line) progressing through 3:1 block (centre) to complete block (lowest line). Note that the ventricular rate hardly alters.

**257**

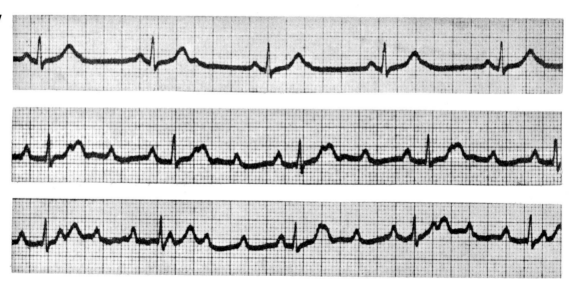

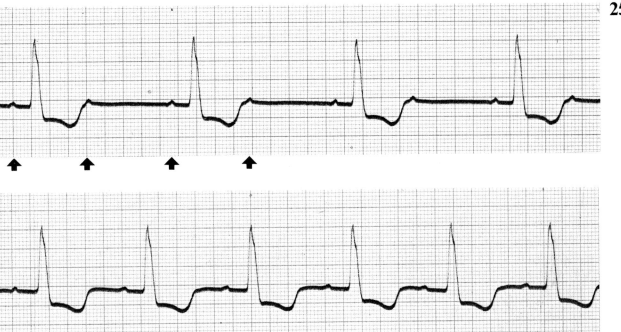

**258 Grade 2 heart block, type 2; effect of vagal stimulation.** The effect of an increase in atrial rate on the degree of block in type 2 partial heart block is described in **257**. The reverse process, atrial slowing (conveniently achieved by carotid sinus massage) produces a paradoxical effect on ventricular rate which can provide valuable bedside diagnostic information. As the atrial rate slows, a reduction in the degree of block may initiate 1:1 conduction and a faster heart rate. On the upper line 2:1 block is present with an atrial rate of 70/minute and a ventricular rate of 35/minute. After carotid massage (below) the atrial rate is reduced to between 50 and 60/minute but 1:1 conduction has returned. A short series of P waves are arrowed on the upper line.

**259**

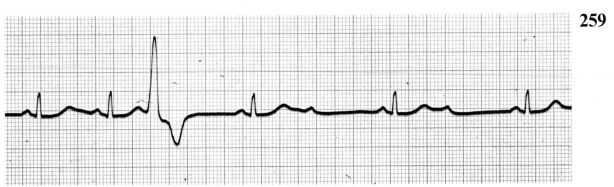

**259 Grade 2 heart block precipitated by an extrasystole.** In this trace, a ventricular extrasystole appears to initiate 2:1 heart block. Presumably this is the effect of poor coronary perfusion induced by the inefficient pressure generated by the extrasystole.

**260**

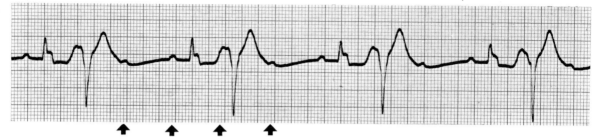

**260  Partial heart block and extrasystoles.** As with complete block (see **267**) extrasystoles may interrupt partial heart block. In the example illustrated there is 3:1 block with coupled unifocal ventricular extrasystoles. Note that despite the P wave preceding each extrasystole, the latter cannot be in reality a conducted beat with aberration, for the PR interval would be too short. A short series of P waves are arrowed.

**261**

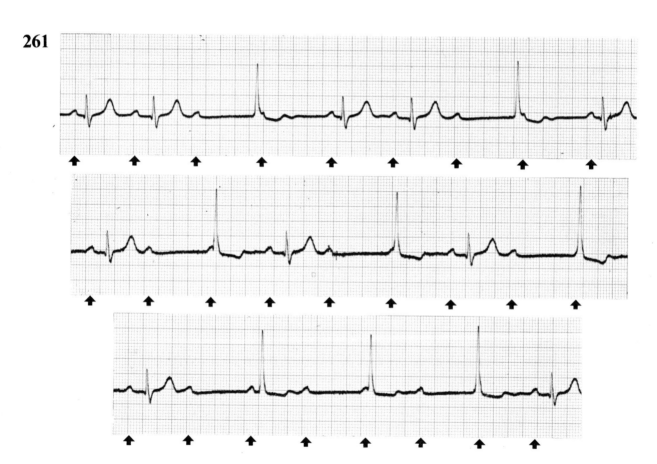

**261  Partial heart block and escape beats.** The recurrent long gaps caused by dropped beats in Wenckebach block may be interrupted by escape beats, which upsets the repetition of cycles. In these three strips, all taken from the same patient, the escape beats occur 1.42 seconds after the preceding beat. They have a different contour but are narrow, so they are junctional in origin. Above, there are Wenckebach periods of 3:2 block; in the centre, 2:1 (or should it be 3:2?) block; and below, a short period of ventricular standstill. (Note that it is impossible to be dogmatic about the underlying degree of block because the escape beat renders the ventricle refractory at the crucial moment.) N.B. interestingly, in the lowest trace, the escape beat is enclosed by a shorter P–P interval, as in 2:1 block sometimes. (See **249**.) All P waves are arrowed.

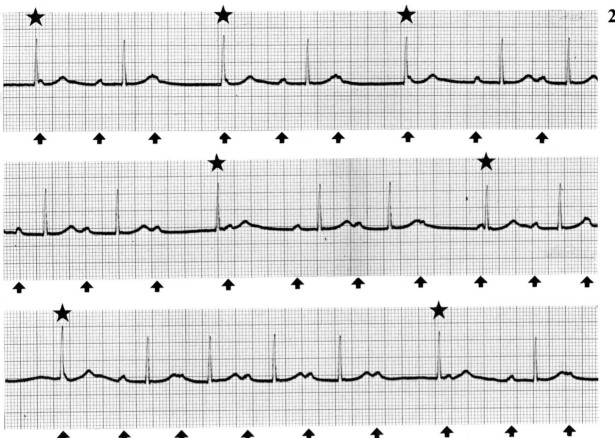

**262 Partial heart block and escape beats.** This situation is described in detail in **261** and is easy to identify when the escape beats have a different contour; but in the trace illustrated opposite (a continuous strip in three rows), the escape beats are identical with the rest*, and the result is confusing and liable to be misdiagnosed for complete block. The P waves are arrowed for clarity, and the escape beats are starred above. Some of the Wenckebach cycles are only 2:1. As in **261**, there is a tendency for P–P intervals enclosing a QRS complex to be shorter (**249**), but this is not seen everywhere.

*Except spuriously, when P coincides with QRS and increases its height, e.g. the first beat on the third line.

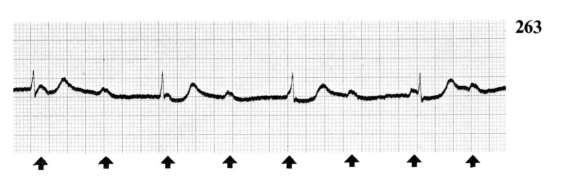

**263 Complete heart block (grade 3).** The atria and ventricles beat independently of each other. No relationship is discernible between P waves and QRS complexes. If they cannot be seen clearly, P waves must be sought inside QRS or T. The P waves are arrowed to assist analysis. The QRS complex in this example is narrow and suggests a ventricular pacemaker high in the bundle of His above the bifurcation, or in the atrioventricular junction.

263

**264**

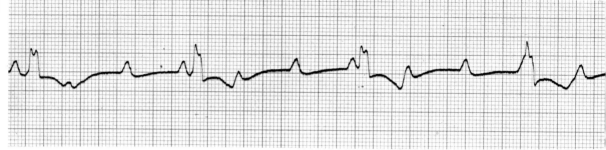

**264 Complete heart block.** When the ventricular pacemaker is situated lower in the bundles of His or in the ventricular muscle itself, the QRS is wide and bizarre in shape and the rate tends to be slower. Of course, a higher focus with aberrant conduction will produce a similar pattern but the rate will usually be faster. The majority show the pattern of right bundle branch block because the pacemaker is on the left side. In the example illustrated, the ventricular rate is 33/minute. Note how the large P waves produce considerable distortion of the last QRS.

**265**

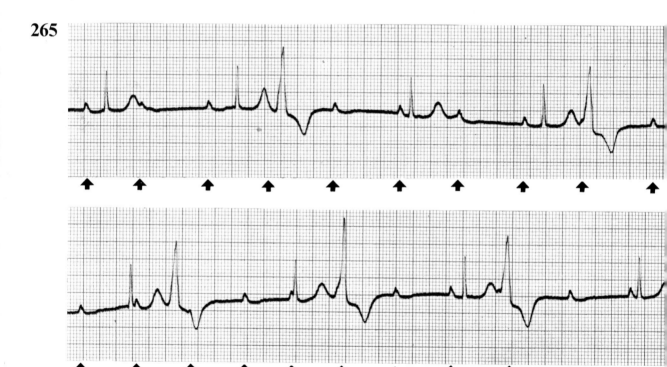

**265 Complete heart block and extrasystoles.** If extrasystoles arise in the ventricle during complete heart block they produce irregularity. They are identified as extrasystoles by the fixed time relationship they have to the preceding QRS, the period being constant (as usual) for each separate focus if more than one is present. Obviously, only ventricular extrasystoles are seen. In the example opposite, analysis is made easy because the idioventricular pacemaker is high in the bundle of His or in the atrioventricular junction and the complexes are narrow. All P waves or their positions are arrowed. Note the inconstant atrial rate in this trace (**266**). The upper strip shows occasional extrasystoles; the lower one, taken later, shows a coupled rhythm. The other causes of an irregular ventricular rhythm in complete heart block are illustrated next—i.e. two competing foci (**268, 269**), an unstable pacemaker (**270**), and occasional conducted beats (**271, 272**).

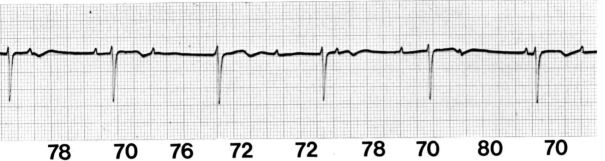

78  70  76  72  72  78  70  80  70

**266, 267  Complete heart block, atrial irregularity.** Although it is usual to find relative constancy of the atrial rate in most traces showing complete heart block, the sinus node is still subject to the usual factors which influence it and atrial irregularity may be seen. Two examples are illustrated, one showing modest irregularity (266), and the other (267), marked irregularity (the two rows represent a single continuous strip). P–P intervals are given below both traces (hundredths of a second). In both, it is noteworthy that the ventricular pacemaker is 'high' (i.e. the QRS is narrow) and that the P–P intervals which include a QRS are shorter than the others, so that part of the atrial irregularity is due to a vagal effect (as in 2:1 block). (See **249** and also atrial behaviour in Stokes–Adams attacks, **277, 278**.)

267

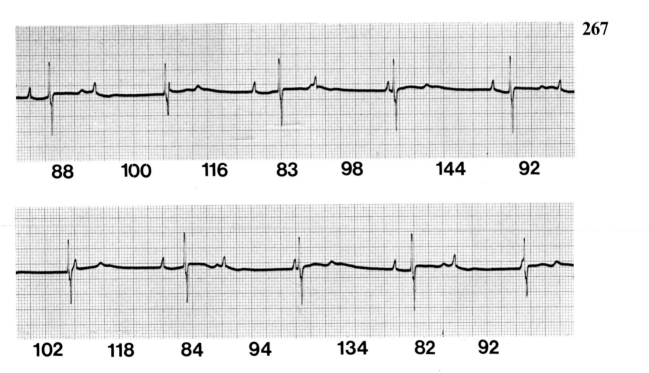

88  100  116  83  98  144  92

102  118  84  94  134  82  92

**268**

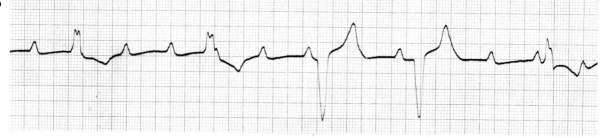

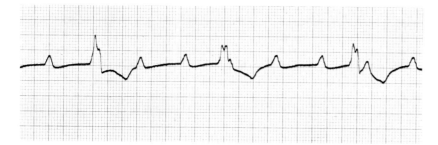

**268, 269 Complete heart block, competition for control.** Occasionally in complete heart block, two or more foci in the ventricles compete for control. Obviously this will happen only if the faster of the two is subject to exit block from time to time. Two examples are illustrated, both continuous strips cut up. In **268** the faster focus appears for two beats only, while in **269**, the slower focus emerges as an escape rhythm. See also **274**.

**269**

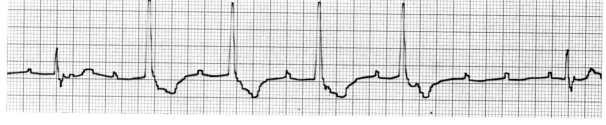

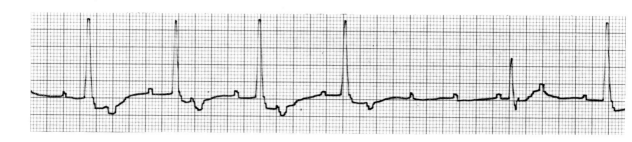

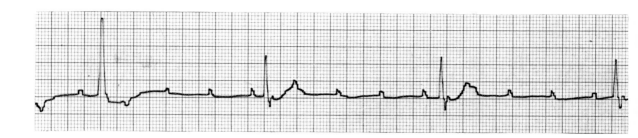

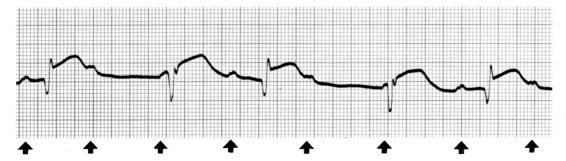

**270  Irregular ventricular rhythm in complete heart block.** Usually the ventricular rhythm is regular in complete heart block. Irregularities may occur however, if extrasystoles are present (**265**), if there are occasional conducted beats (**271, 272**), or if there are two foci competing for control (**268**) and occasionally, as in this example, the idioventricular pacemaker fails to produce a regular discharge. To assist analysis the P waves are arrowed. At a first glance one might suspect Wenckebach periods but it is clear that these are not present, for the 'PR' intervals after the gaps are too short and inconstant.

**271**

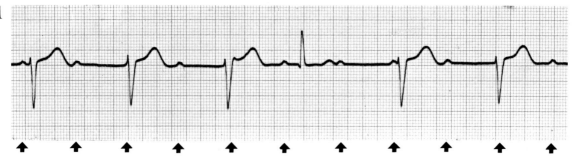

**271, 272  Occasional conducted beats in complete heart block.** From time to time tracings of complete heart block are seen in which there are occasional complexes of apparently supraventricular origin. One is seen in **271**—the fourth QRS being narrow and different in shape from the rest. Note that it is preceded by a P wave with a timing suitable for conduction. P waves are arrowed to assist analysis.

In the longer trace from which **271** was taken, the same sequence was seen several times (**272**). Note that each time there is the same PR interval before the narrow complex and that the P wave itself occupies the same position in relation to the preceding T wave. Note too that P waves falling slightly 'earlier' or 'later' are not conducted. The explanation is probably the existence of a brief phase of supernormal conduction following the T wave.

**272**

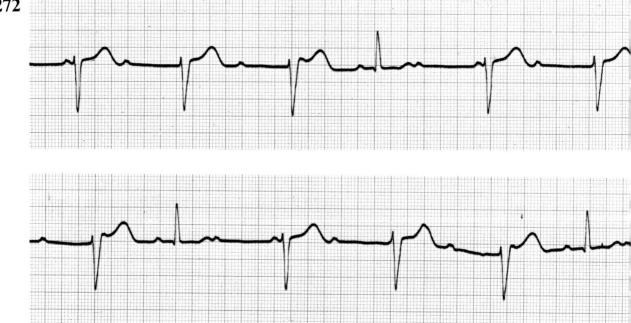

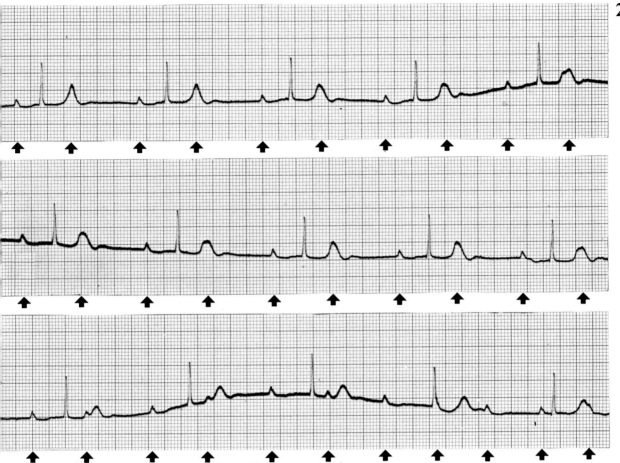

**273  Complete heart block masquerading as a lesser degree of block.** It is not uncommon to find the atrial rate is nearly an exact multiple of the ventricular rate so that, if only a short strip is examined, complete heart block may be missed or mis-diagnosed. An example is shown. The atrial rate is almost twice the ventricular rate and, as the record begins (the three rows are one continuous strip) there is apparently sinus bradycardia with grade 1 heart block; then, as the trace proceeds, it becomes clear that the correct diagnosis is complete heart block, and that P waves have been hidden in T waves. At first, with a slower atrial rate, P–P intervals vary considerably (**266, 267**); then the atrial rate speeds up and this gets less obvious. All P waves are arrowed.

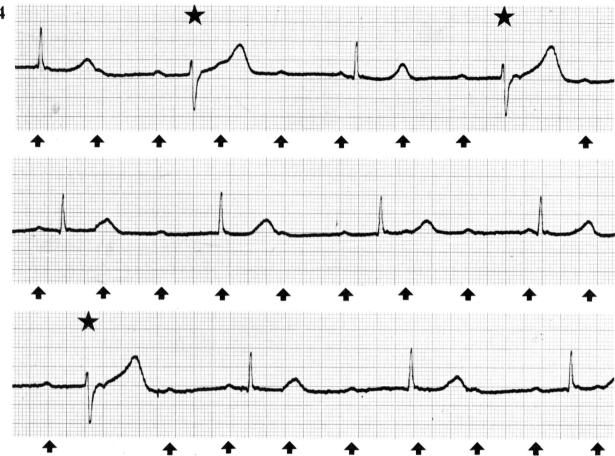

**274** **Retrograde conduction with atrial capture in complete heart block.** Although in theory the atria and the ventricles are isolated from each other in complete heart block, occasionally, retrograde capture of the atria is seen—i.e. the paradoxical situation that conduction occurs in one direction but not in the other. The illustration shows complete heart block. P waves are arrowed for ease of analysis. Two ventricular foci compete for control of the ventricles (**268**). Both are relatively slow. One focus is identified by a star above each complex. The second and third of these complexes are followed by a tiny blip in the ST segment which is an inverted (i.e. retrogradely activated) P wave of atrial capture. Note that in each instance the atrial capture causes no interruption in the fundamental timing of the other P waves though the very next P wave fails to appear in its expected place (no arrow). This cannot be because it is lost in the ST segment because elsewhere in this situation it is clearly visible. The explanation is that the impulse from the atrial capture beat has rendered the atrium refractory at the crucial moment but has failed to penetrate the sinus node itself because of entrance block protecting it.

**275** **Complete heart block complicating myocardial infarction.** Complete heart block (or lesser grades) are seen more often with inferior infarctions. The illustration shows an acute inferior infarction in the earliest hours. The rhythm strip below confirms the presence of complete block.

**276** **Congenital heart block.** This is uncommonly of any grade other than complete. The QRS complexes are narrow since the idioventricular pacemaker is situated high in the bundle of His or in the atrioventricular junction. The ventricular rate is usually faster than in acquired heart block—often as much as 50–60/minute. The example opposite has a relatively slow rate of 40/minute. Although no rhythm strip is provided, the varying relationship of the P waves to the QRS complexes can be clearly seen. (See also **341** and **451**.)

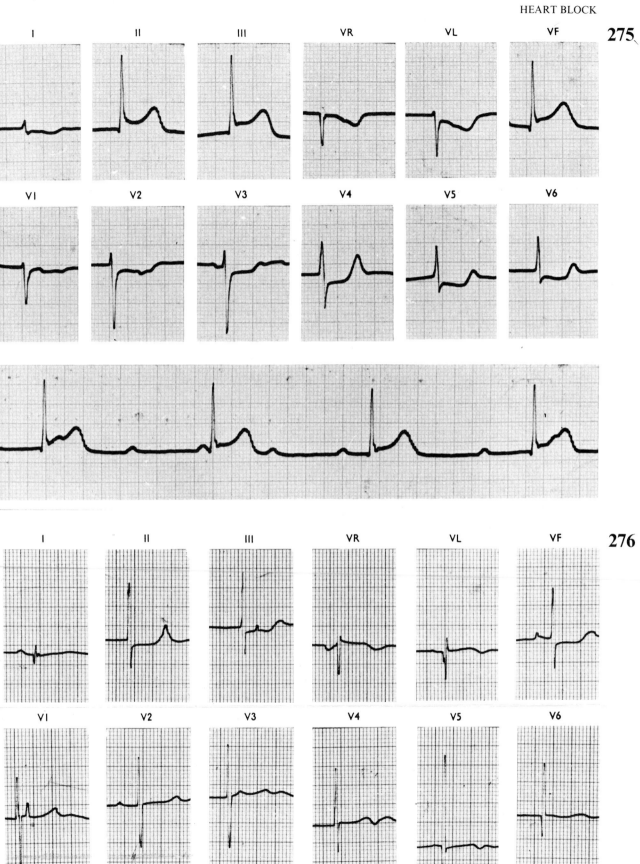

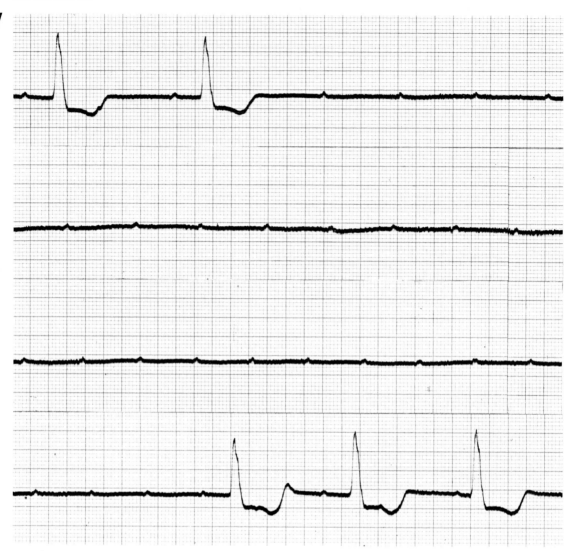

**277 Stokes–Adams attack.** The classical Stokes–Adams attack is caused by the unheralded onset of ventricular standstill with continuing atrial activity in a patient with established, or intermittent, heart block, but clinically similar episodes can accompany rapid ventricular dysrhythmias or the cardiac arrest seen in carotid sinus hypersensitivity (**66**). The duration of an attack varies from a few seconds (when it may escape the patient's attention) to a minute or more. The attack illustrated in this example develops on the basis of 2:1 block and when the ventricle restarts, complete block is seen. Note how the atrial rate speeds up as the attack proceeds (the four lines are a continuous strip); this is because the patient is aware of what is happening and is alarmed. (See **265**).

**278 Stokes–Adams attacks.** Although, as illustrated in **277**, Stokes–Adams attacks occur during the higher grades of heart block (grades 2 and 3), they may occur without warning in patients with normal sinus rhythm who get intermittent attacks of complete heart block. The illustration does not quite show this situation, for the patient has the combination of left bundle branch block and a prolonged PR interval, indicating impaired conduction in the right bundle or atrioventricular junction or main bundle too, but it does show two short episodes of ventricular standstill occurring in the absence of grade 2 or 3 block and serves to document the possibility. Note that each episode begins with a ventricular extrasystole, which is not necessarily the case. During the second attack idioventricular beats of similar contour to the rest occur; in the first attack, such a beat is followed by an extrasystole and terminates the attack. The marked complex was caused by chest percussion (**197**). Note once again (**277**) the way the atrial rate speeds up in the second attack (of which the patient was aware) but not in the first (which was too brief to reach his attention). The five rows are one continuous strip.

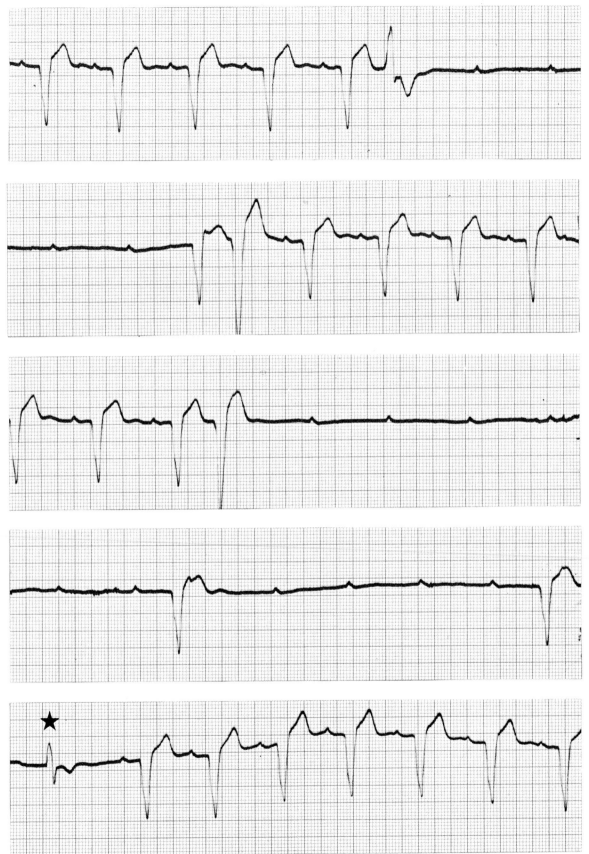

**279**

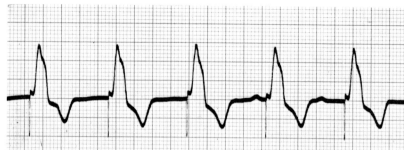

**279   Endocardial pacing, unipolar pacing catheter.**
The tip of the pacing electrode catheter (the negative or 'active' electrode) is situated at the apex of the right ventricle and the circuit is completed via a distant electrode (the positive or 'indifferent') which is usually a plate on the pacemaker itself (**718, 719**). The result is a large pacing artefact either above or below the isoelectric line (or both), depending on the lead studied. The artefact is a thin vertical line immediately preceding the paced complex and is the brief duration electrical impulse emitted by the pacemaker. In the example shown it points downwards.

**280**

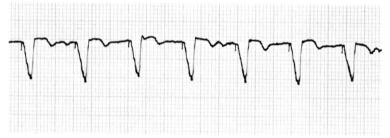

**280   Endocardial pacing, bipolar pacing catheter.**
Both electrodes are contained in the catheter and emerge about 1cm apart at the tip. The circuit is completed via the blood in the ventricle. The result is a tiny pacing artefact which can just be seen in the illustration, pointing downwards in this instance; sometimes it is invisible.

**281**

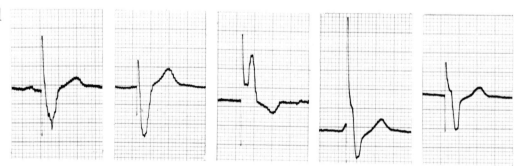

**281   The electrocardiogram during pacing.** Paced beats are simply a series of controlled ventricular ectopic beats and little can be learned from the electrocardiogram while pacing proceeds. To emphasise this point, the illustration shows five different paced complexes recorded in the same ventricle by moving the tip of the pacing catheter into several different positions.

**282**

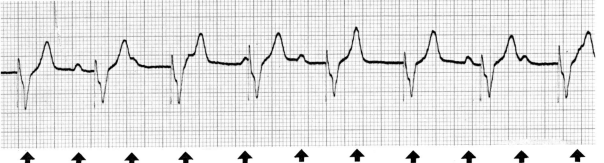

**282 Fixed rate pacing and continuing atrial activity.** The P waves, or their presumed positions, are arrowed. Note how they distort the paced complexes.

**283**

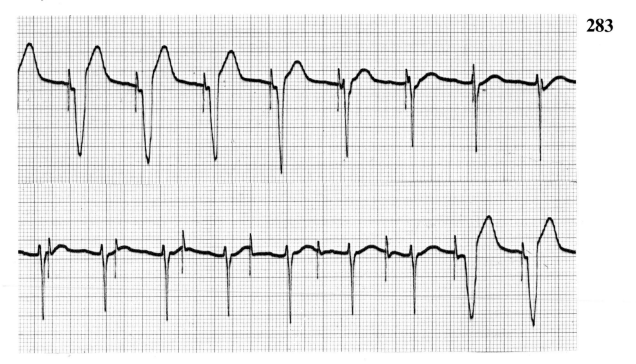

**283 Fixed rate pacing competing with sinus rhythm.** If sinus rhythm returns while fixed rate pacing is in progress, there is competition between the sinus node and the pacemaker for control of the heart. The illustration shows a continuous strip in two rows. The record begins with a series of paced beats but in the centre of the upper row sinus rhythm returns (the P waves are not easy to see) since the sinus rate is marginally faster than the rate of the pacemaker. Sinus rhythm persists but so do the pacing artefacts. Because of the difference in rate, the artefact moves progressively through the QRS complex and T wave of the sinus beats. In the centre of the second row it reaches the peak of the T wave—the point at which the heart is most vulnerable to the development of ventricular fibrillation (**183**). Eventually, the pacing artefact moves beyond the refractory period of the sinus beat and captures the ventricles to restart the entire cycle. The dangers of this situation are obvious and for this reason demand pacemakers have been introduced. Note the fourth and fifth complexes on the upper row; these are fusion beats activated by both sources simultaneously and therefore intermediate in shape between paced beats and sinus beats.

**284**

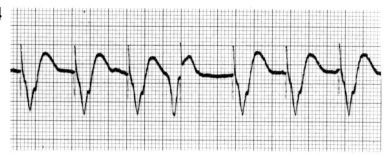

**284 Fixed rate pacing and extrasystoles.** The situation is analogous to that outlined in **283**. Extrasystoles interrupt the smooth sequence of pacing and there is a risk that the next pacing artefact will fall upon the peak of the T wave of the ectopic itself. The illustration shows a ventricular extrasystole occurring after the first three paced beats.

**285**

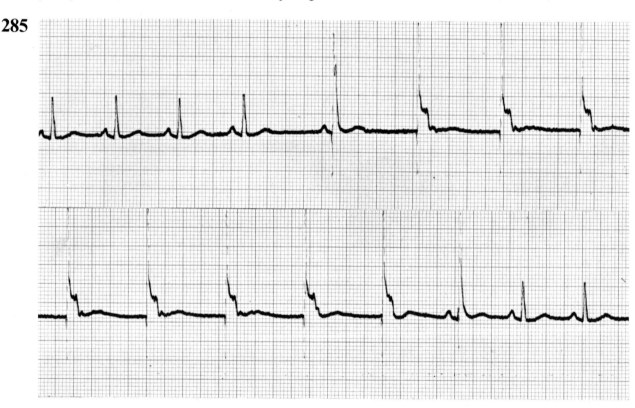

**285 Demand pacing with an inhibited demand pacemaker.** The pacing catheter is used to sense spontaneous ventricular activity as well as delivering the pacing stimulus. When the pacemaker detects this, it is inhibited from discharging itself, thus avoiding competition. If, however, after a pre-set interval, no further spontaneous activity is detected, the pacemaker discharges once more. The upper row of this continuous strip begins with sinus rhythm. Then sinus rhythm slows and stops, and pacing commences. At the end of the lower row sinus rhythm returns and the pacemaker shuts off. The third complex from the end is a fusion beat (**283**).

**286**

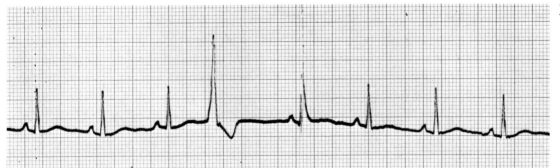

**286   Pacing induced by an extrasystole.** This record was taken from a patient with a demand pacemaker in situ. After the third sinus beat, a ventricular extrasystole occurs. The pause following the extrasystole is sufficiently long to trigger the pacemaker and a paced (actually a fusion) beat occurs (see **283**).

**287**

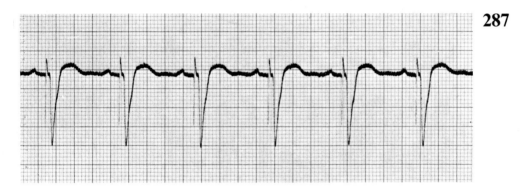

**287   Atrially triggered pacing.** A separate electrode is used to pick up atrial activity from the right atrium and the P wave is fed into a pacemaker which introduces a PR interval and then paces the ventricle in the usual way. The advantage is that the heart rate can increase normally with exercise. Note the P wave, the PR interval of 0.2 second, and the pacing artefact before each QRS.

**288**

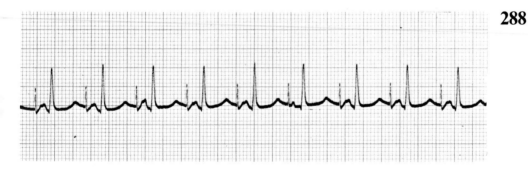

**288   Atrial pacing.** The pacing electrode is situated in the right atrium and the artefact is followed by a normal P wave and QRS complex.

**289**

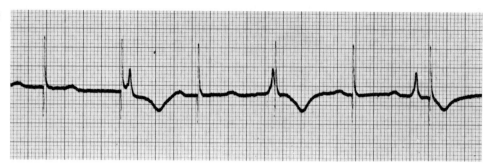

**289  Failure of pacing due to loss of electrode contact.** The pacing artefacts are not followed by ventricular activity. It is true the second artefact has a close relationship to one of the three idioventricular beats on the record but it is clear by reference to the others that this is not a paced beat, for it has the same contour as the others and they are obviously unrelated to the pacing artefacts. Complete heart block is present. Exit block produces the same appearance, as will impending generator failure.

**290**

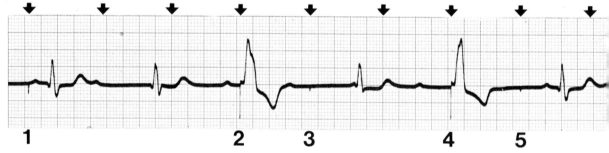

**290  Failure of fixed rate pacing due to breakage of the pacing electrode.** If a pacing electrode breaks the two ends may make intermittent contact*. As a result, sometimes the pacing stimulus is transmitted successfully but on other occasions only part of the stimulus crosses the break and of course, frequently, the circuit is completely broken. Thus, while pacing artefacts and paced beats are seen, they do not occur regularly. This illustration shows five pacing artefacts at different intervals apart. They are numbered below the trace. Numbers 2 and 4 are large, and pace the ventricle normally. Numbers 1, 3, and 5 vary in size and do not pace the heart—i.e. only part of the stimulus has crossed the catheter break and is insufficient to stimulate the ventricle. Some artefacts do not appear at all, having failed altogether, and this is demonstrated by the arrows, which show the position or the expected position of all pacing artefacts. N.B. when the heart is not being paced, complete heart block is present.

*A faulty connection may have the same effect.

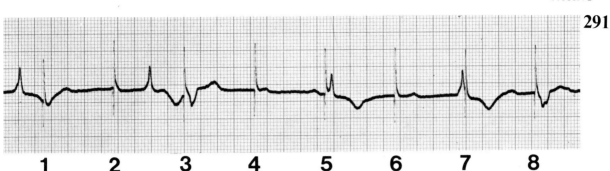

**1  2  3  4  5  6  7  8**

**291 Intermittent pacing due to poor electrode contact.** If the tip of the pacing electrode makes intermittent contact with the myocardium, not every pacing artefact stimulates the heart. In the example shown, only the third and eighth artefacts pace the heart. The first and seventh may have failed because they fall within the refractory period of the idioventricular rhythm, but the second, fourth, and sixth artefacts are not followed by ventricular capture. At first sight the fifth artefact might be conducted but comparison with the two definitely paced beats and the patient's own complexes reveals the true state of affairs. Pacing artefacts are numbered for convenience.

N.B. exit block will produce the same appearances if the electrode tip is firmly anchored.

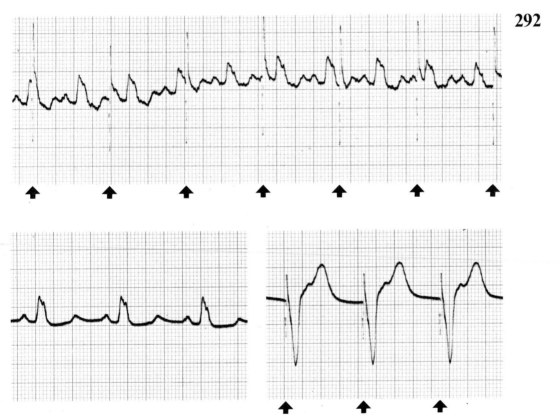

**292 Failure of inhibited demand pacing.** If the tip of the pacing catheter loses contact with the myocardium when an inhibited demand pacemaker is in situ, the pacemaker fails to appreciate that spontaneous activity is taking place and will discharge regularly. Continuing pacemaker artefacts in a patient who has temporarily returned to sinus rhythm is a sign of failure of the pacing system. This situation is illustrated on the upper line of the example. On the lower line, to assist analysis, the traces show, on the left, normal sinus rhythm in the lead shown above, and on the right, successful pacing in the same lead. All pacing artefacts are arrowed.

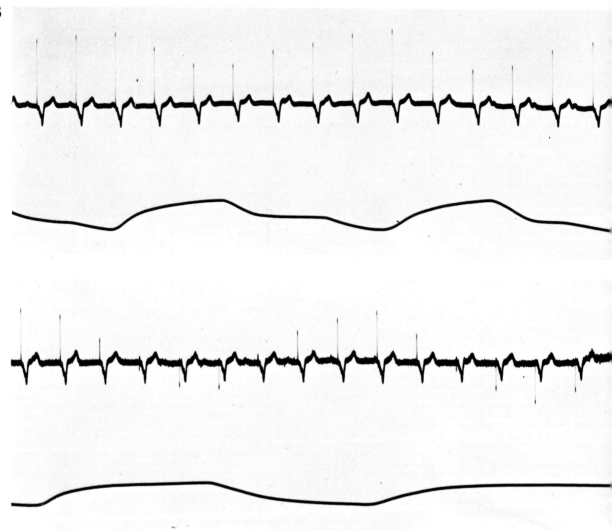

**293   Alteration in the sign of the pacing artefact due to respiration.** Usually, the pacing artefacts are constant in size. Sometimes, due to the direction of the vector of the pacing artefact in a particular lead, it will vary in size with breathing, as the hearts shifts in the chest. The upper illustration shows this occurring in lead II, the line beneath indicating respiration. The lower illustration shows the effect of deeper respiration; now the artefact becomes actually negative.

**294   Left ventricular hypertrophy.** This is present when, in an adult of normal build, the R wave in V5 or V6, or the S wave in V1 or V2 exceeds 25mm. These figures require amendment for body fat and for age, younger adults normally having larger voltages (**11**). Voltage changes may or may not be

reflected in limb leads (see later). In this example the heart is semi-vertical, and changes are seen in inferior leads. Note the tall rather pointed T waves in V5 and V6—sometimes referred to as the 'diastolic overload' pattern, e.g. in dominant aortic regurgitation or severe mitral regurgitation, as opposed to 'systolic overload' pattern (see **296**) seen in aortic stenosis or coarctation, though this is not a reliable distinction clinically.

**295   Left ventricular hypertrophy, early T wave changes.** There is T wave inversion in V6, and flat T waves in V5, VL, and I. Voltage changes are reflected in VL and I as the heart is semi-horizontal. Note that the maximum height of R wave is in V4 because of anticlockwise rotation.

# VENTRICULAR HYPERTROPHY

294

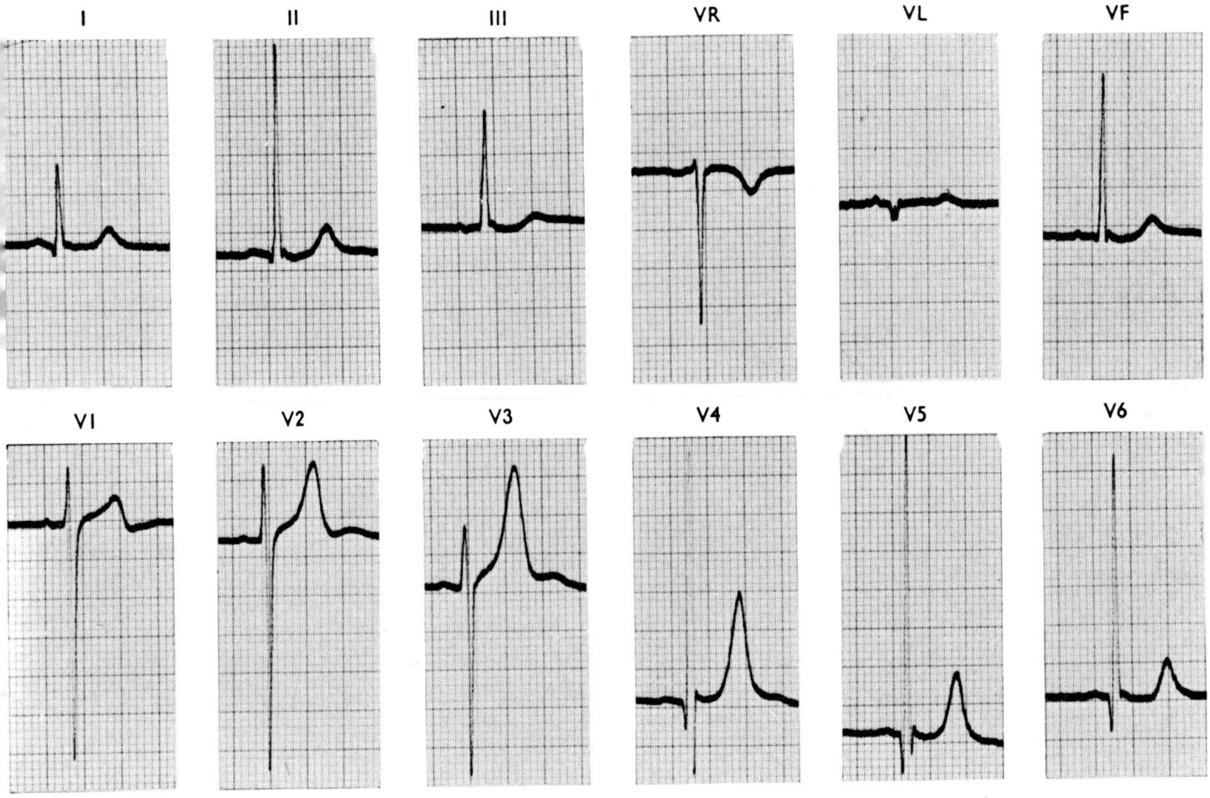

295

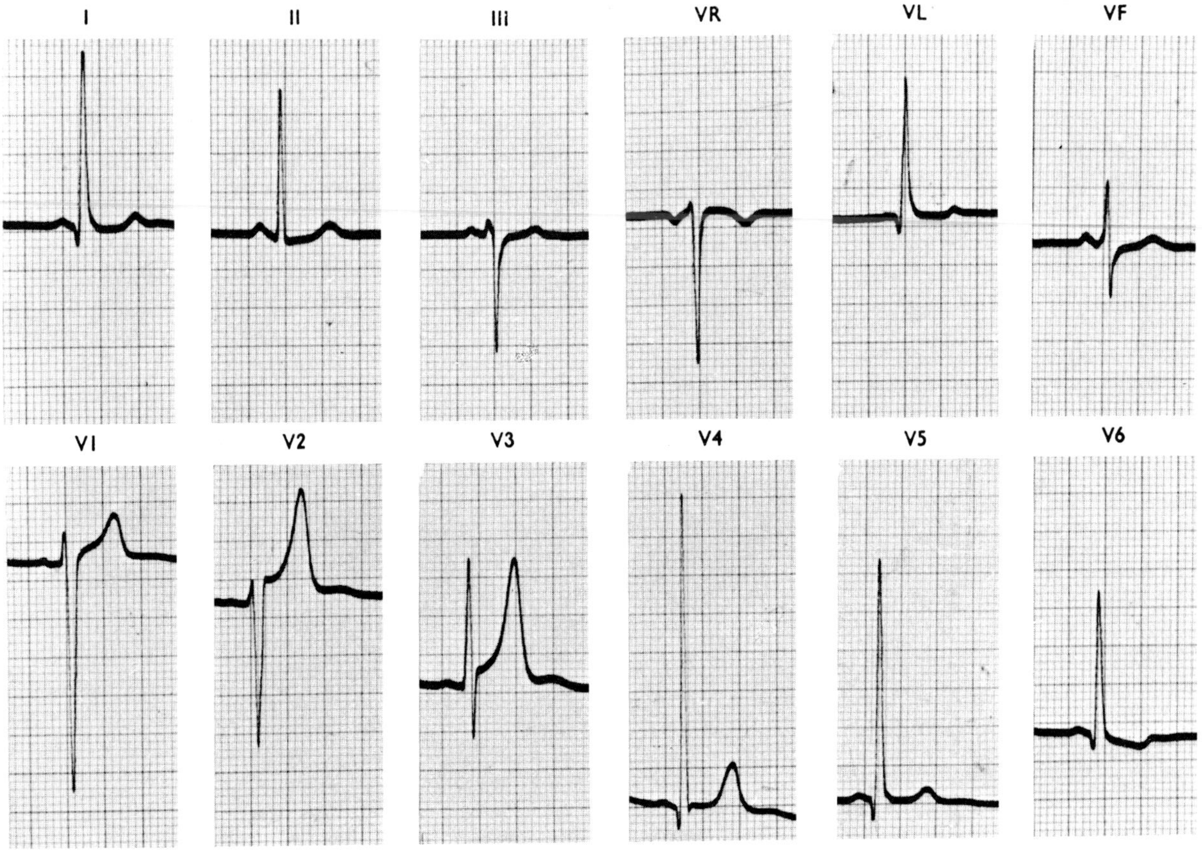

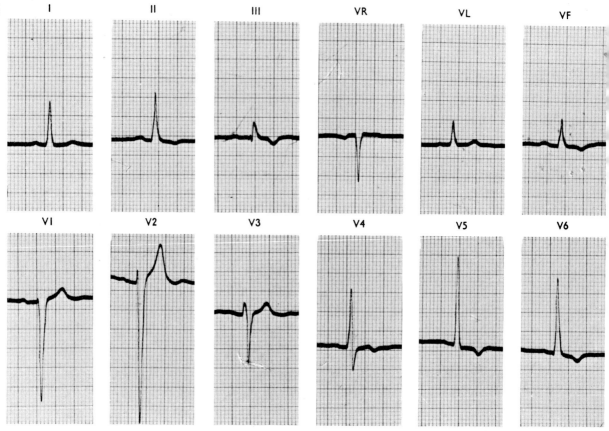

**296  Left ventricular hypertrophy, a later stage.**
Frank T wave inversion (or 'strain') is present in
V4–6 and is reflected in the inferior leads. This is
the so-called 'systolic overload' pattern. Note the
distribution of voltage changes in this case—absent
in limb leads (see **299**) and only borderline in V6,
with maximum voltage in V2. Unimpressive R
waves in V6 are often associated (as in this case)
with clockwise rotation, and V7 or V8 might show
more, but there can be no doubt from V2 that left
ventricular hypertrophy is present. The trace also
shows slight prolongation of QRS to 0.1 second in
the most favourable leads, which is another sign of
left ventricular hypertrophy (**324**) as long as septal
Q waves can still be seen (tiny one in V6). See **327**.

**297, 298  Left ventricular hypertrophy, severe.** Two
examples are shown, both illustrating the full-
blown picture of 'strain', with steep T wave
inversion over the left ventricle.

Figure **297** shows the classical pattern with a
gently sloping descent of the ST segment, often a
little convex upwards, followed by a sharper rise of
the far limb of the T wave. There is often a small
overshoot before the baseline is regained. These
changes are well seen in V5, V6, and, the heart being
horizontal, in 1 and VL.

Figure **298** shows very steep T wave inversion
indeed, and the temptation is to speculate about the
possibility of additional myocardial ischaemia, but
it is impossible to diagnose this in left ventricular
leads in the presence of 'strain'. The same is true
about the right praecordial leads, which in both
examples show exuberantly tall T waves (especially
in **297**) and a high ST take-off; these changes simply
mirror the T inversion on the other side of the heart
(often in areas not recorded in conventional
tracings) and must not be mistaken for infarction.

N.B. in **298**, the heart is semi-vertical, so changes
in V4–6 are seen well in II, III, and VF, in addition
to I and VL.

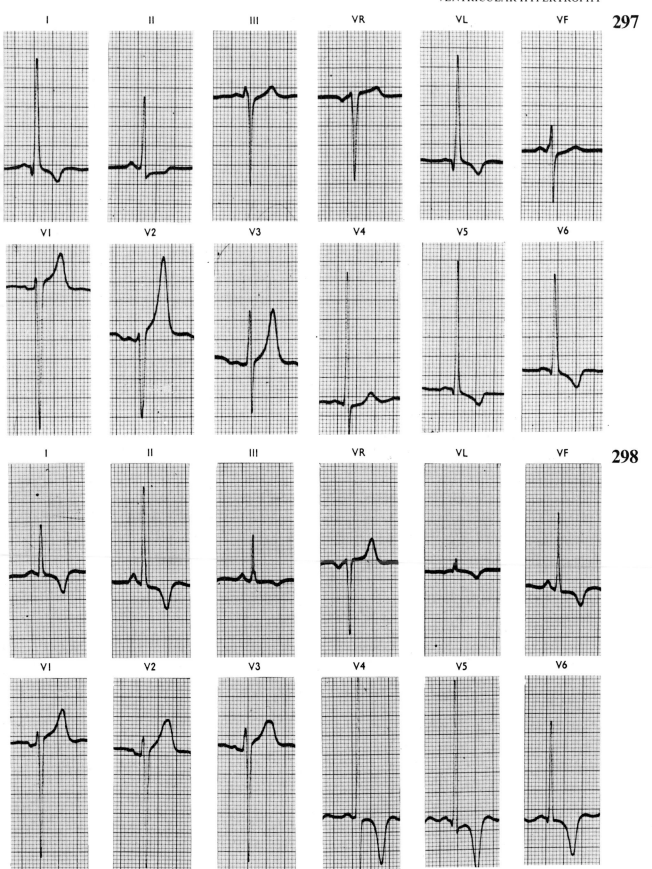

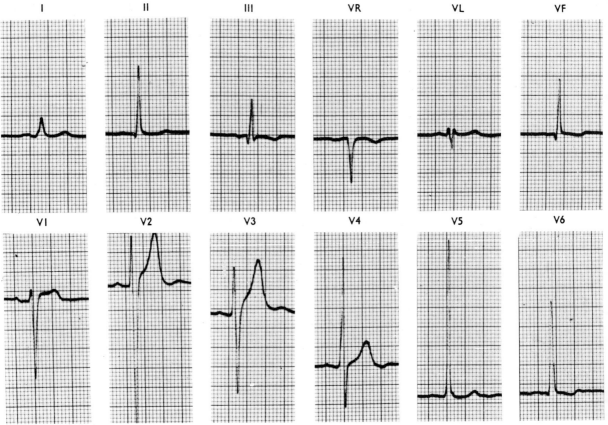

| I | II | III | VR | VL | VF |

| VI | V2 | V3 | V4 | V5 | V6 |

**299 Left ventricular hypertrophy, unremarkable limb leads.** The pattern shown is not uncommon, i.e. voltage changes confined to the chest leads. This occurs when the QRS vector is more posteriorly directed than usual. Other examples are seen in **296** and **301**.

N.B. in this trace the heart is vertical.

**300 Left ventricular hypertrophy seen in limb leads only.** An occasional presentation of left ventricular hypertrophy in which, because of the direction of the QRS vector (markedly leftwards and parallel with the frontal plane), the voltage changes are seen in the limb leads rather than the chest leads. (Also see **305**.)

**301 Left ventricular hypertrophy, clockwise rotation.** Another pattern of left ventricular hypertrophy in which the transitional zone in the chest leads is shifted to the left. The result is an absence of tall R waves in V5 and V6, though V7 or V8 might show them. This too is due to posteriorly directed QRS forces as in the trace illustrated in **299**, and once again, the limb leads are unremarkable.

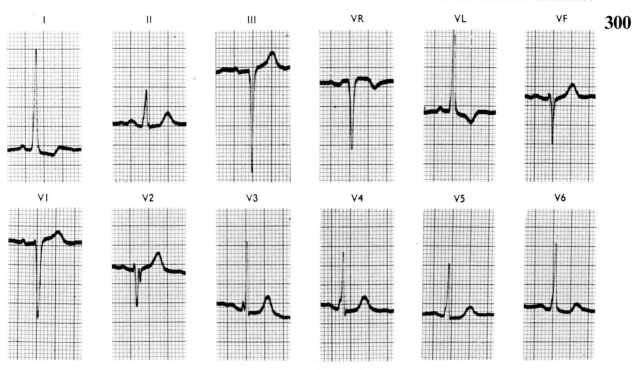

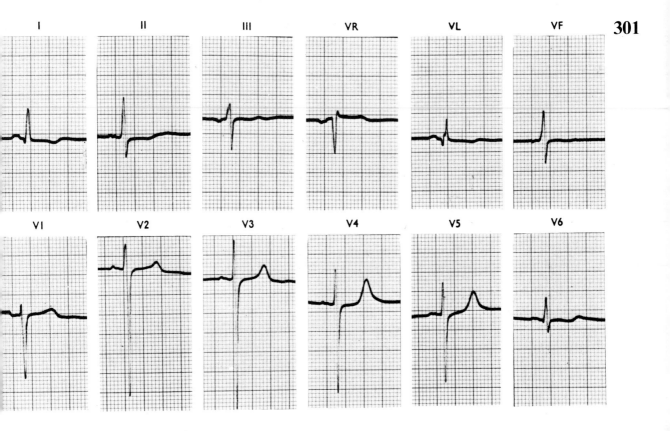

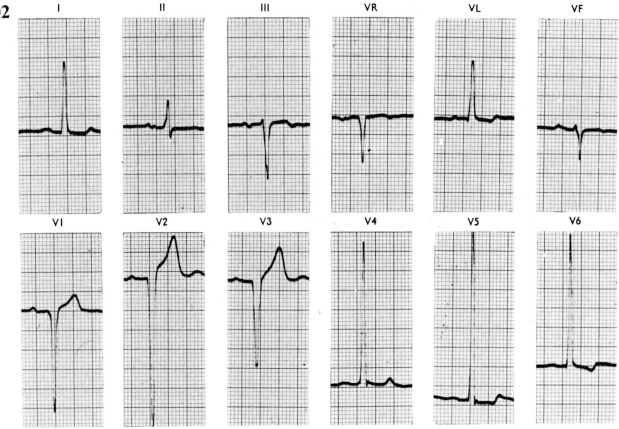

**302  Antero-septal leads in left ventricular hypertrophy.** It is not uncommon to see apparent QS complexes in V2 and V3 in the presence of left ventricular hypertrophy. Often, as in this case, the septal Q waves are not large and possibly this accounts for the absence of an R wave to the right of the septum. Whatever the explanation, myocardial infarction should not be inadvertently misdiagnosed. (See **411**.)

**303  Left ventricular hypertrophy and incomplete right bundle branch block.** The combination of these two patterns is not uncommon, especially in children.

**304  Left ventricular hypertrophy and left anterior hemiblock.** There is left ventricular hypertrophy with maximum voltage in V2 and QRS prolongation to 0.11 second in the face of septal Q waves in I and VL. In addition, left axis deviation (just beyond − 30°) indicates left anterior hemiblock. Although associated with left ventricular hypertrophy in many instances, left anterior hemiblock is not a constant feature even in severe cases and should be regarded as indicating additional myocardial disease or damage. See **330**.

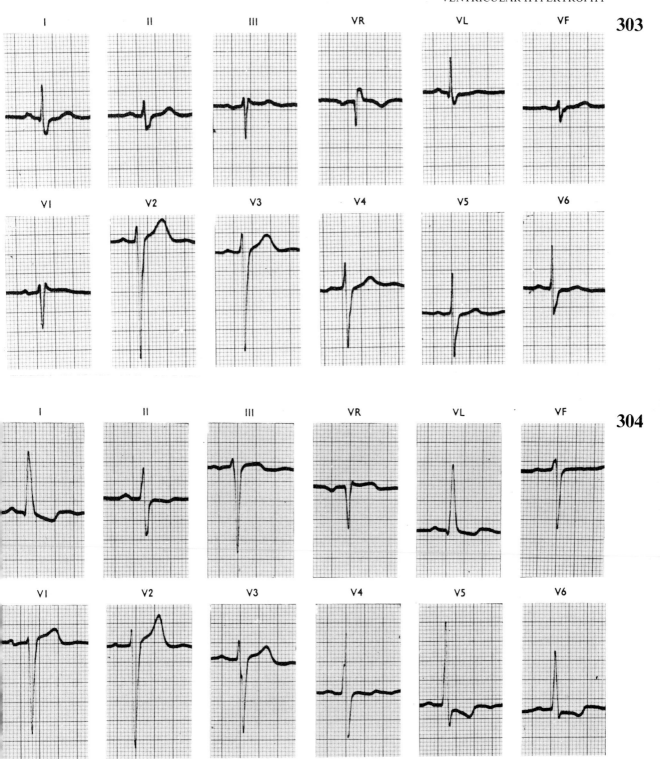

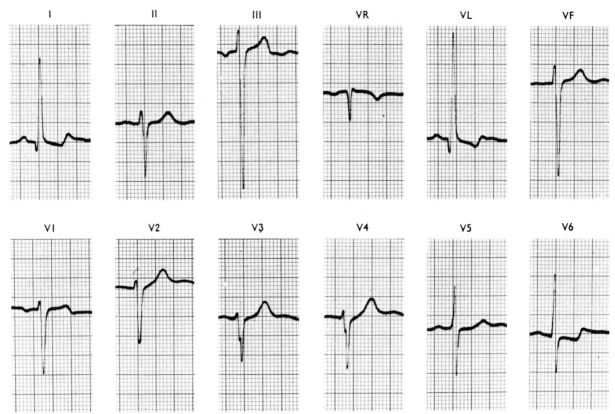

**305 Left ventricular hypertrophy and left anterior hemiblock.** Another example with much more marked left axis deviation. The trace also shows voltage changes confined to the limb leads (see **300**), and clockwise rotation.

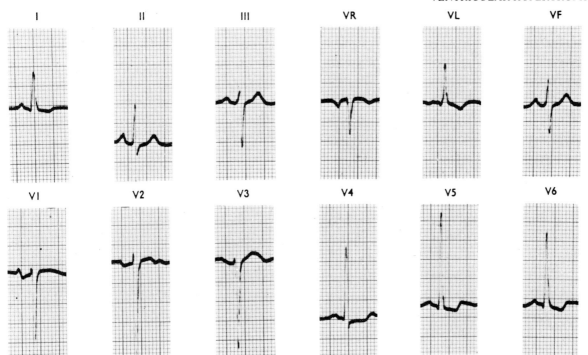

**306 Acute left ventricular diastolic overload.** In acutely acquired aortic or mitral regurgitation of some magnitude the electrocardiogram takes some weeks to develop voltage changes, though ST–T changes may occur early. The unremarkable electrocardiogram makes a striking contrast to the impressive physical signs of valvar disease and the symptoms of heart failure, and furnishes a valuable clue to the presence of a recently acquired lesion. The trace illustrated was taken a month after acute chordal rupture of the mitral valve with severe regurgitation for which urgent valve replacement was needed. There is early left ventricular and left atrial hypertrophy. Another significant feature of acute mitral regurgitation is the presence of numerous ventricular extrasystoles (not illustrated). See **593**.

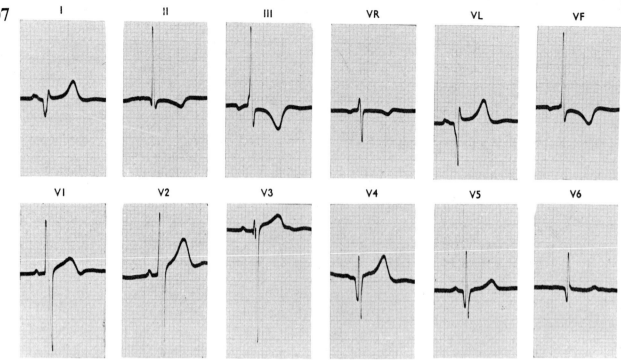

**307, 308 Hypertrophic cardiomyopathy.** The classical findings are the combination of left ventricular hypertrophy and deep, wide, pathological Q waves. The latter are probably produced by massive hypertrophy of the interventricular septum and are seen either in the antero-lateral leads (**307**) or inferior leads (**308**). Myocardial infarction is mimicked but is unlikely to cause confusion since most of these patients present in childhood or early adult life. In many proven cases, however, the Q waves are not seen.

In **307** the deep Q waves in I and VL result in right axis deviation—it is doubtful if this genuinely indicates right ventricular involvement. Note the tall broad R waves in V1 and V2; again, these are merely the septal Q waves in mirror image, not the voltage changes of right ventricular hypertrophy (note the absence of an S wave in V6). In **308** the Q waves in the inferior leads produce left axis deviation; deep S waves in V5 and V6 probably *do* represent right-sided involvement.

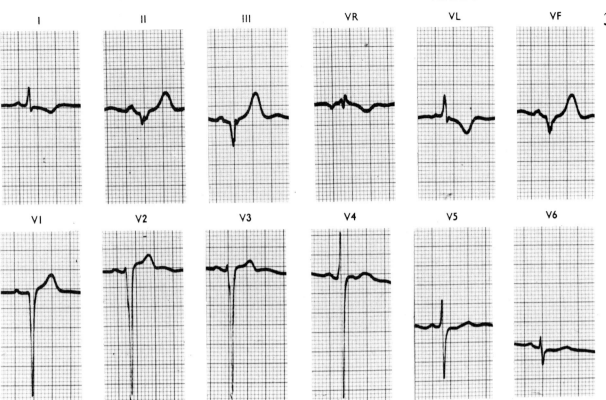

**309**

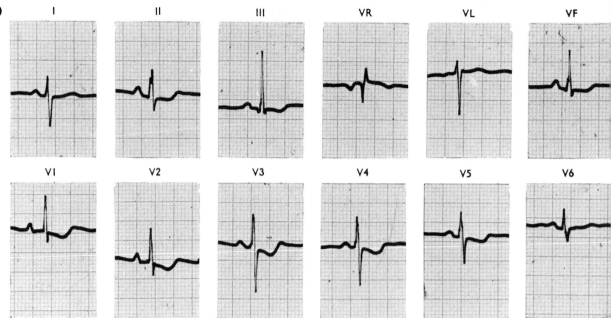

**309, 310 Right ventricular hypertrophy.** The criteria include: an R wave of 7mm or more in V1 (or V4R), a combined voltage of R in V1 and S in V6 of 10mm or more, an R wave taller than the S wave in V1, an S wave deeper than the R wave in V6, and right axis deviation. Right bundle branch block may accompany right ventricular hypertrophy and partly mask it (316), and of course, P pulmonale is a frequent finding. Right ventricular 'strain'

manifests itself as ST depression and T wave inversion from V1 to V4 or beyond. Naturally, not all these features are present in every case. Two broad patterns emerge—tall R waves over the right ventricle with equiphasic complexes across to V6; and dominant S waves right across the chest leads. These two traces are examples of the first pattern. Note the presence of a qR complex in V1 in **310**; this is a sign of severe hypertrophy. See **311** and **51**.

**310**

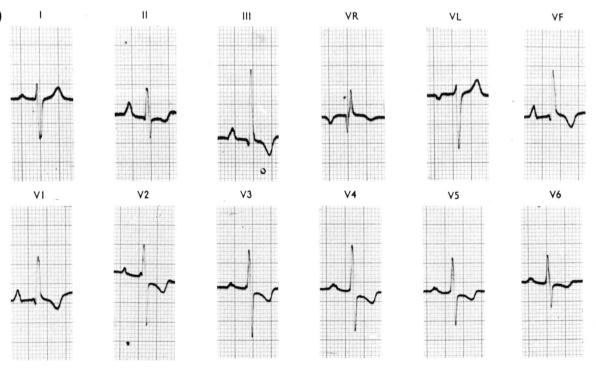

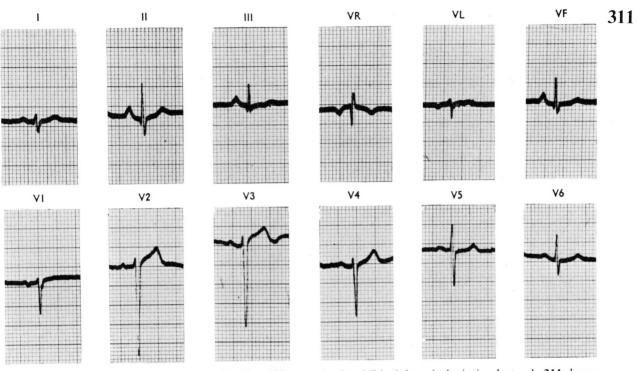

**311, 312   Right ventricular hypertrophy.** See **309**, **310**. These traces are examples of the pattern showing dominant S waves across the chest leads.

Both exhibit right axis deviation but only **311** shows P pulmonale; **312**, despite obvious right ventricular hypertrophy, does not. See also **58** for similar trace.

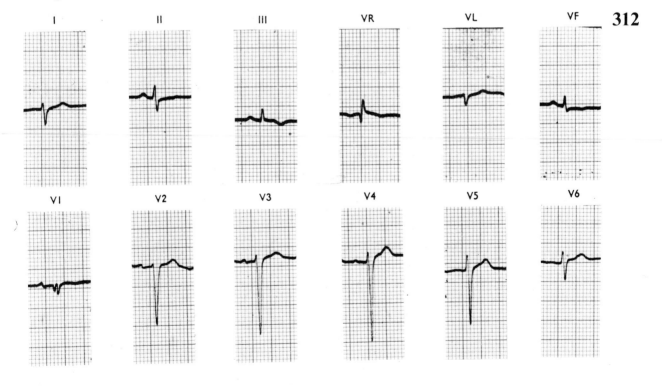

**313**

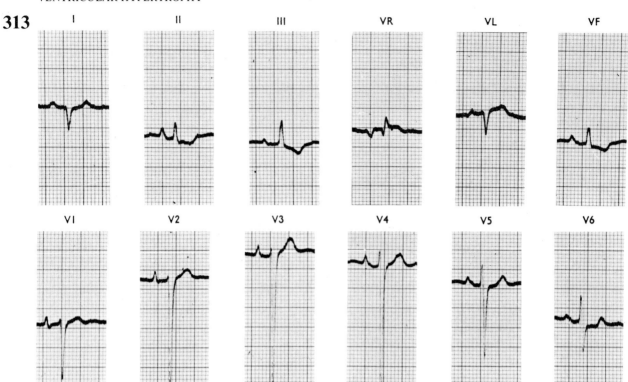

**313  Cor pulmonale.** The pattern of right ventricular hypertrophy in cor pulmonale tends to be that showing dominant S waves in the chest leads and their voltage is sometimes so great (as in this trace) that left ventricular hypertrophy may be suspected in error. P pulmonale helps to avoid the mistake as does right axis deviation (but some cases show left axis deviation). (See **311**, **312** and also **46**, **422**.)

**314  Right ventricular hypertrophy in a neonate.** Right ventricular dominance is normal in neonates, and the range of normality is very wide, so it is difficult to be sure when excessive right ventricular hypertrophy is present. In this trace, taken from an infant with severe pulmonary stenosis, suggestive points are an R in V2 above 20mm, an S in V6 greater than 9mm in depth, an axis of about −120° (normal +75 to +150°), and P pulmonale.

**315  Severe right ventricular hypertrophy in a young child.** Enormous voltages may be seen in this age group. In this trace for instance, V2 and V4, although impressive, are actually recorded at half standardisation, so that the height of R wave in these leads is around 80mm, while the height of P in V2 was 6.5mm. Note the extreme right axis deviation.

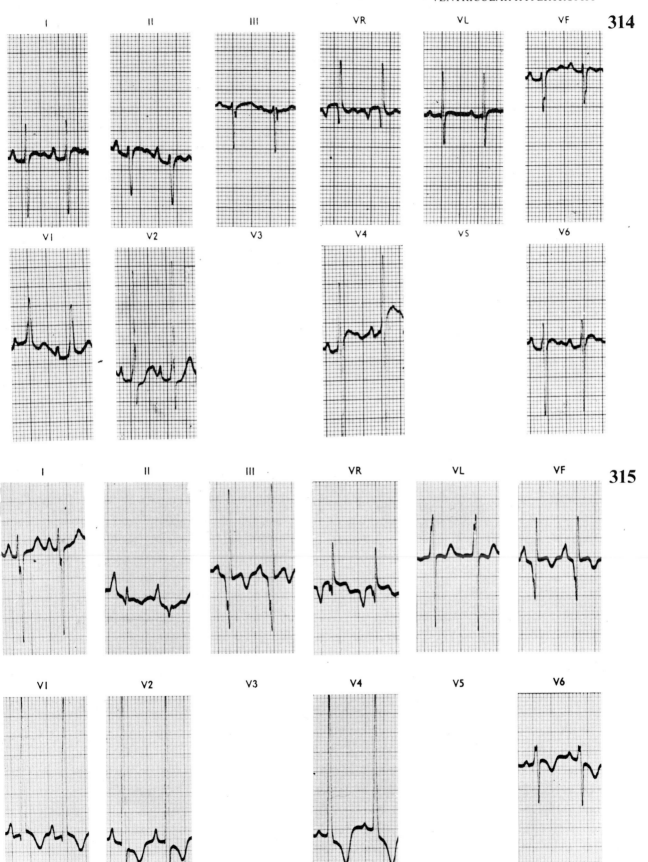

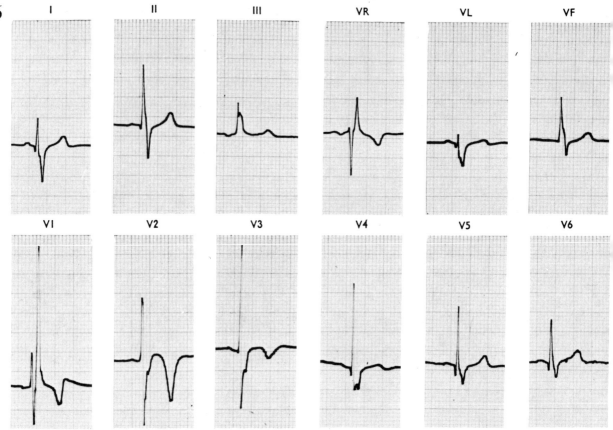

**316** **Right ventricular hypertrophy and right bundle branch block.** The diagnosis of right ventricular hypertrophy is difficult in the presence of right bundle branch block but a secondary R wave in V1 of more than 15mm enables it to be made. See also **50**.

**317** **Biventricular hypertrophy.** Left ventricular hypertrophy is indicated by a tall R wave in V4 and a deep S wave in V1. Right ventricular hypertrophy is indicated by a tall R wave in V1, an S wave in V6 (especially in the presence of anticlockwise rotation), and by right axis deviation. Note too, P pulmonale. Another trace of this kind is illustrated under 'combined P mitrale and pulmonale' (**59**).

**318** **Biventricular hypertrophy.** In many cases when left ventricular hypertrophy is present, additional right ventricular hypertrophy (usually the result of long-standing pulmonary hypertension) can be inferred from the finding of right axis deviation, as in this trace taken from a patient with aortic and mitral valve disease. The rhythm is atrial fibrillation.

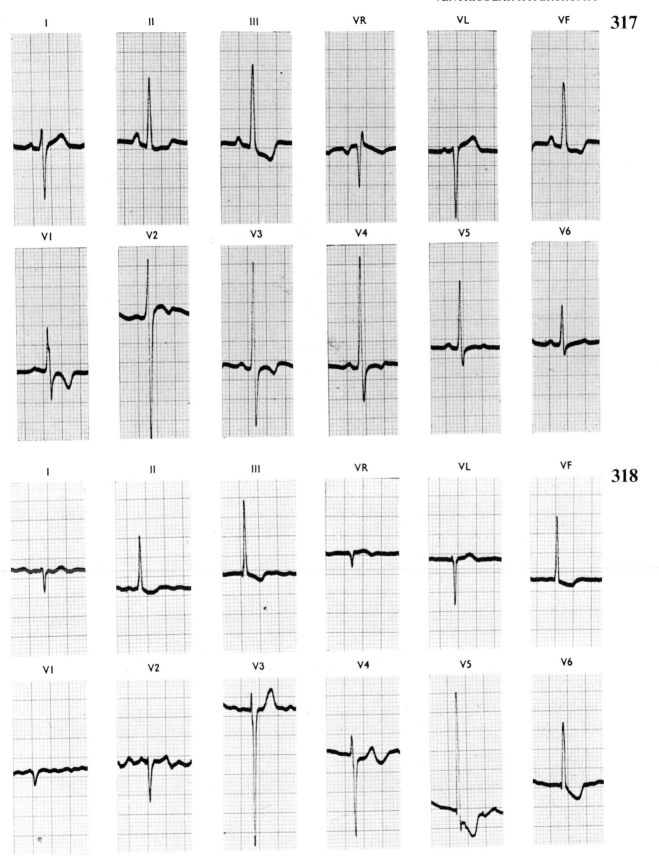

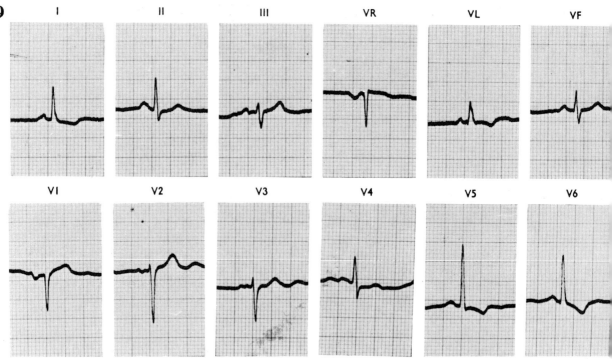

| I | II | III | VR | VL | VF |

| VI | V2 | V3 | V4 | V5 | V6 |

**319 Balanced ventricular hypertrophy.** This term is used for tracings which, though taken from patients showing clear clinical evidence of both left and right ventricular hypertrophy, show no convincing voltage or axis abnormality. The hypothesis is that relatively equal forces in the two ventricles have cancelled each other out. The electrocardiogram illustrated for instance was taken from a patient with severe mitral regurgitation and pulmonary hypertension close to systemic level. The presence of biventricular hypertrophy was later confirmed at post-mortem. Note the presence of P mitrale; P pulmonale is not seen. The lateral T wave changes were due to the left ventricular strain pattern. In the circumstances the absence of right axis deviation is note-worthy.

**320 Left bundle branch block.** Over the left ventricle the QRS complex is widened (duration of 0.12 second or more) and notched. The abnormal activation is followed by equally abnormal repolarisation so T waves are sharply inverted in these leads. In V6 the normal tiny Q wave is lost because the septum is no longer activated initially from the left side. In right praecordial leads a mirror image pattern is seen—tiny or absent R waves, poor R wave progression, tall T waves, and a high ST segment take off—which must not be mis-diagnosed as myocardial infarction (but see 350, 351). Note the mean QRS axis which is just within the normal range. (See 322.)

**321 Left bundle block, primary T wave abnormality.** As stated in 320 the T waves are normally opposite in sign to the QRS complexes in left bundle branch block—the so-called 'secondary' T wave change. The absence of this finding with T waves pointing in the same direction as the QRS complexes indicates T wave changes due to myocardial disease independent of the bundle branch block—'primary' T abnormality. Again, the QRS axis is just less than −30°.

# BUNDLE BRANCH BLOCK, HEMIBLOCK,
## MULTIFASCICULAR BLOCK

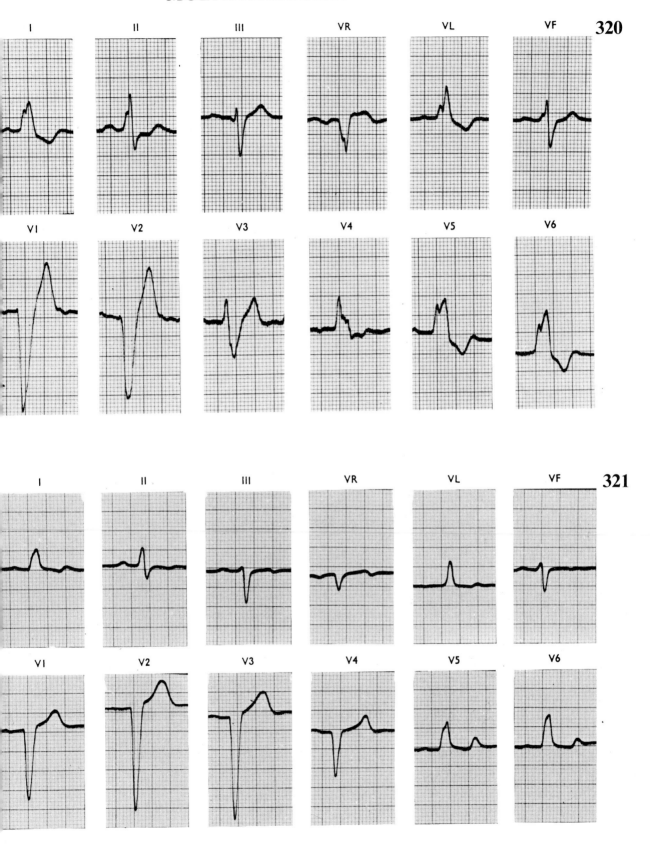

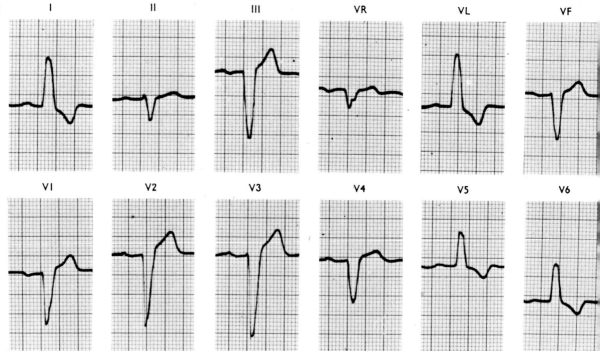

**322   Left bundle branch block, left axis deviation.** Unlike the previous two examples of left bundle branch block, the one in **322** shows definite left axis deviation. Since left axis deviation is due to a block of the anterior division of the left bundle branch only, the inference is that so-called 'complete' left bundle branch block is not in fact complete, and a further degree of block distally is possible. Evidence to support this is provided in the behaviour of the mean QRS axis before and after the development of left bundle branch block (**323–325**) and tracings showing widening of the QRS complex *after* apparently complete left bundle branch block has occurred (**326**).

**323   Development of left bundle branch block, effect on mean QRS axis.** The upper row shows the limb leads of a patient before the development of left bundle branch block and the lower row the same leads afterwards. There is no fundamental change in axis (approximately —20°). And see **324**.

**324   Left bundle branch block and pre-existing left axis deviation.** The points have been made (**322, 323**) that the development of left bundle branch block has no effect on QRS axis, and that the presence of left axis deviation in complete left bundle branch block indicates an additional, separate, distal conduction fault in the anterior hemi-division. Both are reinforced by the trace illustrated. The upper row shows the limb leads of a patient with left ventricular hypertrophy and left axis deviation. Note the prolongation of QRS duration to 0.1 second—a sign of left ventricular hypertrophy in this instance (**296**)—and the presence of septal Q waves in I and VL. The lower line shows the same leads after left bundle branch block has occurred; the axis is unchanged.

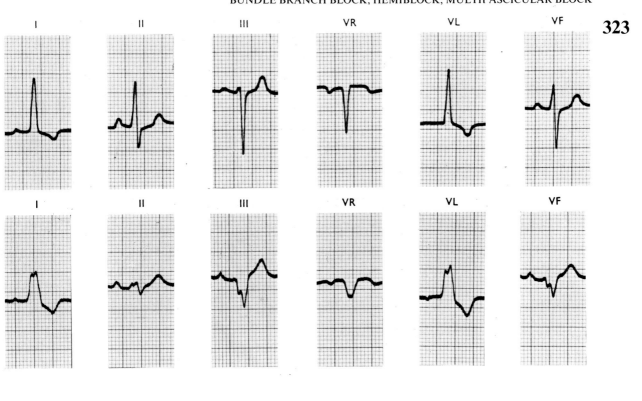

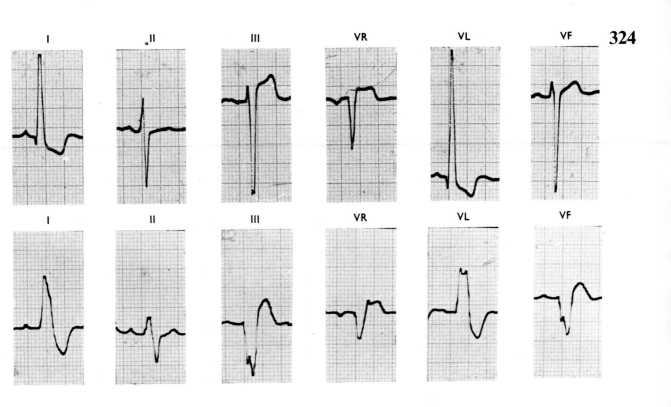

**325**

| I | II | III | VR | VL | VF |
|---|----|-----|----|----|----|

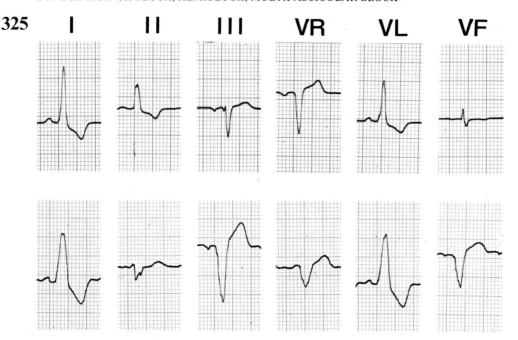

**325 Development of left bundle branch block and left anterior hemiblock.** See **322–324**. The upper row shows the limb leads of a patient before the development of complete left bundle branch block. The QRS duration is 0.10 second and there are no septal Q waves in I or VL so incomplete left bundle branch block may be present (see **327**). The lower row shows the same leads in a later trace. There is now 'complete' left bundle branch block and in addition, left axis deviation, indicating a further peripheral block of the anterior division of the left bundle.

**326**

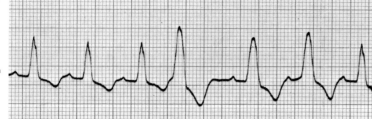

**326 Completeness of left bundle branch block.** The completeness of left bundle branch block has been discussed above (**322–325**) in relation to the presence or otherwise of left axis deviation, but the existence of traces showing a much greater QRS duration than the minimum of 0.12 second (e.g. **320**) also points to the possibility of an increase in the degree of apparently complete left bundle branch block. Figure **326** provides support for this.

It shows V6. The first three beats have a QRS duration of 0.12 second. An extrasystole follows and the two beats which succeed it show a QRS duration of 0.16 second. The last beat returns to 0.12 second. Presumably, the lower pressure generated by the extrasystole has caused transient ischaemia and increased the 'completeness' of the block.

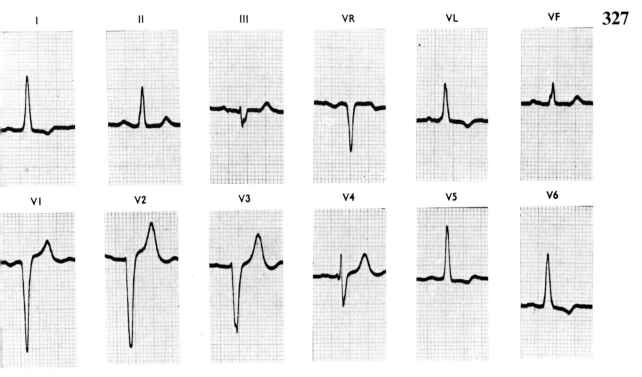

**327 Incomplete left bundle branch block.** The pattern of left bundle branch block is suggested particularly by the absence of the 'septal' Q wave in V6 (and in VL and I) and by an absent R wave in V1 but the QRS complex is not necessarily notched. The duration of QRS is between 0.1 and 0.12 second. Note the abnormal T waves in left ventricular leads; these could, of course, have another explanation.

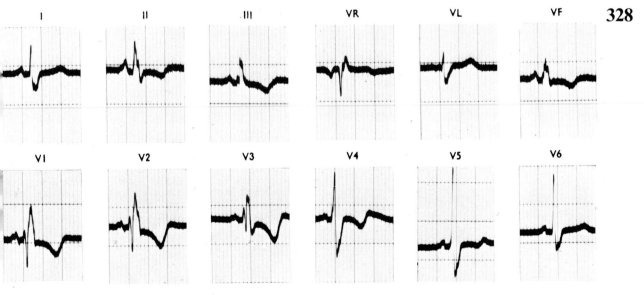

**328 Complete right bundle branch block.** The QRS width is 0.12 second or more. In right praecordial leads there are RSR complexes, with broad secondary R waves, while over the left ventricle a normal, narrow R or qR is succeeded by a wide, notched S wave representing, like the broad secondary R wave in V1 and V2, late and unopposed right ventricular activation. T wave inversion over the right ventricle completes the pattern. The mean QRS axis of the initial forces remains normal but the later portion shows right axis deviation. (See **346**.)

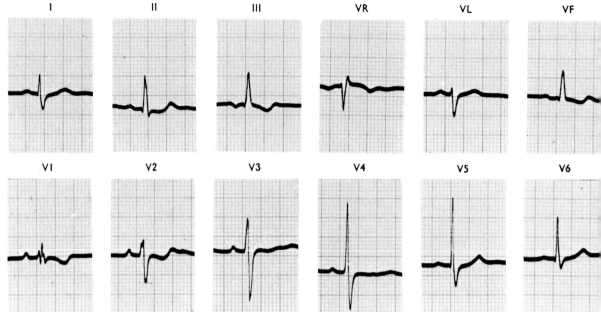

**329 Incomplete right bundle branch block.** This term is applied to electrocardiograms showing the pattern of right bundle branch block, with an RSR in V1 and a wide slurred S wave in V6, but with a QRS duration of only 0.1 second or less. It is often found in normal subjects but is also a feature of some diseases, notably secundum atrial septal defect. See also **341, 453**.

**330 Left anterior hemiblock.** Left axis deviation is present at approximately −40°. In the absence of inferior or anterior infarction (see **390** and **393**) or the W.P.W. syndrome (**168, 169**) left anterior hemiblock is the only likely explanation.

**331 Left posterior hemiblock.** Isolated interruption of conduction in the posterior division of the left bundle branch is uncommon. Furthermore, the pattern (right axis deviation, an rS complex in lead I, and small, narrow Q waves in leads II, III and VF) is seen in right ventricular hypertrophy. It is therefore easiest to diagnose when a previous electrocardiogram is available, as in the case illustrated. Only the limb leads are shown. The upper line shows the usual appearances of this patient's electrocardiogram; the lower line, taken from a trace recorded ten days later, shows left posterior hemiblock. Reversion to normal conduction occurred shortly afterwards. See also **376**.

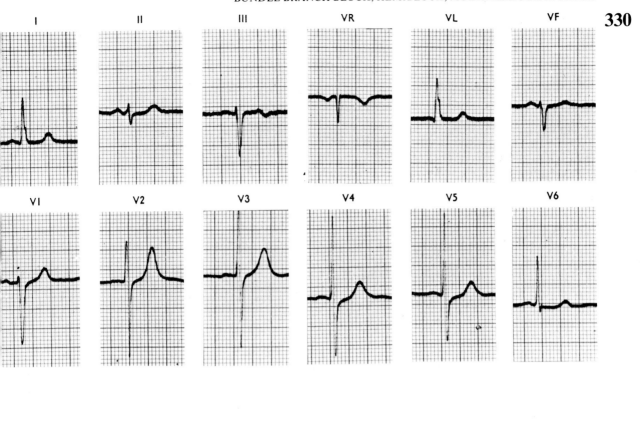

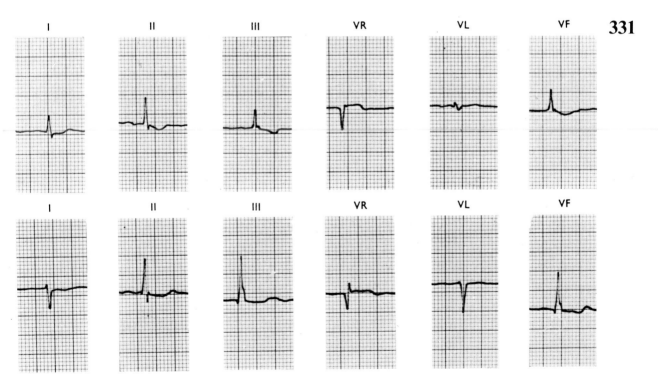

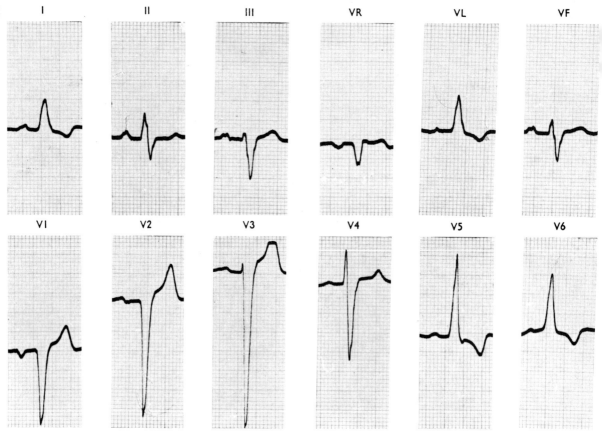

**332 Bifascicular block.** Left bundle branch block is present and the PR interval is just above the upper limit of normal at 0.24 second, which indicates first degree block in the right bundle and/or the atrioventricular junction or main bundle as well. The flattening of the T wave in V3 is artefactual.

**333 Bifascicular block.** Right bundle branch block is present and the PR interval is well above normal at 0.30 second, indicating first degree block in the left bundle and/or the atrioventricular junction or main bundle as well. (See **332**.) Despite the tiny Q waves in II, III and VF the axis of initial forces is normal (**336**).

**334 Bifascicular block.** Right bundle branch block is present and in addition there is left axis deviation, indicating blockage of the anterior division of the left bundle branch. The tall secondary R wave in V1–3 of this example suggests the presence of right ventricular hypertrophy (**316**).

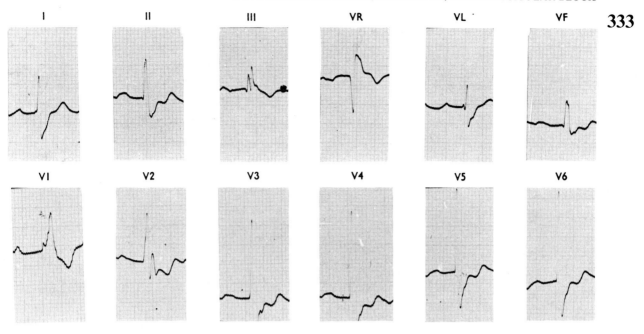

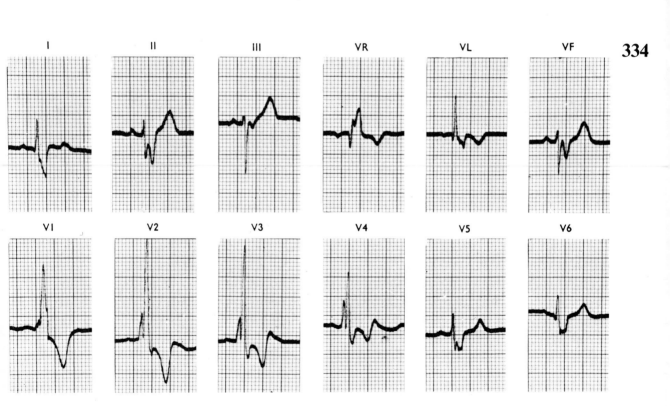

**335**

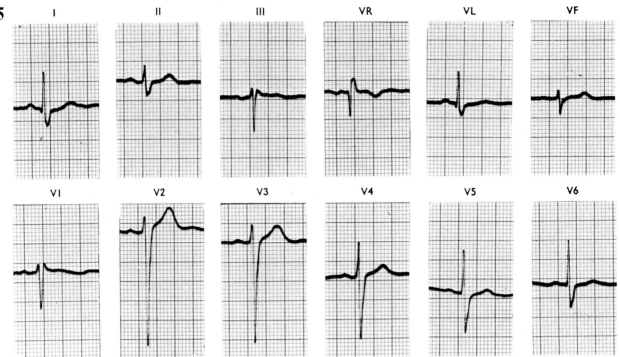

**335  Bifascicular block.** As in the previous example there is the combination of right bundle branch block and left axis deviation but in this instance the right block is incomplete. The deep S wave in V2 suggests left ventricular hypertrophy.

**336  Bifascicular block.** Right bundle branch block is present. There is right axis deviation which affects not only the latter portion of the QRS complex (as is the rule in right bundle branch block) but also the early portion. Small narrow Q waves are seen in the inferior leads, II, III, and VF. This pattern combination suggests blockage of the posterior division of the left bundle branch as well as of the right bundle branch. (See **331**.)

**337  Bifascicular block.** The changes described in **336** as suggestive of right bundle branch block and left posterior hemiblock may be seen in patients with right ventricular hypertrophy so that, as with isolated left posterior hemiblock (see **331**), diagnosis is facilitated when a previous tracing is available. The illustration shows the limb leads of a patient before (upper line) and after (lower line) the development of this particular combination of bifascicular block. The right bundle branch block in this instance is incomplete. Note the appearance of tiny Q waves in II, III, and VF, and the axis shift affecting both the initial and the terminal portions of the QRS. The rhythm is atrial fibrillation.

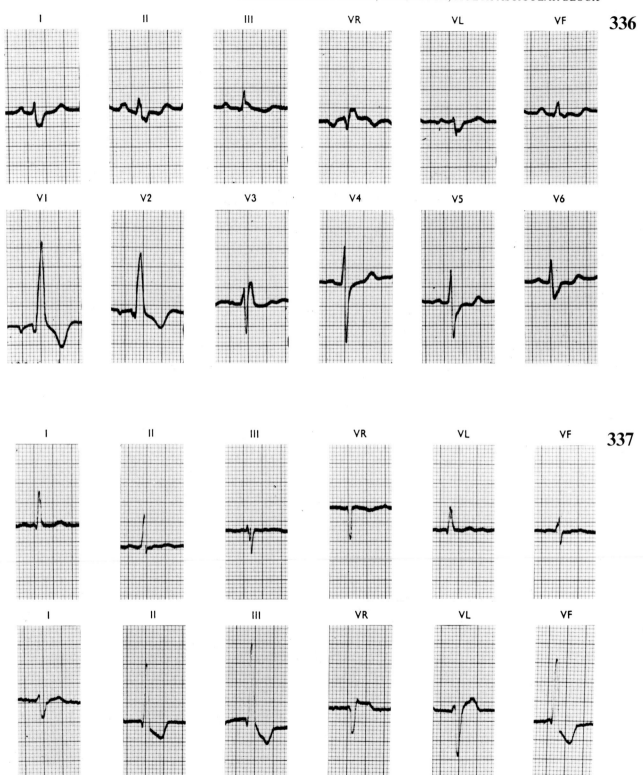

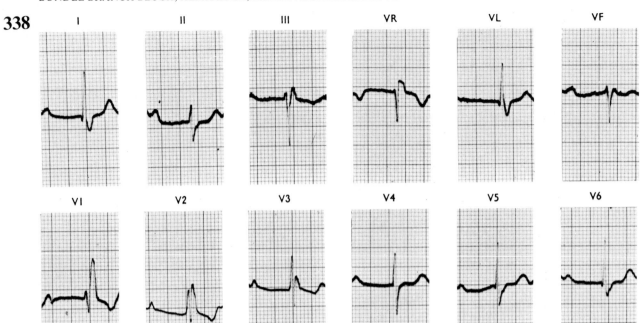

**338 Trifascicular block.** The right bundle is blocked. There is left axis deviation, indicating interruption of the anterior division of the left bundle branch, and the PR interval is prolonged at 0.4 second, demonstrating impairment of conduction in the remaining fascicle and/or the atrioventricular junction or main bundle. If the degree of block increases in the latter, complete heart block will occur. See also **353**.

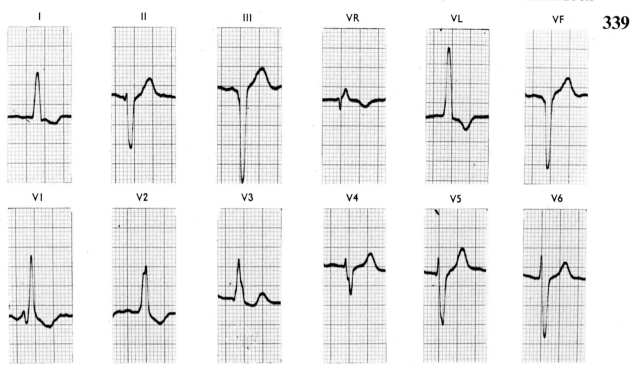

**339 Trifascicular block.** The right bundle branch is blocked as shown by the RSR in V1 and the wide S wave in V6. Left axis deviation is present indicating left anterior hemiblock. Lastly, there are no Q waves in V6, VL, or I, which is very suggestive of some degree of block in the left main bundle. In this case atrioventricular conduction is of no help in diagnosis because atrial fibrillation is present.

**340**

**341**

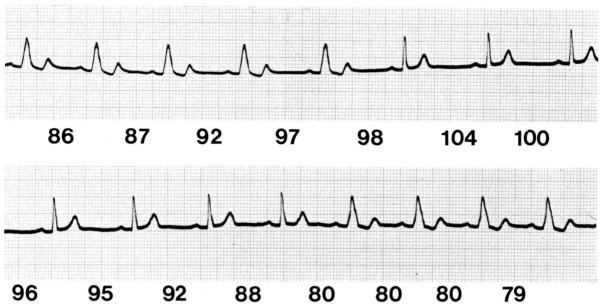

86    87    92    97    98    104    100

96    95    92    88    80    80    80    79

**340, 341 Atrioventricular cushion defects.**
Bifascicular or trifascicular block is the characteristic finding in ostium primum atrial septal defect and in atrioventricular canal, and these diagnoses may be suspected in patients with left to right shunts by this feature alone. If the electrocardiogram is viewed in isolation a congenital origin for the pattern is suggested by the presence of ventricular hypertrophy, P pulmonale, or a splintered S wave in lead II. Figure **340** shows incomplete right bundle branch block and left anterior hemiblock; the PR interval is normal. Figure **341** shows a more florid example with complete right bundle branch block, left anterior hemiblock, and a PR interval at the upper limit of normal. However, the PR interval diminishes with tachycardia, and is lower in children—upper limit 0.16 second at 14 years and under, 0.14 second in infants—so that in fact, this is really a prolonged PR for the 8-year-old child from which **341** was taken.

**342 Rate-dependent bundle branch block.**
Aberrant conduction due to incomplete recovery from the refractory state in the bundles of His is a common finding during paroxysmal tachycardia (see **148, 149**) or atrial flutter or fibrillation (**212, 234**) but the same phenomenon may be seen at normal rates. The illustration is a continuous strip in two rows. The figures underneath are interbeat intervals in hundredths of a second. The record starts with bundle branch block but, as the heart slows down, normal conduction is restored. On the lower line the heart speeds up again and aberrant conduction returns. Note that the rate at which bundle branch block is lost is slower than the rate to which the heart has to accelerate for it to return. The explanation appears to be prolongation of the refractory period by late activation during bundle branch block, and the tendency of refractory periods to alter in direct relationship to the length of the preceding cycle.

**343**

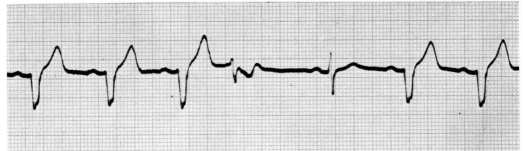

**344**

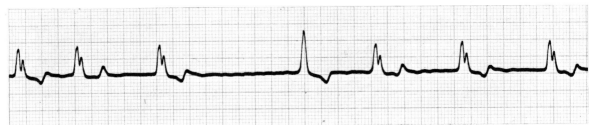

**343, 344  Rate-dependent bundle branch block.** This phenomenon is explained in **342**. These two traces illustrate another presentation. Figure **343** shows sinus rhythm with aberrant conduction interrupted by an extrasystole which is followed by a pause. The extra period of rest enables the bundle to recover and normal conduction returns—for one beat only.

Figure **344** shows an analogous situation during atrial fibrillation when a long diastolic pause provides the same opportunity for a reduction in the QRS duration of the subsequent beat (it may be conducted, or a junctional escape beat). (Also see **232–234**.)

**345**

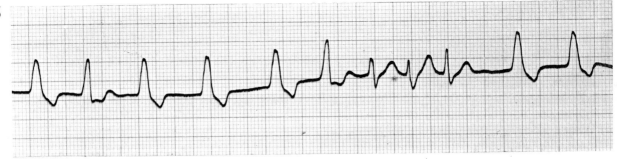

**345  Paradoxical rate-dependent bundle branch block.** The occurrence of aberrant conduction with tachycardia, prematurity, or critical rate are illustrated elsewhere and the phenomenon depends on the heart speeding up. The reverse, bundle branch block appearing only at slower rates, is rare, and the explanation for it obscure. The trace shows atrial fibrillation (which, with its varying cycle length affords good opportunities for rate-dependent aberration to occur). Bundle branch block is present but the second and sixth beats, which are preceded by the shortest cycles, show less aberration than the rest—the reverse of what would normally be expected (see **342**). Beats 7–9 are probably extrasystoles.

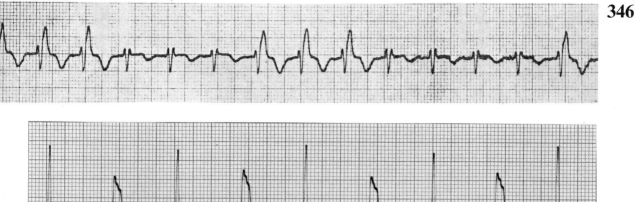

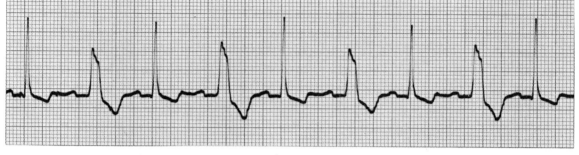

**346 Intermittent bundle branch block.** The upper trace shows V1. Complete right bundle branch block appears and disappears without any alteration in heart rate. The underlying QRS shows an rSr configuration. The illustration also demonstrates the fact that only the terminal portion of the QRS is affected by the development of right bundle branch block, initial forces remaining unaffected, as would be expected on theoretical grounds. The lower trace shows V6 in another patient. Alternating left bundle branch block is present.

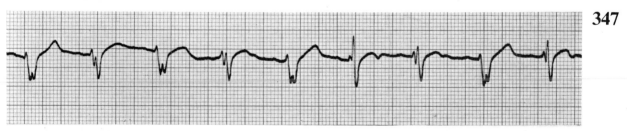

**347 Aberrant conduction, varying patterns.** The trace shows sinus rhythm (the P waves are not easy to see). Aberrant conduction is present throughout but there are three different patterns of complexes reflecting three differing paths of conduction.

**348**

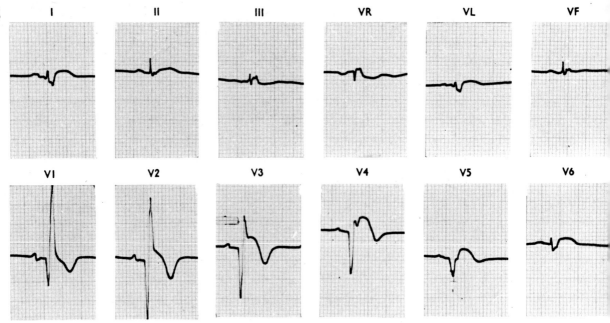

| I | II | III | VR | VL | VF |
| V1 | V2 | V3 | V4 | V5 | V6 |

**348, 349  Right bundle branch block and myocardial infarction.** In right bundle branch block, the initial forces are left unaffected and only the terminal portion of the QRS complex is changed (see **346**), so the diagnosis of myocardial infarction is still possible because abnormal Q waves can be identified. The two illustrations are from the same patient. Figure **348** shows right bundle branch block, and in addition, pathological Q waves in V1–5, indicating myocardial infarction. There is further evidence of infarction in the raised ST segments in V2–5. This patient had indeed sustained an acute infarction the day before admission. In **349**, taken a week later, bundle branch block has disappeared, leaving the changes of infarction.

**349**

| I | II | III | VR | VL | VF |
| V1 | V2 | V3 | V4 | V5 | V6. |

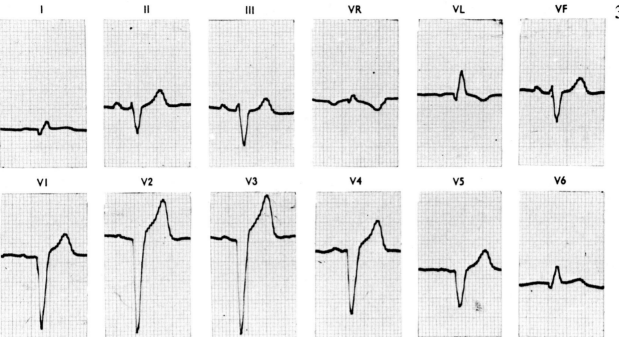

**350 Left bundle branch block, myocardial infarction.** The difficulty of diagnosing myocardial infarction in the presence of left bundle branch block is mentioned elsewhere (**320**). It is however possible to do so if Q waves appear in left ventricular leads in which they should be absent in left bundle branch block. In this example they are seen in V6, VL, and I. Note the left axis deviation (−75°).

**351 Masking of infarction by left bundle branch block.** The difficulty of diagnosing myocardial infarction in the presence of left bundle branch block (**320**) is underlined by this short trace. It is a strip of V2 in a patient with an antero-septal infarction. The first three beats are sinus beats; note the QS complexes and ST segment elevation of acute infarction. The fourth beat is an atrial extrasystole (note the different P wave and PR interval) which manifests fatigue block of the left type because the bundle has had insufficient time to recover. The infarct pattern is lost.

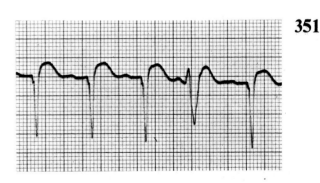

**351**

**352**

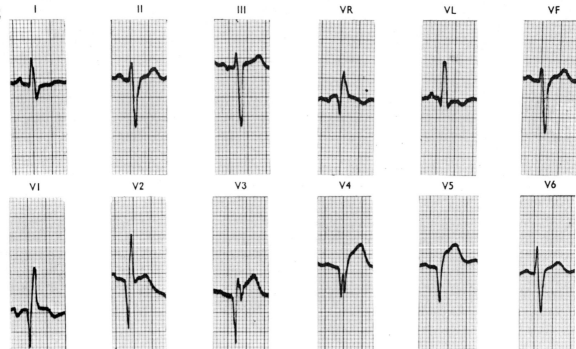

**352 Bifascicular block and myocardial infarction.** There is left axis deviation, and right bundle branch block as evidenced by a QRS duration of 0.12 second and a wide S wave in V6. In the anteroseptal leads a broad Q wave is present. See **334**.

**353**

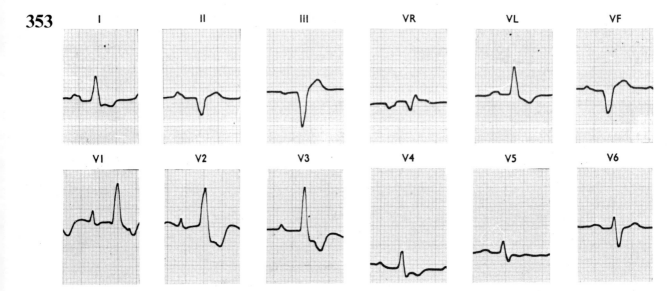

**353 Bifascicular block and myocardial infarction.** There is QRS prolongation and a wide S wave in V6, so right bundle branch block is present. The PR interval is 0.24 second. QS complexes are present in II, III, and VF, indicating inferior infarction. Since the latter produce left axis deviation, the temptation is to diagnose trifascicular block but the absence of any R wave in the leads mentioned makes this unlikely; however, such traces can cause real difficulty. See **338**.

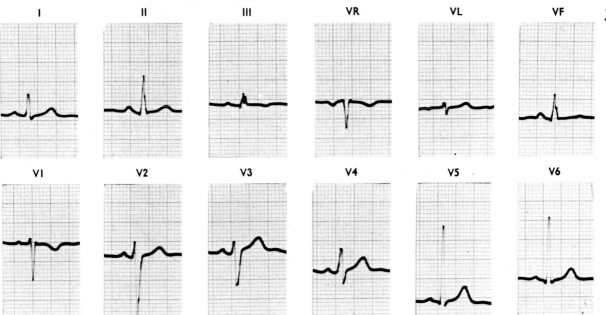

**354 Coronary heart disease, normal electrocardiogram.** This trace was taken from a patient with disabling angina and is included to make the point that it is very common to find no abnormality in the resting electrocardiogram in such patients.

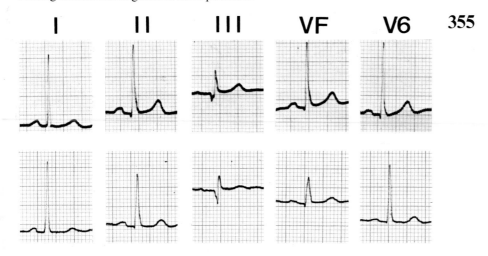

355

**355 Coronary heart disease, horizontal ST segments.** Normally, the ST segment slopes gently upwards to meet the T wave with a slight concavity. Horizontally running ST segments for 0.12 second or more with an abrupt angulation between them and the T wave are a minor sign of ischaemia when they occur in several leads grouped together in one of the localised combinations which suggest ischaemia. The illustration shows leads I, II, III, VF and V6 on a patient with coronary disease before (upper row) and after the development of this sign. Later, ST segments become depressed, and T waves flatten and invert. See **357, 359–373**.

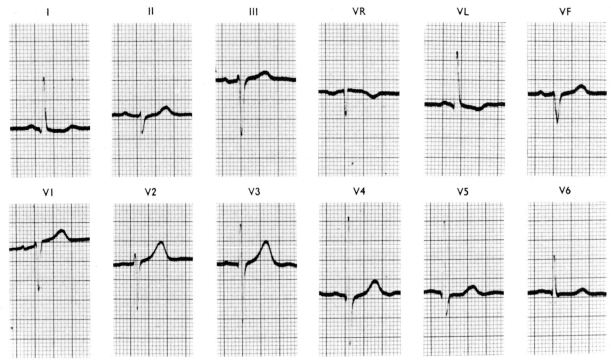

**356  Myocardial ischaemia, left axis deviation.** Left axis deviation (indicating left anterior hemiblock) as an isolated finding is very suggestive of myocardial ischaemia in otherwise likely subjects. In the particular trace illustrated there are other minor signs of ischaemia as well—T wave inversion in VL; flat T waves and I and V6 (lower than the T waves in III and V1 respectively); horizontal ST segments in V5 and V6, and I.

**357  Non-specific T wave flattening.** The interpretation of widespread T wave flattening must be cautious because, although the majority of cases will be due to ischaemia, there are several other possibilities, e.g. pericarditis, myxoedema, electrolyte disorders, etc. The trace illustrated falls into this non-specific category, though the relative sparing of I and VL may be suggestive that the changes are localised (and therefore probably ischaemic). (See **12, 15, 27, 131, 162, 415–417, 424, 429, 437, 440–442, 445.**)

**358  Myocardial ischaemia, inverted U waves.** U wave inversion is one of the minor signs of ischaemia which can nevertheless be useful when the cause of T wave flattening is in doubt. It can just be seen, for instance, in V4–6 of the preceding trace. In this electrocardiogram it is more marked (in V4–6, and VL). U wave inversion should not be misinterpreted as T wave inversion—a glance at other leads should prevent this. Note that the degree of inversion is usually slight. See **376.**

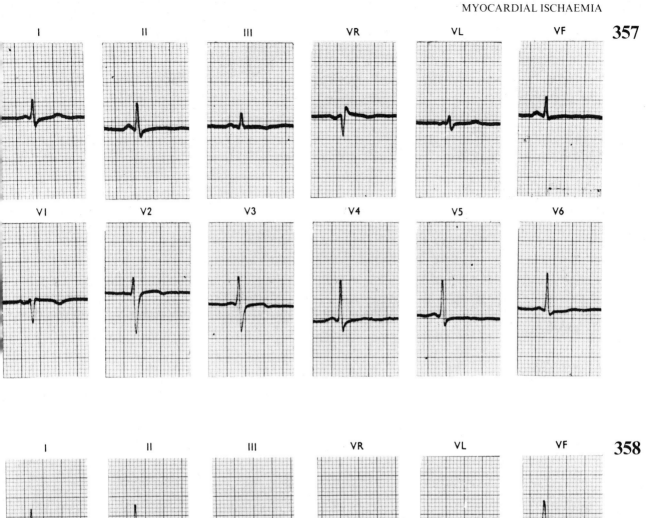

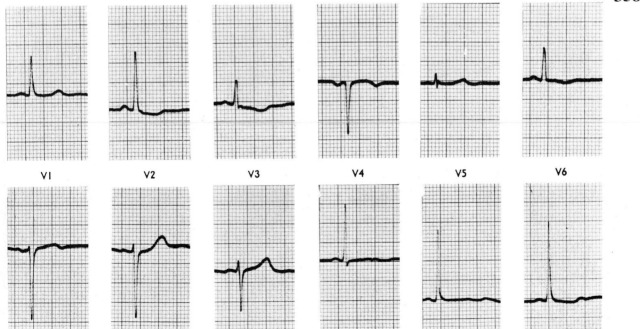

**359**

| VI | V2 | V3 | V4 | V5 | V6 | I |
|----|----|----|----|----|----|---|

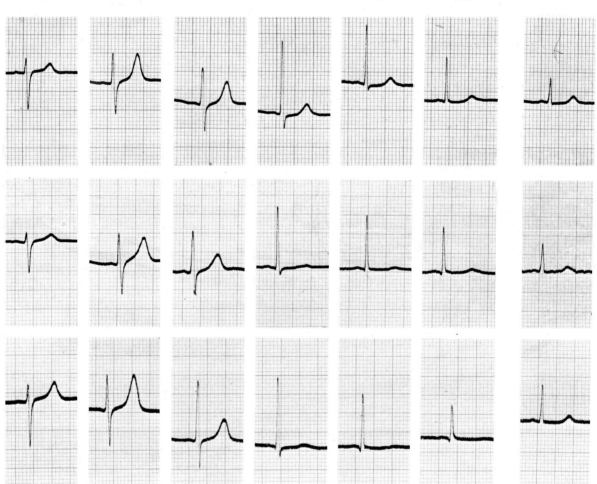

**359 Myocardial ischaemia.** In this example, T waves in V4–6 are normal in the first trace taken (top line) but show increasing flattening in the other two electrocardiograms which were taken from the patient six and thirteen months later respectively.

Such T wave flattening is not diagnostic but the localised nature of the changes and their progressive appearance are suggestive of myocardial ischaemia. (See cross references in **357**). Note the horizontal ST segments in I and V6.

**360**

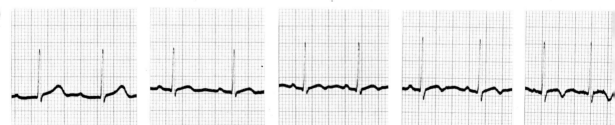

**360 Myocardial ischaemia, T wave inversion.** The development of T wave flattening progressing to inversion is shown in these five traces taken over a

period of hours from a monitoring lead in a patient with acute coronary insufficiency. The first trace shows grade 1 heart block.

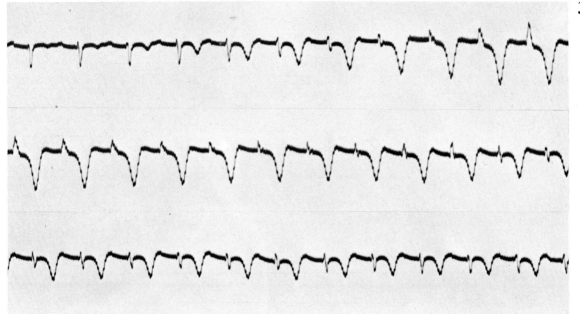

**361, 362 Acute myocardial ischaemia, T wave alteration.** Demonstration of the ischaemic aetiology of T wave changes in patients with coronary heart disease is neatly obtained during coronary arteriography, when the injection of radio-opaque contrast into the vessels produces transient myocardial ischaemia. Both the traces illustrated were obtained in this way. Both are continuous strips cut up. Figure **361** shows the development of gross T wave inversion, and **362** the appearance of taller T waves—the mirror image of T inversion on the opposite side of the heart. Note the change in QRS shape, especially in **361**, suggesting a swing in axis. Note too the extrasystole induced in **362** at the moment of injection.

**362**

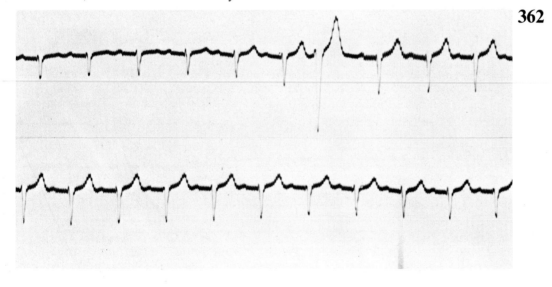

**363**

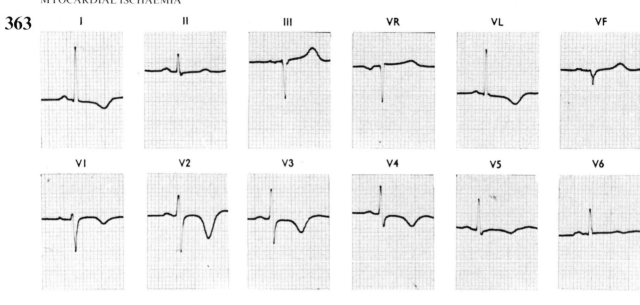

**364**

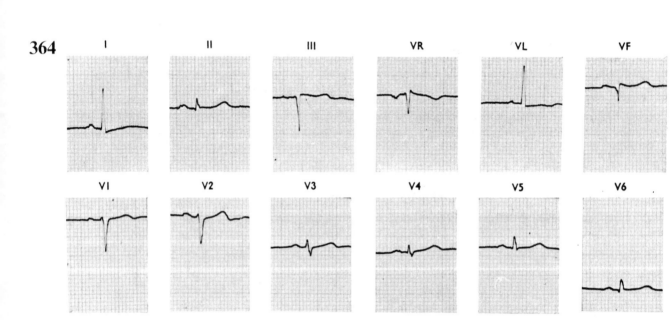

**363, 364 Acute myocardial ischaemia.** Symmetrical inversion of T waves is part of the pattern of recent or old infarction, and, in a partial thickness lesion, may be the only sign. Nevertheless, cases are seen in which such T waves seem to be due to reversible ischaemia. Figure **363** shows symmetrical T wave inversion in the antero-septal leads. Figure **364** was taken only days later; T waves have reverted to normal in V2–6, though they remain abnormal in I and VL. The lower voltage of the second trace may be a technical fault in recording.

**365 Acute myocardial ischaemia.** Three traces are illustrated. The limb leads are mounted above, and the chest leads below. In each set the top line shows the appearances prior to pain, and the centre and lowest lines the changes during and after the ischaemic episode respectively. Initially, there is T inversion in I and VL. During ischaemia, the axis shifts to the left and ST depression appears in anterior and inferior leads. On recovery, ST depression is lost but now there is T inversion persisting in anterior leads; the axis returns to normal.

I    II    III    aVR    aVL    aVF

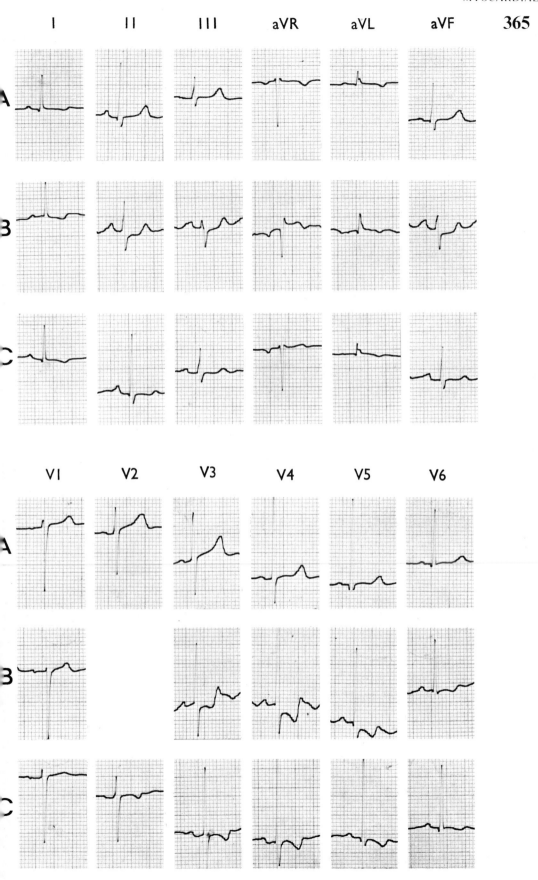

V1    V2    V3    V4    V5    V6

**366**

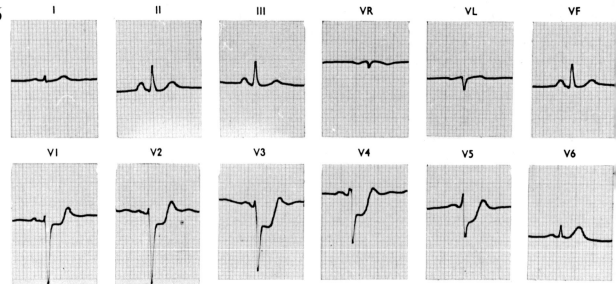

**366, 367 Acute myocardial ischaemia or sub-endocardial infarction?** Figure **366** shows marked ST depression with horizontal ST segments and upright T waves in V2–5. This pattern is described in subendocardial infarction but could simply be due to ischaemia. Clinical and laboratory findings may help to decide, but the progression or otherwise of the changes may also furnish evidence. In this instance, a trace taken a day or so later, **367**, shows resolution of the ST depression. However, T wave inversion is now present in V4–6, II, III, and VF, indicating infero-lateral ischaemia.

**367**

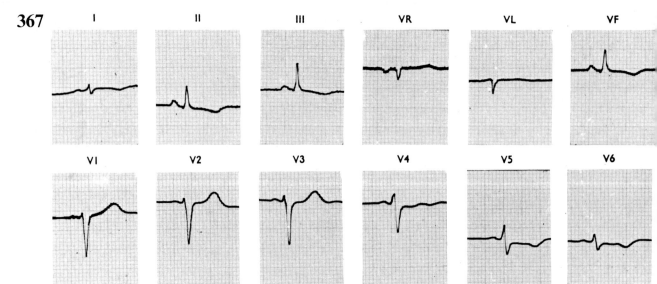

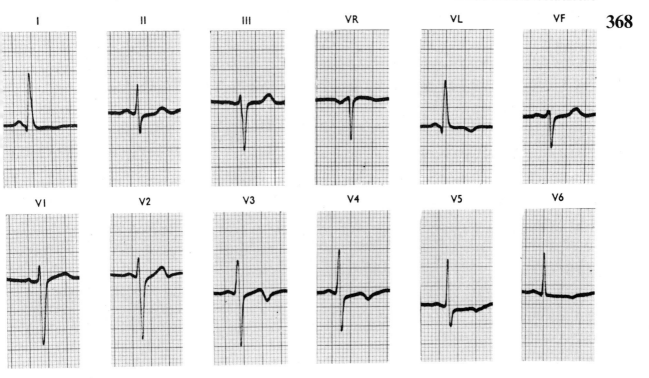

**368    Antero-lateral myocardial ischaemia.** T wave inversion is present in leads V3–6, I and VL.

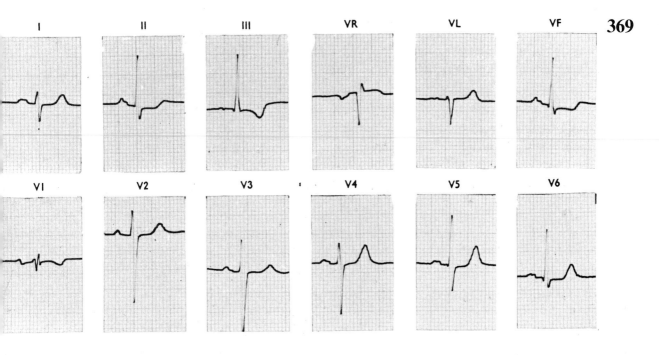

**369    Inferior myocardial ischaemia.** ST depression is present in II, III, and VF. Although not marked, these changes are probably significant.

**370**

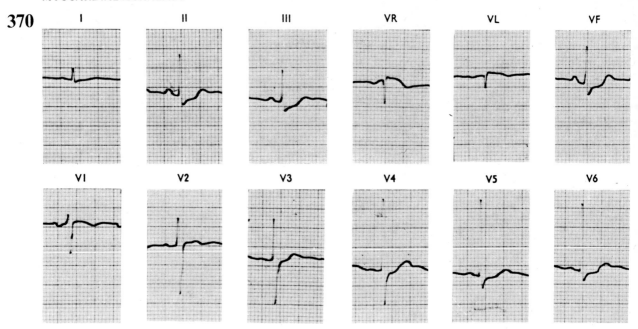

**370 Infero-lateral myocardial ischaemia.** ST depression is present in II, III, VF, and V4–6.

**371 High lateral ischaemia.** Ischaemia affecting the upper lateral portion of the left ventricle may only be seen in VL and I, as in this example; the praecordial leads are normal except possibly for minimal ST depression in V6. The tiny Q in I and the QS complex in VL, together with the symmetrically inverted T waves in these leads raise the question of infarction in this case.

**372 Posterior ischaemia.** The tall peaked T waves in V2–4 are out of proportion to other praecordial T waves and suggest mirror image T wave inversion on the true posterior surface of the heart—a region not directly represented on the conventional electrocardiogram.

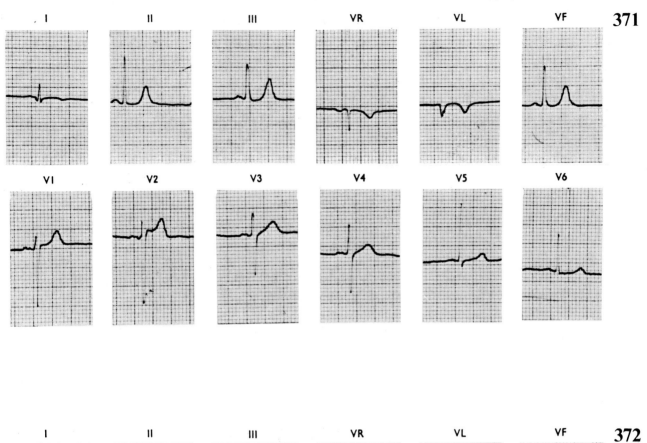

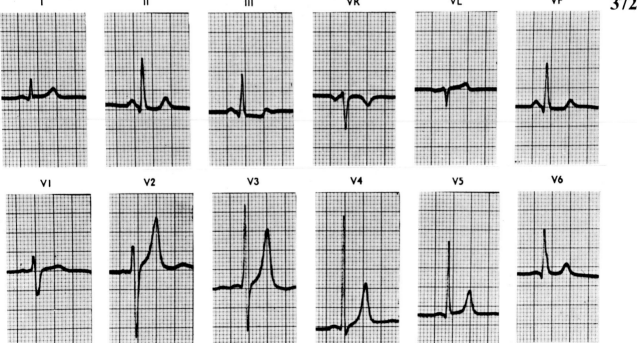

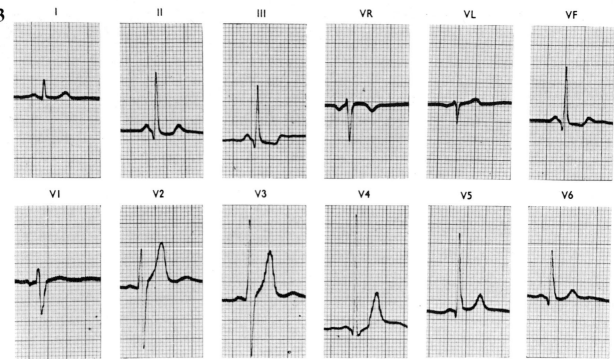

**373  Inferior and posterior ischaemia.** The changes of inferior ischaemia are borderline—very slight ST sagging with rather abrupt angulation between ST and T in II, III, and VF. In addition, tall peaked T waves in V2–4 suggest posterior ischaemia.

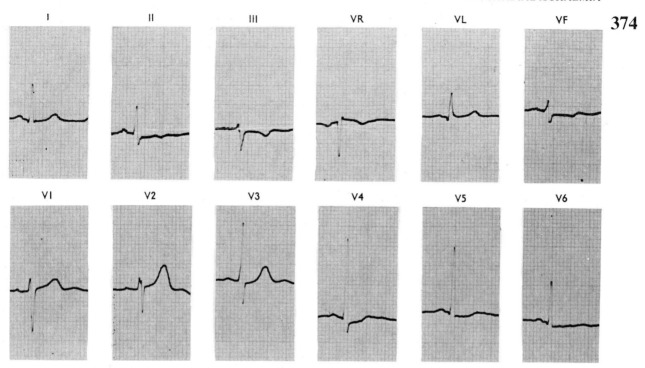

**374, 375  Myocardial infarction following myocardial ischaemia.** Figure **374** shows T wave flattening and slight ST depression in infero-lateral leads—II, III, VF, and V4–6. A week later, infarction occurred in the same leads—**375**.

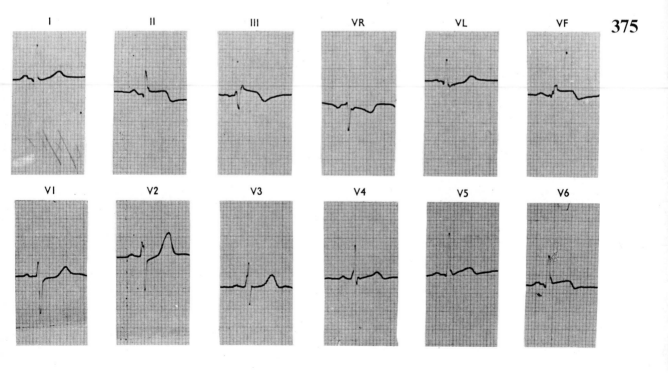

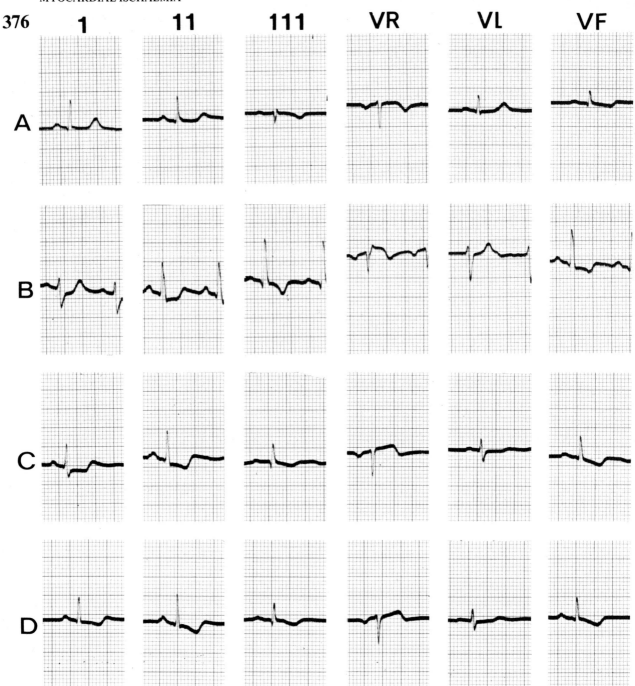

**376  Positive exercise test.** Electrocardiograms are recorded at rest (A), immediately after exercise (B), and twice more during the succeeding four minutes (C and D).

At rest, in the limb leads, there are rather horizontal ST segments and abrupt ST–T angulation in I, VL, II and VF. On exercise, there is a sharp swing in axis to the right together with the appearance of a tiny Q wave in III—the pattern of left posterior hemiblock—and some prolongation of QRS duration (still within normal limits however). ST depression appears in I, II, and VF, and T inversion deepens in III and develops in VF. Note the suggestion of U wave inversion in VL. During recovery, the ST depression resolves and the axis and QRS duration return towards normal but T wave inversion persists.

The chest leads at rest show two possible abnormalities: a horizontal ST segment in V6, and a broad R wave in V1 which may indicate an old

| V1 | V2 | V3 | V4 | V5 | V6 |
|----|----|----|----|----|----|

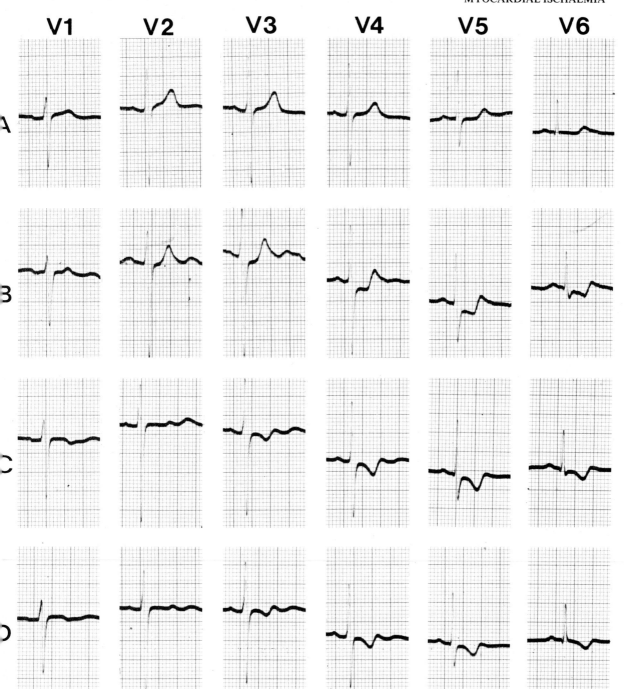

posterior infarction. On exercise, ST depression greater than 1mm appears in V3–6 (note the horizontal or downward sloping direction). During the next four minutes, ST depression slowly resolves but T wave and U wave inversion appear in V1–6.

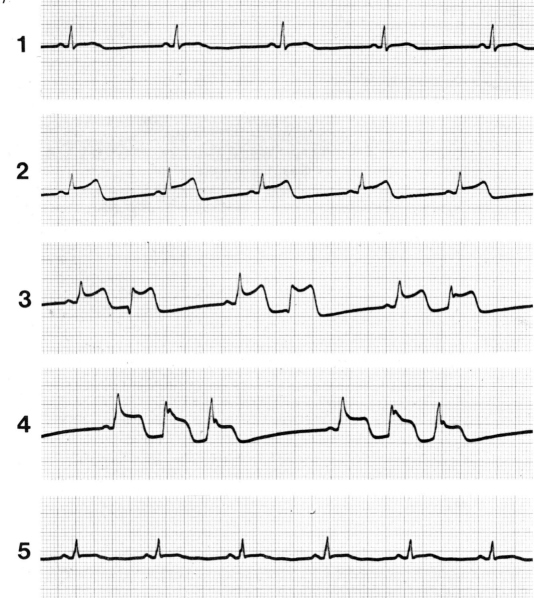

**377 Prinzmetal angina.** In this variety of myocardial ischaemia, pain at rest is associated with ST elevation rather than depression in appropriate leads, though reciprocal ST depression *does* occur as with acute infarction (see **380**). The five rows show the changes in a typical lead during a five minute attack of pain. The ST segment rises, T waves remaining upright. Later, coupled extrasystoles, and then linked extrasystoles appear. Finally, as pain subsides, the ST segment returns towards normal. Other arrhythmias may occur—e.g. ventricular tachycardia, or heart block.

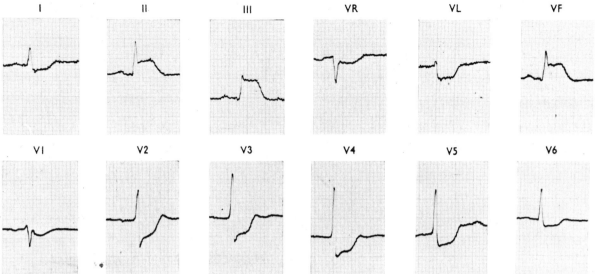

**378, 379 Prinzmetal angina.** Figure **378** shows marked ST elevation in inferior leads with reciprocal depression.in anterior leads. The pattern is indistinguishable from acute infarction not involving the whole thickness of the ventricular wall (i.e. no pathological Q waves). Figure **379** was taken the next day. ST elevation has gone, though conventional inferior and anterior ischaemic changes are seen—organic disease is often present in the vessel in which spasm causes the Prinzmetal pattern.

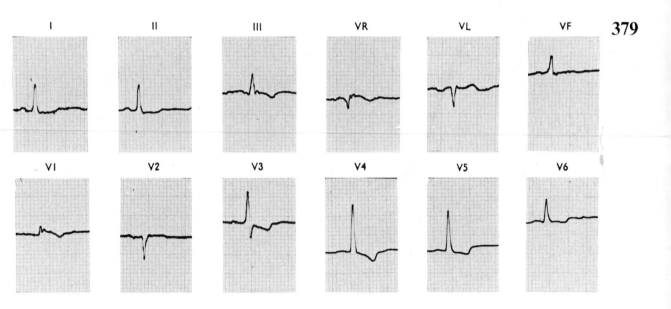

**380**

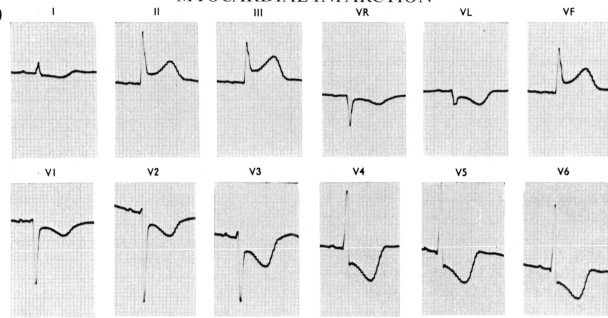

**380 Acute inferior myocardial infarction, the earliest hours.** Immediately after infarction, ST elevation is accompanied by upright, rather than inverted, T waves, the appearances resembling acute pericarditis (**414**). The clue lies in the localised distribution of the changes and the presence of Q waves, if any. Within hours, classical Pardee coving of the ST segments occurs, convex upwards, and the T waves begin to invert (**381**). Note the presence of reciprocal ST depression and T wave inversion on the other side of the heart (in this case, the anterior leads). And see Prinzmetal angina, 377–379.

**381**

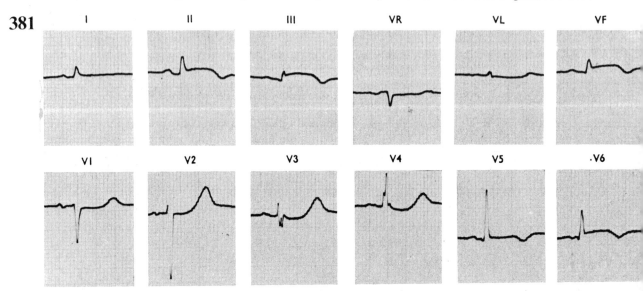

**381 Acute inferior myocardial infarction, the same patient as in 380, 24 hours later.** Classical Pardee coving of the elevated ST segments in the inferior leads is present. There are no pathological Q waves, so the infarction is partial thickness. Note the disappearance of the reciprocal ST depression referred to in **380**. Note too, the extension of the infarction to the lateral leads V5 and V6, and the prolonged QT interval.

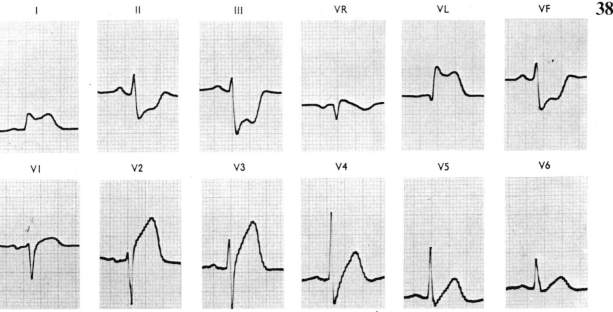

**382** **Acute antero-septal myocardial infarction, the earliest hours.** The pattern of ST segment elevation with upright T waves referred to in **380** is here seen in antero-septal leads V2 and V3, and in I and VL. Reciprocal changes are seen inferiorly, in II, III, and VF. No pathological Q waves are present.

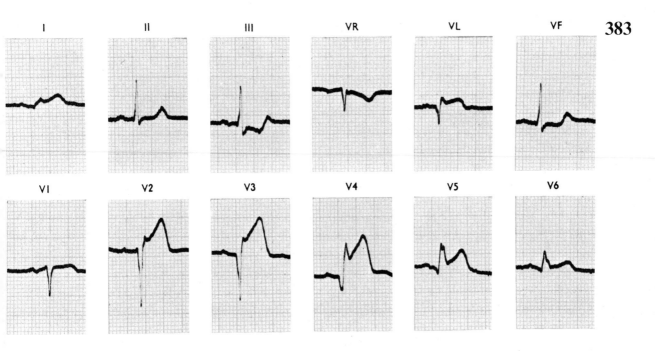

**383** **Acute anterior and lateral infarction, the earliest hours.** The pattern of early acute infarction extends right across the praecordium and is seen in I and VL. Pathological Q waves are present in V2–4, and in VL—a full thickness infarction.

**384**

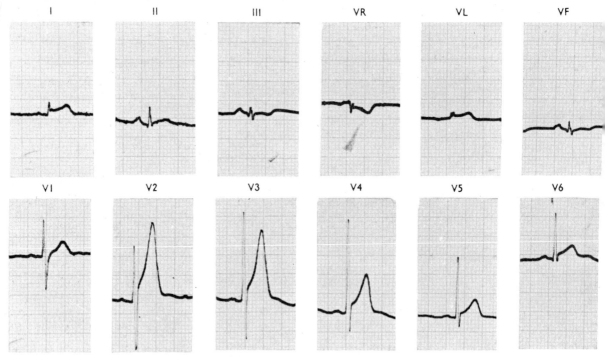

**384, 385   Acute lateral and true posterior myo-
cardial infarction.** Figure **384** shows the hyperacute
pattern of ST–T change in I, VL, and V2–6,
suggesting a recent antero-septal and lateral
infarction, but the very tall peaked T waves and tall
broad R waves in V1–3 raise the probability of true
posterior infarction—i.e. they are mirror images of
T inversion and Q waves that do not appear on the
conventional electrocardiogram. The trace taken

four days later, **385**, lends support to this view.
There is now no suspicion of antero-septal
involvement, but extension appears to have
occurred to the inferior leads and the tall wide R
waves in V1–3 persist. These two traces illustrate
well the point that the extent and location of
infarction are often difficult to judge at the outset.
See also **380** and **381**.

**385**

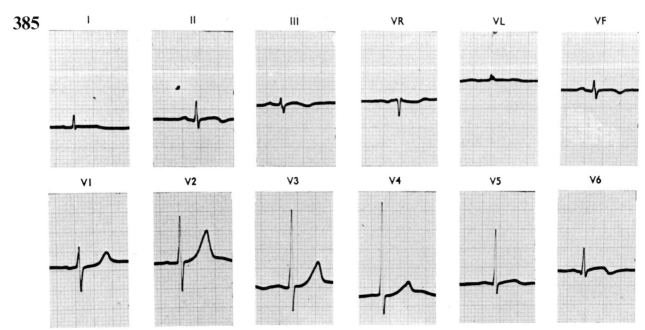

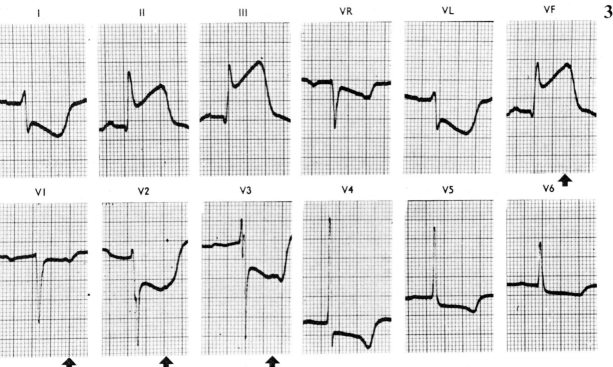

**386  Acute infarction, marked ST segment shifts.**
The displacement of the ST segment in the earliest
hours can be gross and may cause diagnostic
difficulty. For instance, it increases or decreases the
QRS voltage, sometimes to the extent of giving a
false impression of ventricular hypertrophy, and
more important, it can mask, or draw attention
away from arrhythmias. Thus, P waves in the ST
segments of several leads of the trace illustrated
opposite indicate that heart block is present
(arrows).

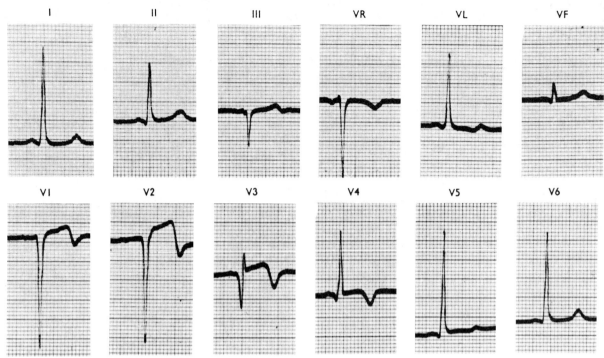

**387   Acute antero-septal myocardial infarction.** In this example, the infarct is not extensive. Changes are localised to leads V1–4. Note the absence of changes in the limb leads, which is frequently the case. The infarction is full thickness, as shown by the pathological Q waves, and relatively recent, as evidenced by the persistence of ST elevation. The symmetry of post-infarction T wave inversion is well shown.

**388, 389   Acute antero-septal myocardial infarction.** The antero-septal leads often normally show some ST elevation, and diagnosis of early infarction in this region can be difficult, particularly if ST shifts are slight and Q waves absent or doubtful. The trace in **388** shows suspicious ST elevation in V3 and V4 but the changes are slight, and the appearance in V2 could be within normal limits. A later trace, **389**, shows the stage of recovery of this infarction; V2 clearly *was* involved. Note the very tiny Q waves in V2–4, unusual in these leads and therefore noteworthy; nevertheless, they do not appear in the second trace. The Q wave in VL *may* be pathological. There is no loss of R wave in the chest leads, so there is minimal myocardial destruction.

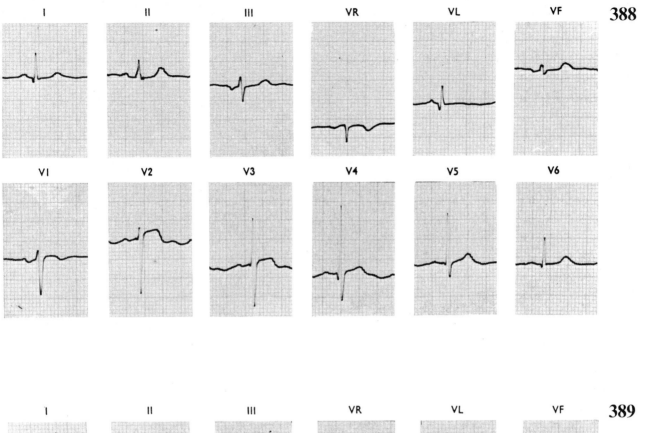

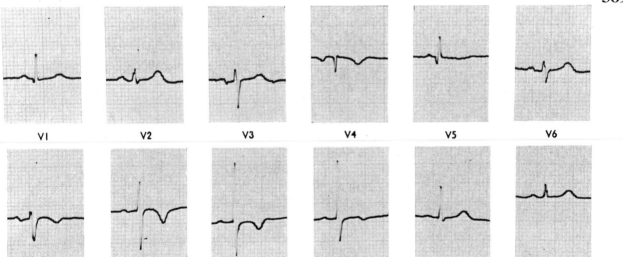

**390**

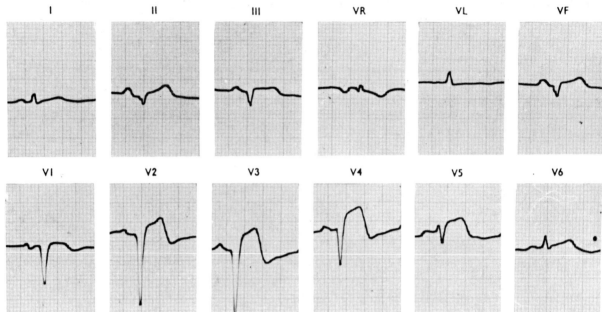

**390 Acute anterior myocardial infarction extending inferiorly.** The changes of acute full thickness infarction are present in the anterior leads and in the inferior leads. This pattern is not uncommon. There is left axis deviation (see **393**).

**391**

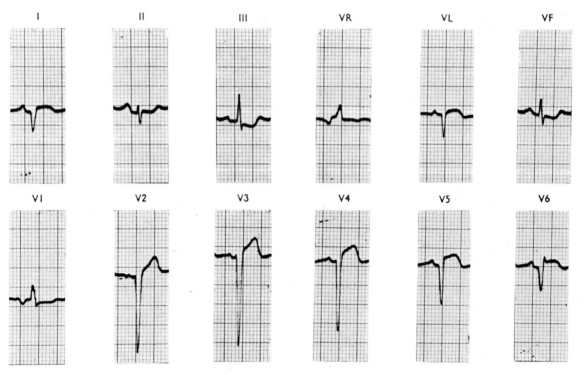

**391 Acute antero-lateral myocardial infarction.** QS complexes are present in I, VL, and V5, a pathological Q wave in V6, and ST segment elevation in all these leads and in V3 and V4. In antero-septal leads tiny R waves precede deep S waves. Note the right axis deviation (residual healthy muscle inferior).

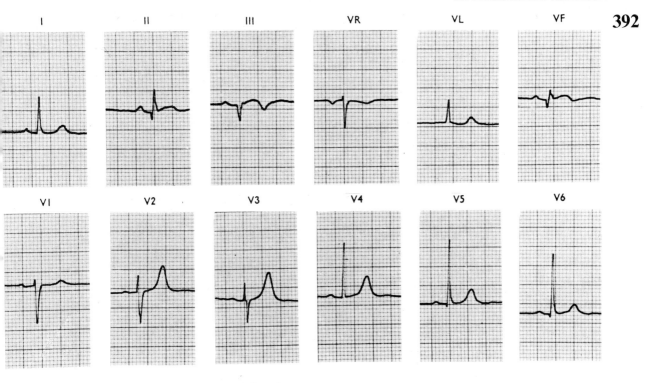

**392 Acute inferior myocardial infarction.** Pathological Q waves and ST elevation in leads II, III and VF.

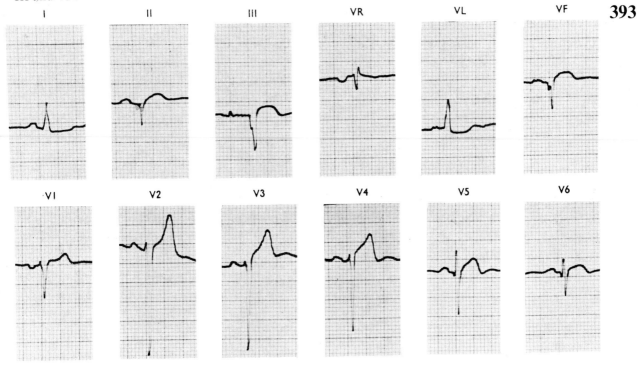

**393 Acute infero-lateral myocardial infarction.** ST segment elevation is present in II, III, VF, and V3–6. Pathological Q waves are seen in II, III and VF, so this is mainly an inferior infarction. Note the left axis deviation seen with inferior QS complexes (residual healthy muscle superior and anterior). See also **168, 169**.

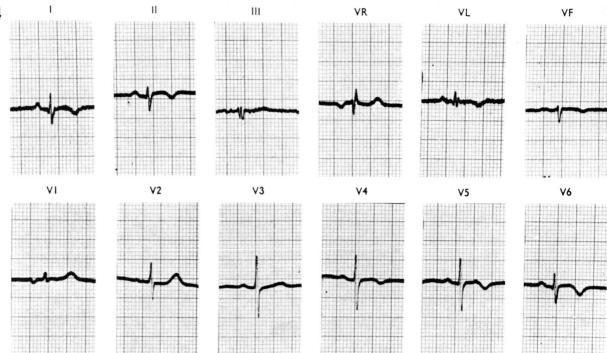

**394    Acute infero-lateral myocardial infarction.** A similar distribution to that in **393**, but ST elevation is slight (perhaps because this infarct is older—note the T wave inversion), and there are no pathological Q waves. Note that although the ST elevation in many leads does not reach even the modest defined limit of abnormality (i.e. 1mm), nevertheless it strikes the eye because *any* ST elevation of this contour is pathological in that particular lead, e.g. I, or V6.

**395    Acute inferior, lateral, and posterior myocardial infarction.** As in **394** ST segment shifts are slight but significant because of their shape and distribution. Inferior and lateral involvement is shown in leads I, II, III, VF, and V4–6. Acute posterior infarction is evidenced by tall, broad R waves in V1–3 with slight ST depression and a slightly pointed T wave in V2.

**396    High lateral infarction.** Infarction high on the lateral wall of the left ventricle may not appear in conventionally sited chest leads, though praecordial recordings taken one space higher may help. In the example illustrated, there are QS complexes in I and VL, but no Q waves elsewhere. ST elevation is present in I, VL, II, and possibly V6. Note the reciprocal ST depression in V1 and V2. The rather broad, tall R waves in V1–3 raise the suspicion that infarction extends onto the posterior aspect of the heart, or alternatively, with a prominent S wave in V6, there is right ventricular hypertrophy. Thus, the right axis deviation seen might have two causes.

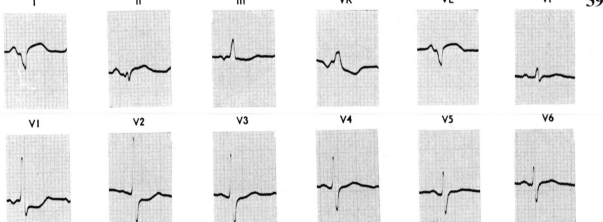

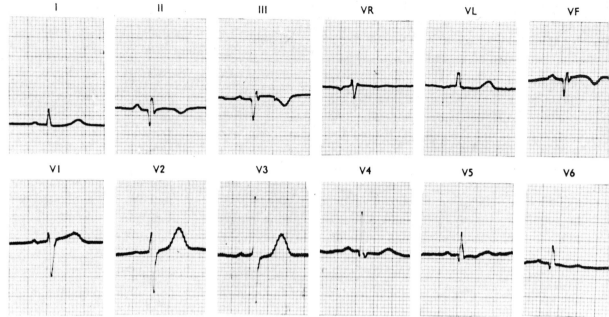

**397, 398 Extension of myocardial infarction.** Both 397 and 398 are from the same patient. Figure 397 shows acute inferior infarction (even slight ST elevation is significant in limb leads—see 394). The trace in 398 was taken later and shows extension of the infarction changes to involve the antero-lateral leads V4–6. Note the absence of infarction changes in I and VL. See also 384, 385.

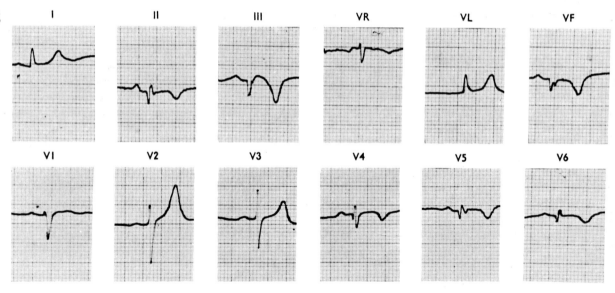

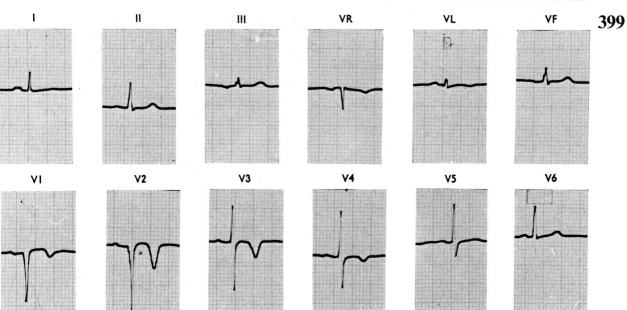

**399 Old antero-septal myocardial infarction.** In this instance, infarction changes are localised to leads V2–4. The T wave inversion in V1 could be normal. Note the loss of R wave in one lead only (V2), interrupting the normal progressive increase in the height of the R wave from V1 to V5. See **389**. Anticlockwise rotation is present.

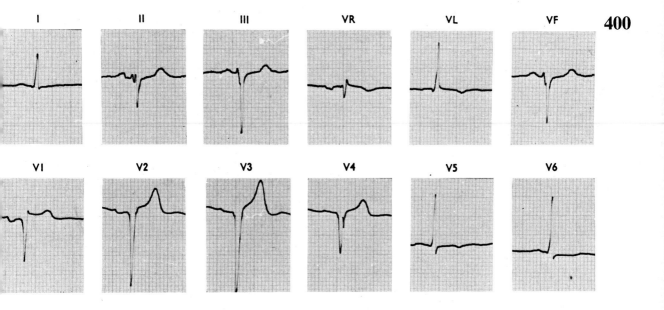

**400 Old antero-septal myocardial infarction.** Pathological Q waves are present in V1–4 (actually QS complexes). T waves have returned to normal, which they may or may not do. Note the absence of pathological Q waves in limb leads. The tracing shows two other features suggestive of ischaemia— left axis deviation and T flattening or inversion in lateral leads.

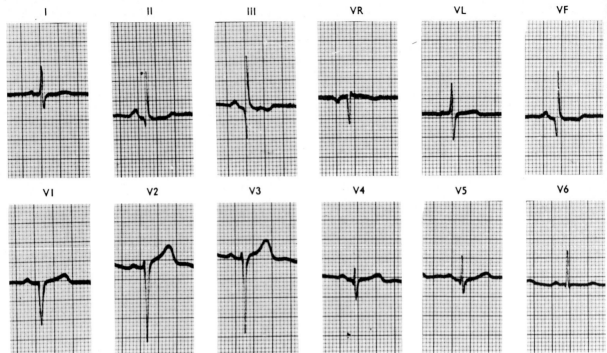

**401**   **The significance of Q waves in limb leads.** The diagnosis of old infarction from the presence of Q waves in the limb leads is not always easy. Accepted criteria are: a duration of 0.04 second, a depth equal to one quarter of the height of the R wave in the same lead or more, the presence of changes in related leads, and, acutely, ST–T changes in the same leads. It should be remembered that Q waves frequently diminish in the inferior leads on deep inspiration (**25**). In the trace shown, deep Q waves are present in II, III and VF and T waves are rather flat. The Q waves however, are less than 0.04 second in duration. This trace was taken from a healthy girl of seventeen. See **403**.

**402**   **Possible old inferior myocardial infarction.** Q waves are present in the inferior leads. In III, the Q wave is wide enough (0.04 second) and deep enough to be considered pathological (see **401**), especially as it is accompanied by smaller Q waves in II and VF. There is non-specific T wave flattening in the same leads. Traces such as this may cause considerable diagnostic disagreement, particularly when the way infarction changes can disappear is kept in mind (see **407–409**).

**403**   **Old inferior myocardial infarction.** There are pathological Q waves and symmetrical T wave inversion in II, III, and VF. See **401**.

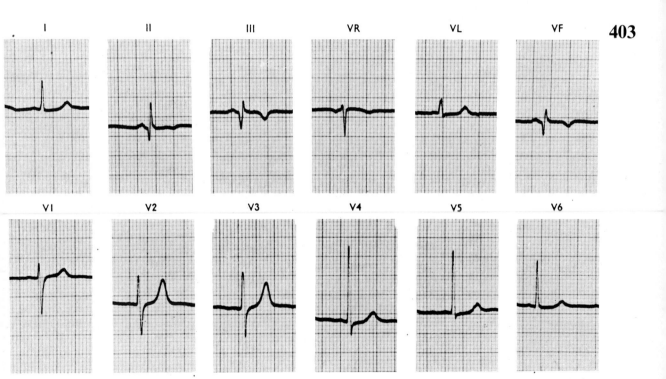

| I | II | III | VR | VL | VF | **402** |
| V1 | V2 | V3 | V4 | V5 | V6 | |

| I | II | III | VR | VL | VF | **403** |
| V1 | V2 | V3 | V4 | V5 | V6 | |

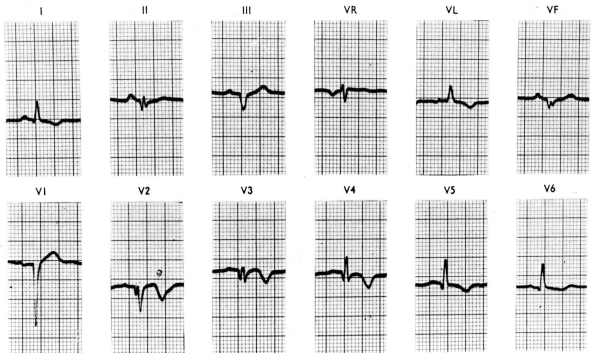

**404  Old antero-septal and inferior infarction.**
Pathological Q waves are present in II, III, VF, and
V2–4. Symmetrical T wave inversion is seen in
anterior leads, but not, in this instance, in inferior
ones.

**405  .Old inferior and true posterior infarction.**
Pathological Q waves are present in II, III, and VF
indicating inferior infarction, but in addition there
are broad initial R waves in V1 and V2 which
indicate mirror image Q waves posteriorly. Often,
the R waves will be abnormally increased in height
as well, and in the acute stages, ST depression in
antero-septal leads mirrors ST elevation, and tall T
waves, T inversion, that do not appear on the
conventional electrocardiogram. (See **395**.)

**406  Old inferior myocardial infarction with lateral
and posterior ischaemia.** There are Q waves in
inferior leads and symmetrically inverted T waves.
The latter are also seen in V6 and may represent
extension of infarction laterally, or ischaemia. The
very tall peaked T waves in V2–4 provide a striking
contrast, and indicate either ischaemia or partial
thickness infarction involving the posterior region
(in the absence of tall broad R waves in these leads it
is impossible to know which). See **372, 384**.

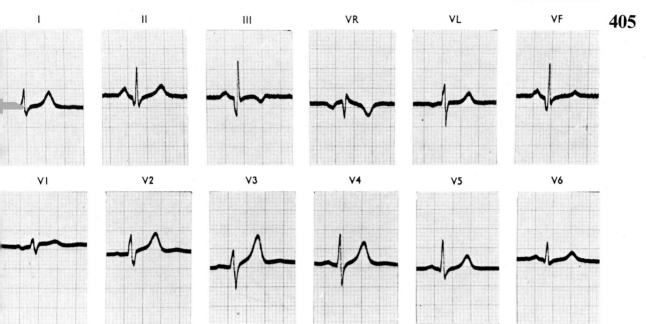

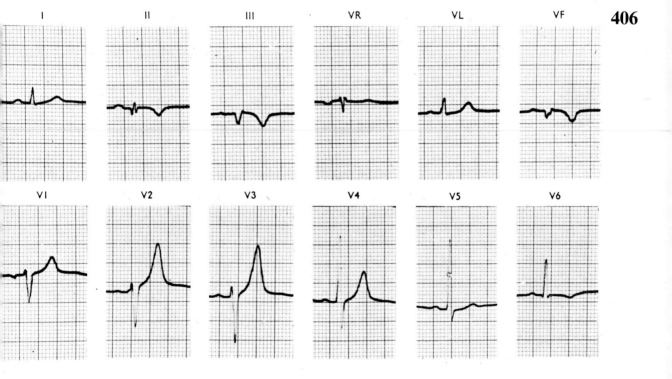

**407**

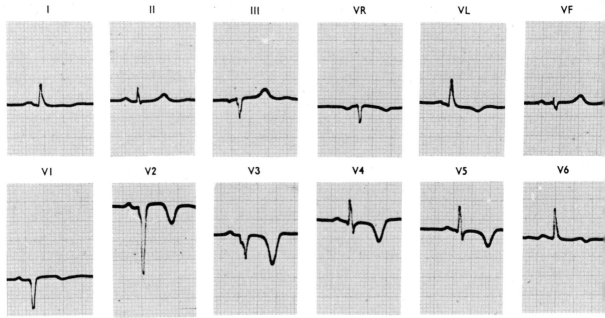

**407   The disappearance of infarction changes, 1.** The three electrocardiograms illustrated in **407–409** were recorded from the same patient. The first was taken at the time of his anterior myocardial infarction in 1965. The infarction is full thickness in the septal region, with pathological Q waves in V2 and V3.

**408**

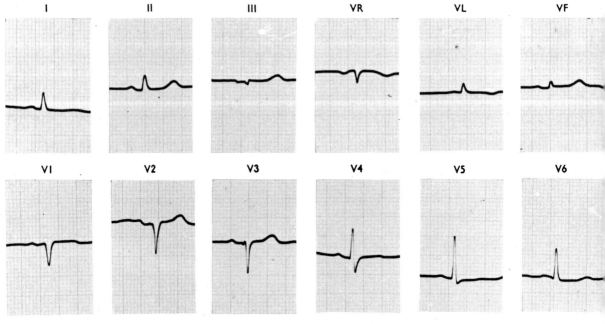

**408   The disappearance of infarction changes, 2.** The same patient as in **407**. Tracing recorded in 1966, one year after infarction. T wave inversion has gone in the septal leads though flattening persists in V4–6, I and VL. Pathological Q waves are still present in V2 and V3.

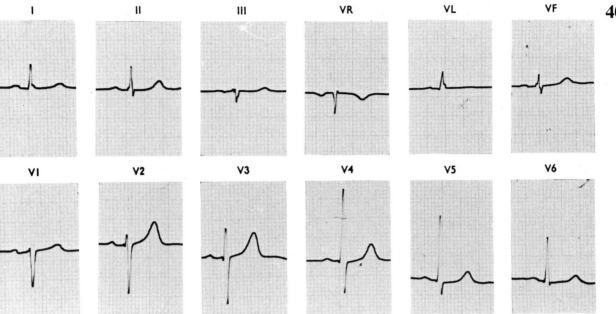

**409 The disappearance of infarction changes, 3.** The same patient as in **407** and **408**. Tracing recorded in 1968, three years after infarction. The only abnormality is a flat T wave in VL. The pathological Q waves have gone and there is even a smooth progression of R waves from V1 to V4. It is a salutary exercise to read this series of electrocardiograms backwards.

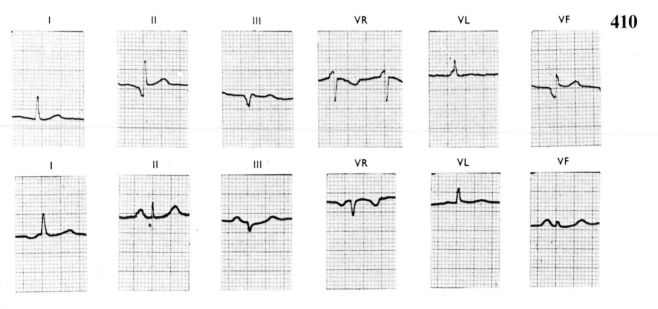

**410 False Q waves in junctional rhythm.** Two sets of limb leads are illustrated, recorded on successive days from the same patient. The upper set show apparent broad Q waves in inferior leads, but a second look reveals that these are in fact inverted P waves, for the patient is in junctional rhythm. Note similar positive waves in VR and VL (in I, presumably the P vector is at right angles in this case). Reference to the lower trace confirms the point.

**411**

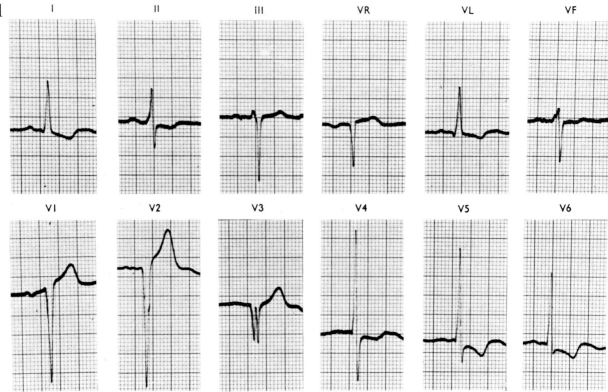

I     II     III     VR     VL     VF

V1     V2     V3     V4     V5     V6

**411 Antero-septal infarction and left ventricular hypertrophy.** The diagnosis of infarction in the antero-septal region can be difficult when left ventricular hypertrophy is present because of the abrupt reversal of polarity of QRS in the septal leads and because R waves over the right ventricle may be diminutive (see **302**). In the trace shown, however, there is an undoubted pathological Q wave in V3.

**412 Ventricular aneurysm.** Persistence of the pattern of acute myocardial infarction long after recovery strongly suggests the existence of an extensive fibrous scar in the ventricular wall, which may be simply an inert segment or which may have yielded to form a frank aneurysm (**520–526**). It is usual to see this with an antero-lateral infarction, but aneurysms do occur elsewhere (**527, 528**). There is no clear rule about the timing of the descent of the ST segment to the isoelectric line, though this will have happened in three weeks in the majority of cases. Occasionally, it takes longer. Persistence of ST elevation beyond six weeks is highly suspicious. Note the presence of QS complexes in all prae-cordial leads; ventricular aneurysms usually follow extensive full thickness infarctions. Most, but not all patients with aneurysms have such an electro-cardiogram.

**413 Atrial infarction.** This is recognised by displacement of the PR segment (upwards in some leads and reciprocally downwards in others) and alteration in the P wave. The upper line shows the limb leads of a patient showing PR depression in II, III, and VF, and elevation in VL and VR, but not in I. Note the prolongation of the PR interval and the P wave vector, which is approximately $+75°$. The lower line shows the same leads before infarction. The PR interval is normal and the P wave vector about $+40°$; the PR segment is isoelectric. Acute pericarditis can produce apparent PR depression but is readily distinguished by the uniform direction of PR and ST segment shifts.

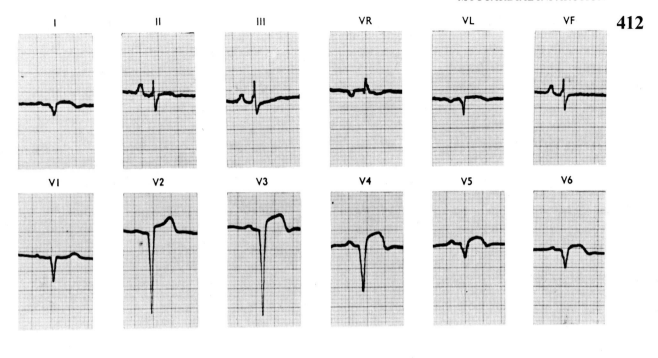

412

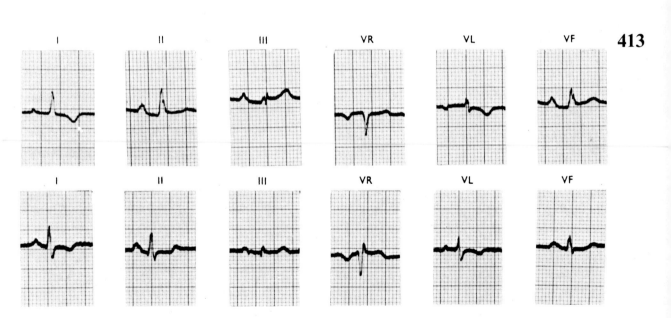

413

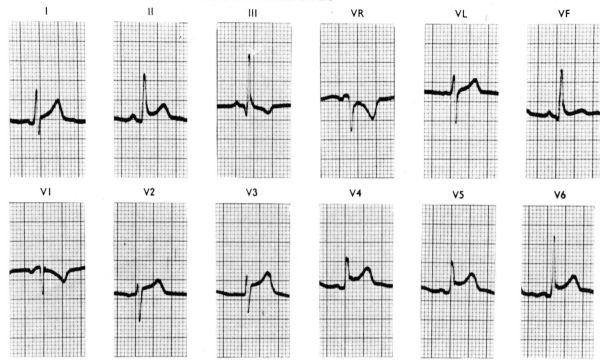

I  II  III  VR  VL  VF

V1  V2  V3  V4  V5  V6

**414  Acute pericarditis.** There is ST elevation, concave upwards, with upright T waves in most, if not all leads. Classically, it is more obvious in lead II than in I or III. There are no pathological Q waves, and the widespread distribution of ST–T changes, without reciprocal depression as is seen in the first hours of myocardial infarction (**380, 382**) distinguishes acute pericarditis from this. The other mimic of acute pericarditis is the sickling pattern—but this is usually associated with only minor ST elevation, and it disappears on effort (see **13, 14**). The changes of pericarditis are due to the superficial myocarditis which accompanies it.

**415  Healing pericarditis.** The raised ST segments and upright T waves of the acute stage give way to symmetrical inversion of T waves in most leads. In the example shown, this is well seen in all limb leads and the lateral chest leads. The slight ST depression in V2 and V3 is principally due to an unstable baseline. Note how the generalised T inversion appears in mirror image in VR. Eventually, the electrocardiogram reverts towards normal with flat and then upright T waves in many cases.

**416  Constrictive pericarditis (see 541).** Widespread T wave inversion or flattening is seen in association with low voltage complexes. Oddly, the P wave is often bifid and prolonged, just as with left atrial hypertrophy and this is well seen in the trace illustrated. Frequently, despite obvious clinical constriction, the electrocardiogram may be surprisingly normal. One third of cases have atrial fibrillation.

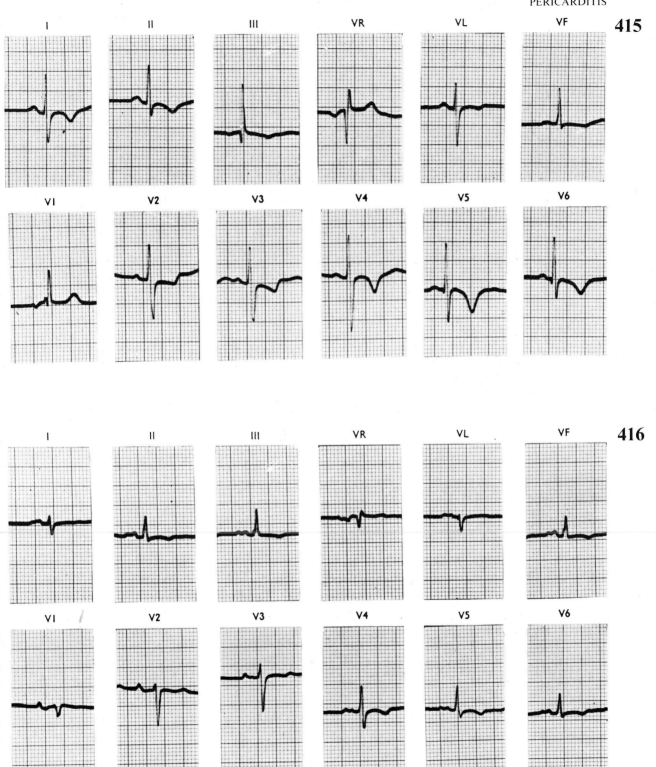

**417**

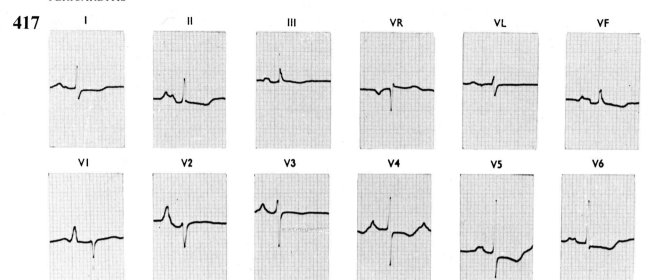

**417, 418   Pericardial effusion.** Large quantities of pericardial fluid (535) produce low voltage curves. Generalised T wave flattening or inversion are partly the result of this insulating effect and partly due to the superficial myocarditis which accompanies inflammatory pericarditis. Figure **417** shows the electrocardiogram of a patient with mitral stenosis and pulmonary hypertension (note the combined P pulmonale and mitrale). Following the development of a massive pericardial effusion there is a striking reduction in voltage (**418**). N.B. the rhythm is now atrial fibrillation.

Another described sign of large pericardial effusions is alternation in the direction of QRS or P (not illustrated).

**418**

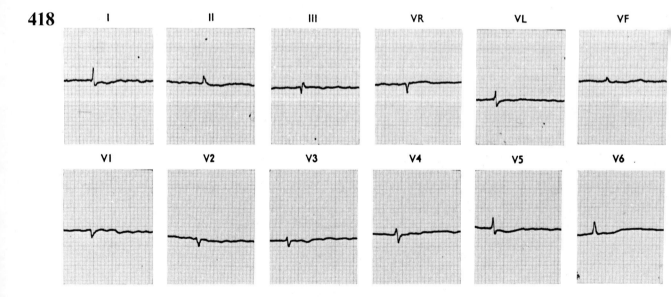

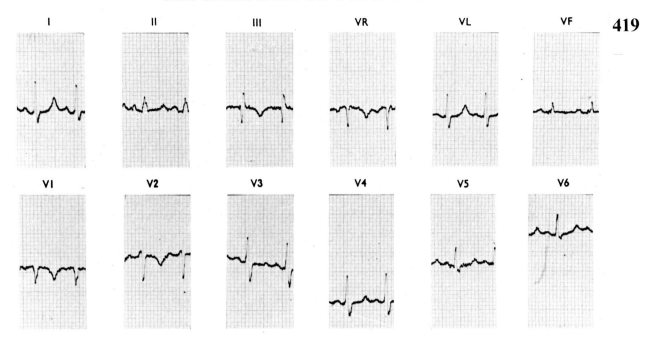

**419, 420   Acute pulmonary embolism (see 618).** The classical changes are: tachycardia, a rightwards shift in axis, the appearance of an S wave in lead I and a Q wave in lead III, T wave inversion in III and over the right ventricle, and incomplete right bundle branch block. Figure **419** shows most of these features, as can be seen by reference to the trace (**420**) taken after recovery. Note that the changes may be slight and easily overlooked; the availability of a previous trace is a great aid to diagnosis of massive pulmonary embolism. See **421**.

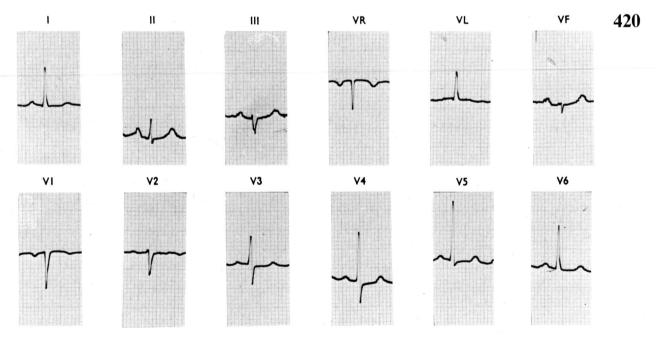

**421**

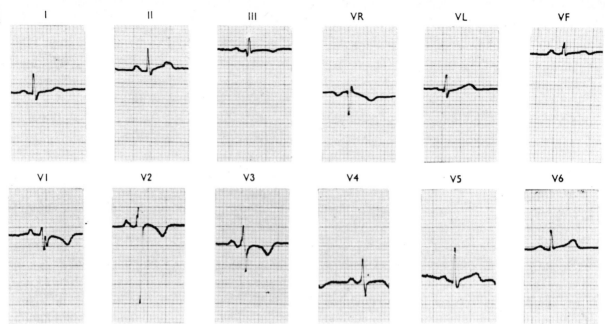

**421 Acute pulmonary embolism.** Another example. The changes are less obvious, only the T inversion in V1–3 is definitely abnormal.

**422, 423 Subacute cor pulmonale.** Figure **422** was taken from a child with upper respiratory tract obstruction due to massive tonsillar enlargement which produced anoxic pulmonary hypertension, and after a few months, frank congestive failure. There is P pulmonale, incomplete right bundle branch block, and secondary R and S wave voltages indicating right ventricular hypertrophy. The trace in **423** was recorded some months after surgical relief of the obstruction. The changes of right atrial and right ventricular hypertrophy have regressed; partial right bundle branch block remains—it may be a normal finding.

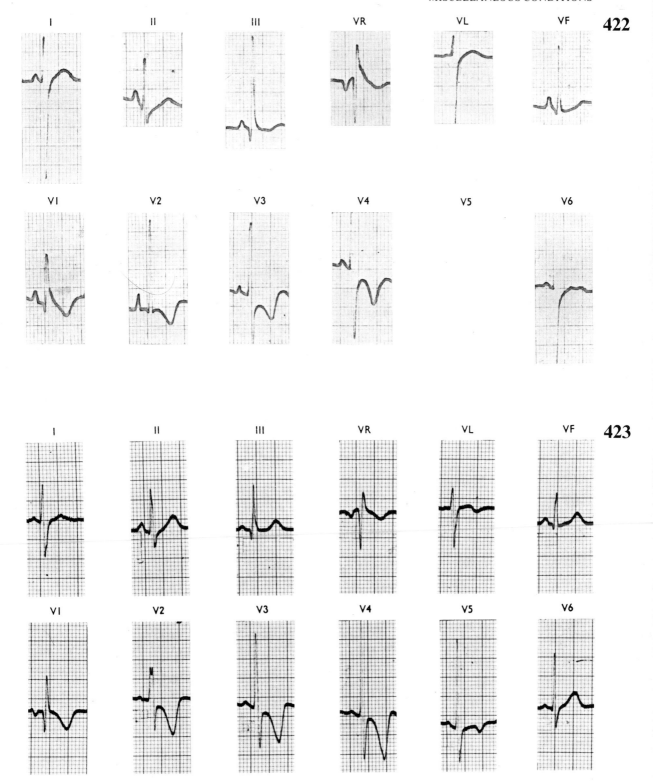

**424**

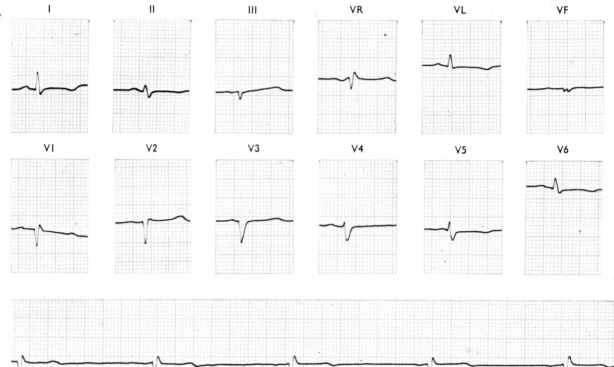

**424 Myxoedema.** All leads shows low voltage with flat or inverted T waves. Sinus bradycardia is present and helps to distinguish such a trace from similar appearances in constrictive pericarditis in which bradycardia would be most unusual. Note the prolonged QT interval at approximately 0.48 second—actually within the normal range for this heart rate, but an eye-catching feature.

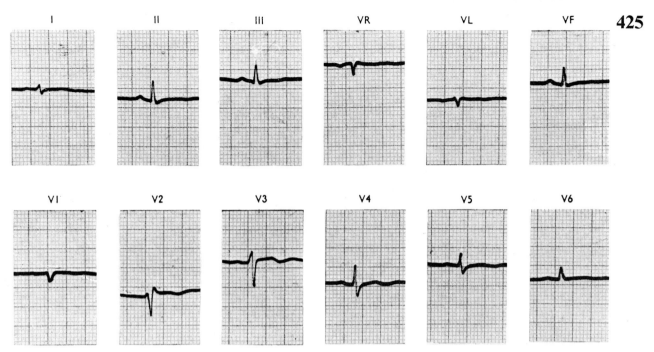

| I | II | III | VR | VL | VF |

| VI | V2 | V3 | V4 | V5 | V6 |

**425, 426   Myxoedema, effect of thyroid.** Figure **425** shows the untreated case; **426** shows the alteration some months after thyroid was started. Voltages have increased, T waves have become upright, and the QT interval is shorter. The heart rates are not available.

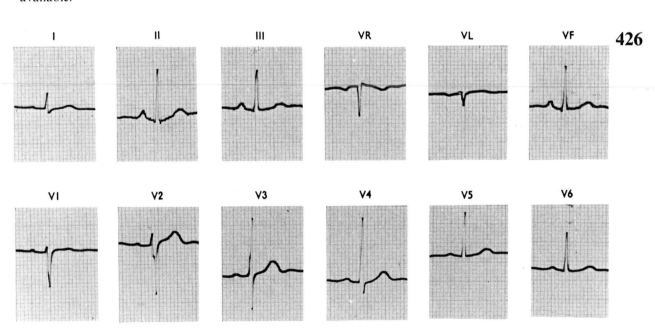

| I | II | III | VR | VL | VF |

| VI | V2 | V3 | V4 | V5 | V6 |

**427**

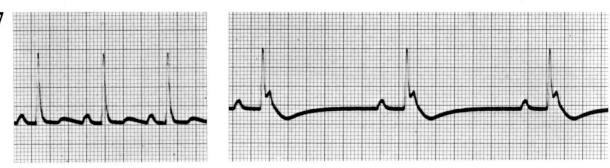

**427 Hypothermia.** The diagnostic finding is the J wave, a positive wave interposed between the QRS and ST segment. It appears in all leads and, as the body temperature drops further, broadens and increases in size, sometimes to amazing dimensions (see **428**). The other changes are sinus, later junctional bradycardia, ST depression and prolongation of the QT interval. The trace on the left shows the normal appearances and the trace on the right, the same lead during hypothermia.

**428 Severe hypothermia.** This remarkable trace was taken from a patient with a rectal temperature of 19.5°C, four hours before death. J waves have become the dominant feature and there are gross ST–T changes and atrial standstill. Note the heart rate of 14/minute.

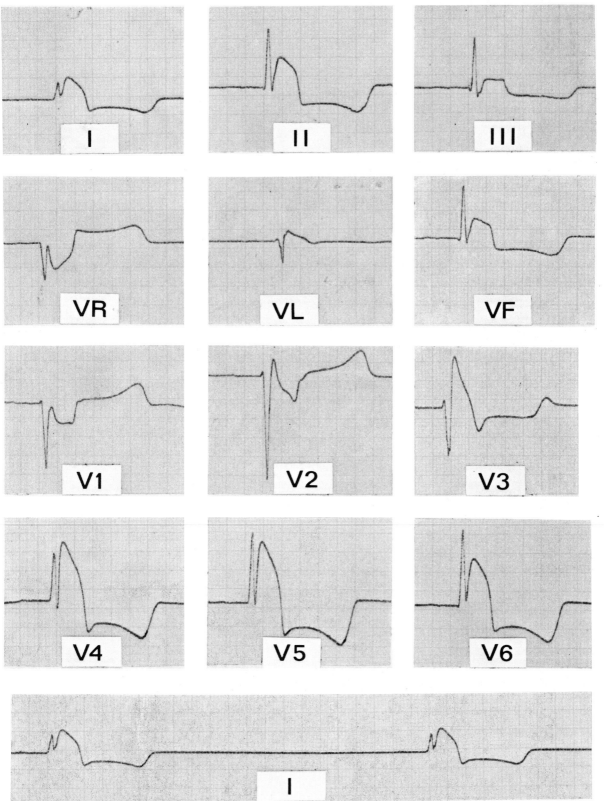

**429**

| I | II | III | VR | VL | VF |
|---|---|---|---|---|---|
| 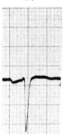 | 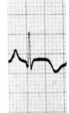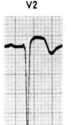 | 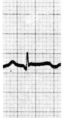 | 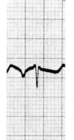 | 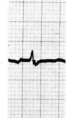 | 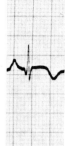 |

| VI | V2 | V3 | V4 | V5 | V6 |
|---|---|---|---|---|---|
| 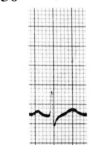 | 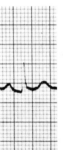 | 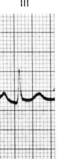 |  | 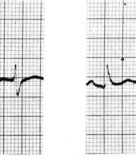 | 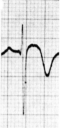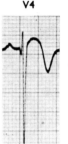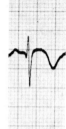 |

**430**

| I | II | III | VR | VL | VF |
|---|---|---|---|---|---|
| | | | | | |

| VI | V2 | V3 | V4 | V5 | V6 |
|---|---|---|---|---|---|
| 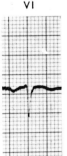 | 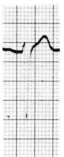 | 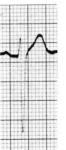 | 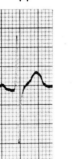 | 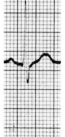 | 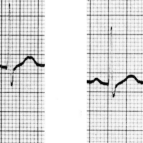 |

**431**

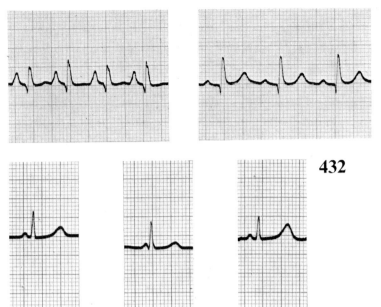

**432**

**429, 430 Subarachnoid haemorrhage.** The electro-cardiographic changes which very commonly appear after subarachnoid haemorrhage are of unproven cause, though there is recent evidence to suggest they are related to catecholamine release. Non-specific T wave changes are frequent, but the appearances may also mimic myocardial infarction. The direct relationship to the haemorrhage is illustrated by the fact that no other evidence of myocardial ischaemia is found (even at post-mortem), and that the changes disappear completely, only to return if bleeding recommences. Figure **429** shows an apparent antero-septal infarction extending inferiorly. It appears acute, with ST segment elevation, and there is a QS complex in V3. Tiny, non-significant Q waves are present in inferior leads and in V3. This trace was recorded in a young woman within a day or so of a subarachnoid haemorrhage. Figure **430** shows the tracing recorded a week later; the abnormal changes have gone. Note the disappearance of the Q waves in the leads mentioned.

**431, 432 Subarachnoid haemorrhage.** In addition to the changes in the QRS complex and T waves described in **429**, abnormalities of the P wave and PR interval occur. Figure **431** shows markedly peaked P waves on the left, recorded during the acute stage of subarachnoid haemorrhage, and on the right, the same lead after recovery with normal P waves. Similar changes are visible in lead II and VF in **429** and **430**. In other contexts, such P waves would be labelled P pulmonale. Note the flat T waves in the left-hand trace of **431**, partly obscured by tachycardia; on the right, these too have returned to normal.

Figure **432** shows alteration in the PR interval. On the left, a week or so after a first subarachnoid haemorrhage, the PR interval is 0.1 second (heart rate 70/minute). A second bleed occurred and the centre example shows an abrupt reduction in the PR interval to 0.07 second (heart rate 88/minute). The complex on the right shows the effect of administering propranolol at this time; the PR interval has returned to 0.1 second (heart rate 60/minute). Although changes in the PR interval occur with changes in rate, this cannot account for the alterations described.

**433**

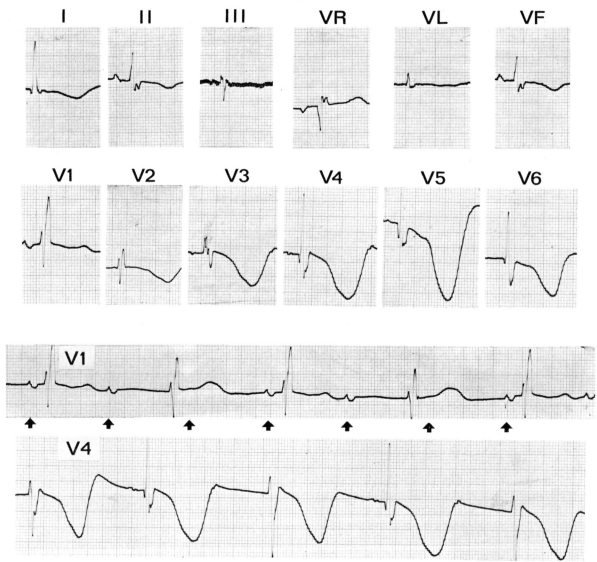

**433, 434  Cerebral haemorrhage.** Another pattern sometimes seen in severe cerebrovascular accidents is that of huge T and U waves fused together. They may be grossly inverted, as in the traces illustrated, or upright. These two traces were recorded in a woman with cerebral haemorrhage. Figure **433** shows the situation on admission. Enormous T–U inversion is present, the junction between T and U being well seen in V1–4. Note that the latter portion of this huge wave is all U wave! The QRS complex shows right bundle branch block.

In this particular case a rhythm disturbance was present. The two strips below show 3:1 heart block interrupted by escape beats which pursue a different conduction path (better seen in the V4 strip). P waves or their expected positions are arrowed under the V1 strip to assist analysis (in the distorted ST segments, they barely show).

Figure **434** shows the electrocardiogram of this patient nine days later. The pattern is still present, but is regressing.

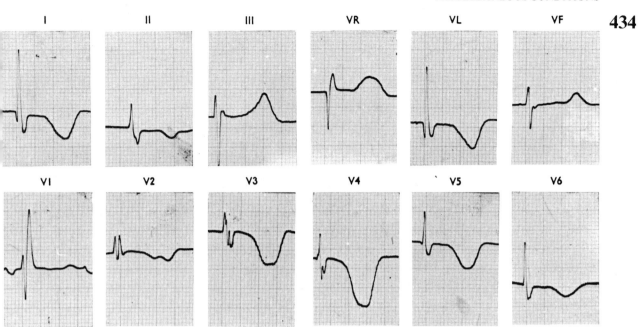

**435**

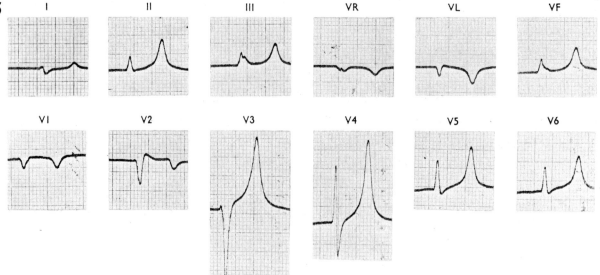

I    II    III    VR    VL    VF

VI    V2    V3    V4    V5    V6

**435, 436 Hyperkalaemia.** The characteristic change is the appearance of tall, peaked, narrow-waisted T waves. When the serum potassium rises above 7 mEq./L., the QRS widens and atrial standstill develops. All these changes are seen in **435**. The rate was 40/minute. Prolongation of the QT interval in these circumstances is attributed to the accompaniment of hypocalcaemia. Figure **436** shows the same patient on return of the serum potassium to normal levels.

Serum levels of potassium of 8 mEq./L. and above cause sudden asystole.

**436**

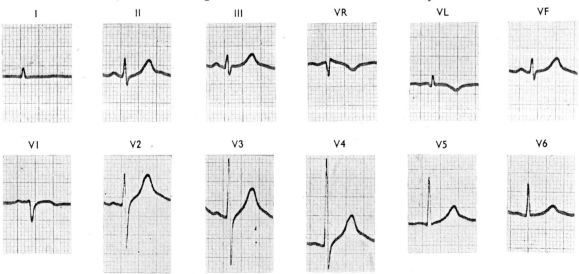

I    II    III    VR    VL    VF

VI    V2    V3    V4    V5    V6

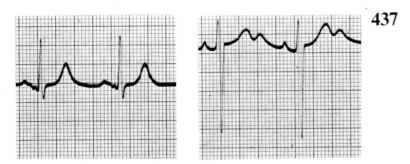

**437**

**437 Hypokalaemia.** Potassium depletion causes the U wave to become prominent. Later, T wave flattening and ST depression appear so that the U wave may be mistaken for the T wave, particularly in chest leads, where U waves are best seen. This may give a false impression of QT prolongation, but this does not occur. The illustration shows lead II on the left and lead V3 on the right in a case with moderate hypokalaemia. The U wave is invisible in lead II and the normal QT is seen. The double hump of T followed by U in the chest lead is characteristic.

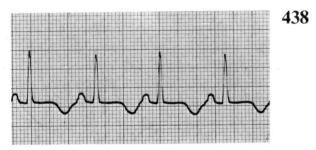

**438**

**438 Hypocalcaemia.** Modest reduction in serum calcium levels produces prolongation of the QT interval. Greater reductions produce further QT prolongation with a horizontal ST segment and T wave inversion—as illustrated here. The serum calcium of this patient was 5mg/100ml.

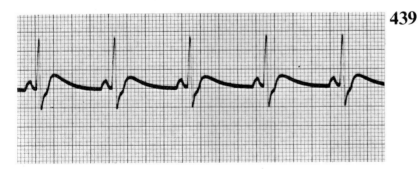

**439**

**439 Hypercalcaemia.** The QT segment is shortened and the T wave has an early peak with a more gradual descent. These changes are best seen in the chest leads.

**440**

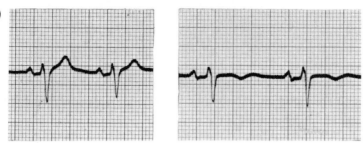

**440   Quinidine effect.** Apart from its influence on atrioventricular conduction, quinidine produces prolongation of the QT interval and T wave flattening and inversion. The left-hand illustration shows the pre-quinidine trace and the right-hand one the same lead after quinidine. Calculation of QT is rendered difficult because of the presence of a prominent U wave but even allowing for the change in rate, the effect on QT is evident. Later effects of quinidine include QRS widening, atrial standstill, heart block, and ventricular fibrillation.

**441**

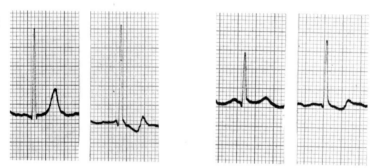

**441   Digitalis effect.** The cardinal change is ST depression. The T waves remain upright but flattened; eventually they may invert. The interpretation of T wave changes is therefore very difficult in patients receiving digitalis. Two pairs of complexes are shown. In both, the complex on the left is before digitalis, and the one on the right, after digitalis.

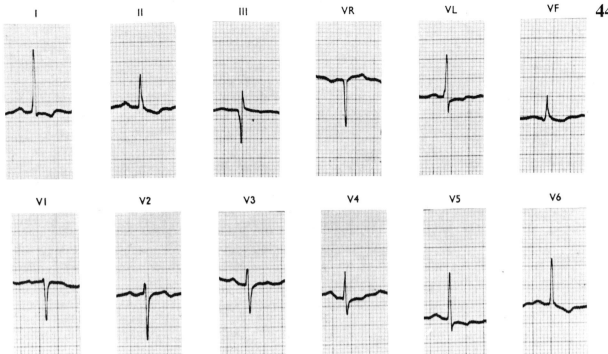

**442 Acute myocarditis.** Non-specific T wave changes in all leads suggest diffuse myocardial abnormality. Other causes of generalised T wave abnormality must not be forgotten. (N.B. the T wave changes of pericarditis are caused by a superficial myocarditis.) This trace was taken from a patient who developed a proven viral myocarditis and later progressed to a chronic myopathic stage. On investigation, normal coronary arteries were demonstrated.

**443**

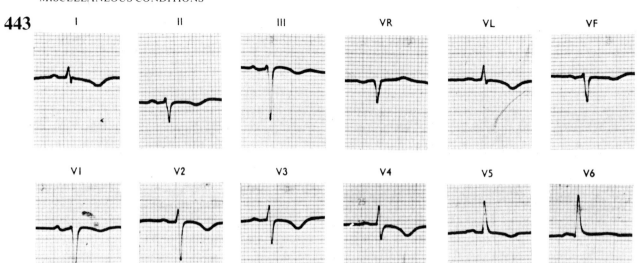

**443, 444  Congestive cardiomyopathy.** There are no diagnostic appearances. The electrocardiographic presentation is so varied that to attempt to illustrate it in depth would be to repeat much material already available elsewhere, but the traces shown are examples of a rather non-specific pattern often seen, which, taken with the clinical picture, and after exclusion of ischaemic heart disease, suggests cardiomyopathy of this type by its very lack of dramatic features. There are low voltage curves with T wave changes which are either generalised (**443**) or localised (**444**). Note the presence of left axis deviation in **443**. Any kind of arrhythmia or conduction defect may be seen.

**444**

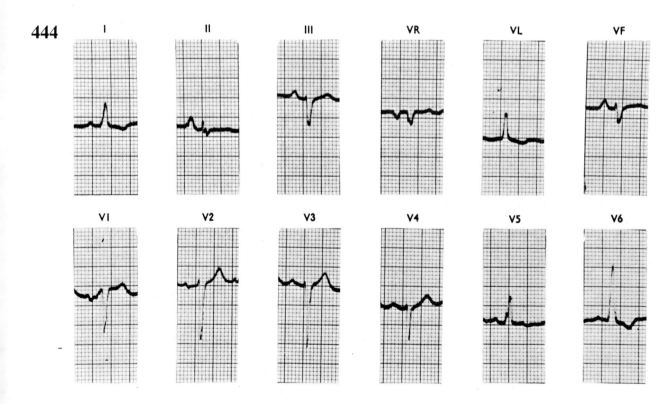

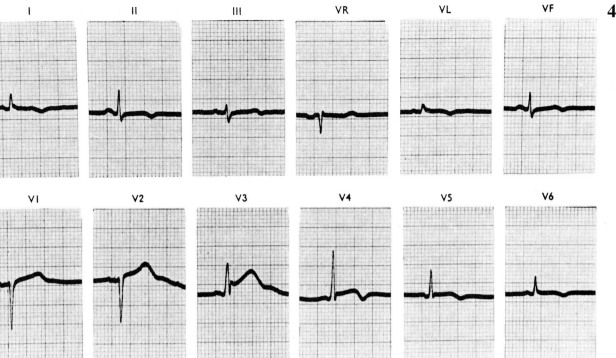

**445 Amyloid disease.** Cardiac involvement in amyloid is perhaps the exception to the rule that primary myocardial disease apart from hypertrophic myopathy (**307, 308**) presents no specific features (**443, 444**). As in other cardiomyopathies low voltage curves are seen, but changes suggestive of infarction are a notable addition. QS complexes in the chest leads are described, though they are absent from this tracing; ST elevation also occurs. In this particular patient the ST elevation in anteroseptal leads persisted unchanged for four years. Coronary arteriography was normal; there was no ventricular aneurysm. The diagnosis was proved on biopsy of the myocardium.

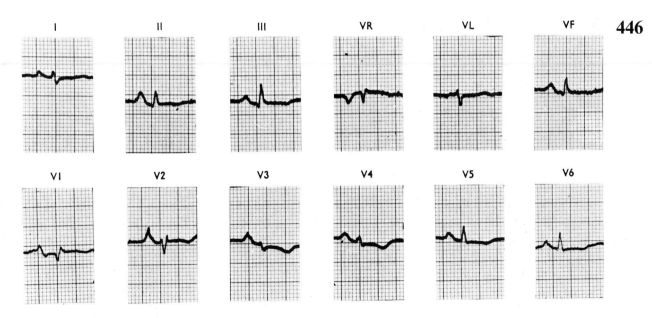

446

**446 Right atrial myxoma.** The striking combination of marked P pulmonale and very low voltage QRS complexes suggests massive enlargement of the right atrium caused by the obstruction to the tricuspid valve. (The same case as in **732–734**.)

# SOME DIAGNOSTIC PATTERNS OF CONGENITAL HEART DISEASE

**447**

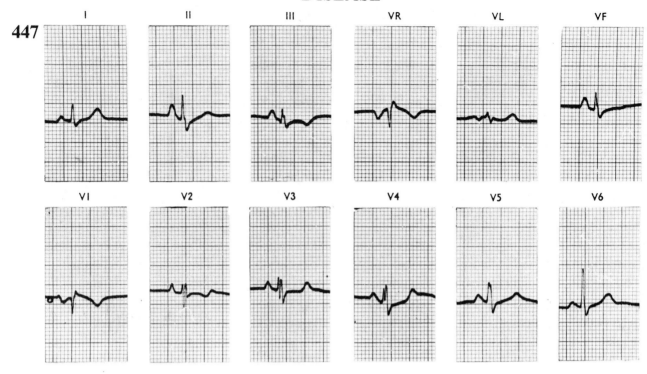

**448**

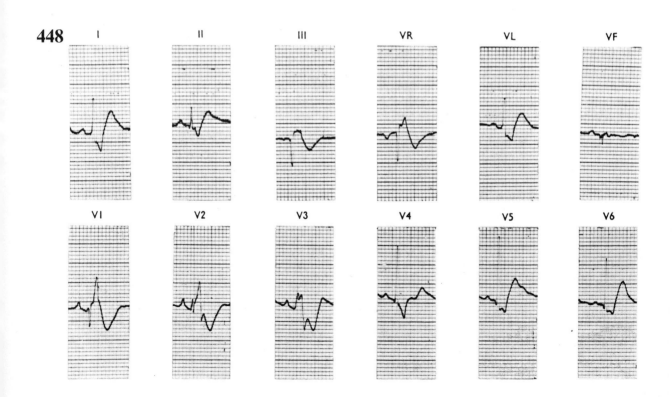

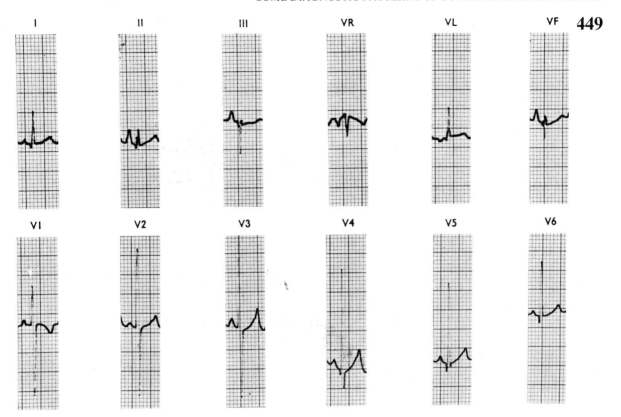

**447, 448    Ebstein's anomaly of the tricuspid valve (see 641).** The combination of P pulmonale and complete right bundle branch block is found, the diagnosis being suggested by the disparity between the tall, rather wide P waves and the low voltage, unimpressive QRS complexes (**447**). The latter characteristically show a complicated splintering over the right ventricle (**448**). Occasionally, type B Wolff–Parkinson–White syndrome is added to the picture (**168**). The PR interval is often prolonged. Arrhythmias are common—paroxysmal supraventricular tachycardia, atrial flutter, atrial fibrillation, extrasystoles, junctional rhythm, and sometimes, heart block.

**449    Tricuspid atresia (see 640).** The classical findings are P pulmonale, left axis deviation, and left ventricular hypertrophy. Since most cases present in infancy the latter two features must be interpreted in the light of the *right* axis deviation and *right* ventricular hypertrophy normally found at this period. In the trace illustrated for instance, the axis at approximately 0°, and the presence of deep S waves in V1 and V2 and dominant R waves in V5 and V6 are well outside the normal range for the week-old infant in whom they were recorded.

**450**

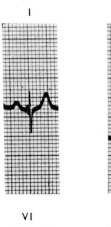
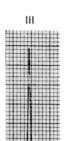
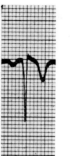
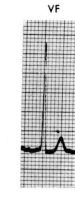

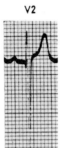
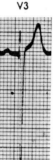
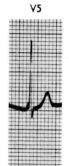
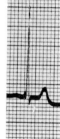

**451**

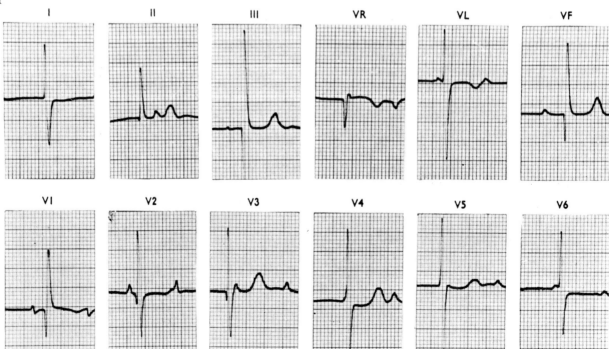

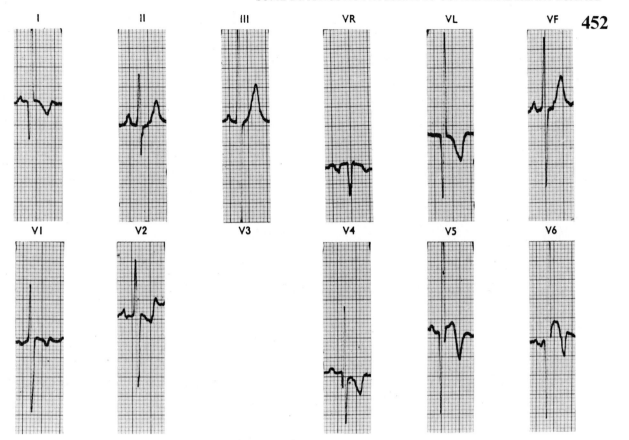

**450, 451 Corrected transposition.** The changes in this condition depend a great deal on which associated anomalies, if any, are present, but two clues may point to the diagnosis—heart block, and reversal of the direction of normal initial activation of the ventricles. All grades of block are described but perhaps complete block is the commonest (**451**). The second feature is due to inversion of the ventricles so that the interventricular septum is activated from the right not the left side. The normal septal Q wave is no longer seen in 'left ventricular' leads and is now to be found over the right praecordium in V1 and V2. Sometimes, the abnormal Q will be found in V4R only (not illustrated). Other common findings are the Wolff–Parkinson–White syndrome, and atrial tachycardias. Figure **450** shows left ventricular hypertrophy, and **451**, incomplete right bundle branch block, probably with additional right ventricular hypertrophy. See **664, 673**.

**452 Anomalous origin of the left coronary artery from the pulmonary artery.** Although very rare, this cause of heart failure and sudden death in children can be readily recognised by the distinctive pattern it produces on the electrocardiogram in classical cases—that of antero-lateral myocardial infarction and left ventricular hypertrophy. The example illustrated shows deep Q waves, ST segment elevation and symmetrical 'arrow head' inversion of the T waves in I, VL, and V4–6. Allowing for the age of the patient from which it is taken (six months) there is also left axis deviation at approximately −5° and left ventricular hypertrophy. ST segment elevation is not transient, persisting for months or years, and may suggest ventricular aneurysm.

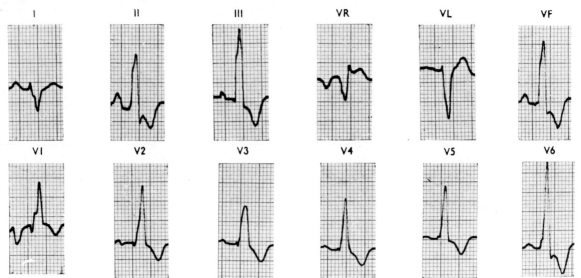

**453  Lutembacher's syndrome.** The coexistence of mitral stenosis (or indeed mitral regurgitation, though this is not the lesion classically described) with a secundum atrial septal defect may be suspected on the electrocardiogram by the presence of P mitrale. In this proven example in a woman of 50 a left atrial component to the P wave is seen in its prolongation to 0.14 second, in its bifidity in some leads, and in the large late negative component in V1 (**56**). P pulmonale is also present and the customary partial right bundle branch block is here complete, with right axis deviation affecting the initial as well as the terminal forces; there is voltage evidence of right ventricular hypertrophy (V leads are at half standardisation except for V1 and V6); these features were due to severe pulmonary hypertension. (See **648**, **649** for chest x-ray appearances.)

# PART 2

# PART 2

## CHEST X-RAYS: INTRODUCTION

In this section, in contrast to the previous one, there is rather more concentration on individual diseases, provided once again that the appearances are distinctive. As with electrocardiograms, some conditions come off badly—there seems little point in illustrating a series of virtually identical cardiac silhouettes, each labelled as having a specific cause, yet occasionally it cannot be avoided, e.g. left atrial myxoma mimicking mitral valve disease. Although angiograms and films taken during catheterisation are outside the intention of this book, some examples have been included where they throw light on the interpretation of a plain film (e.g. kinked aortic arch) and there is a short section on pacing. Once again congenital heart disease in infants has created difficulties because of the variability of appearances at this age and the relative rarity of many of the lesions. The solution has been to illustrate a few readily identified conditions.

**454**

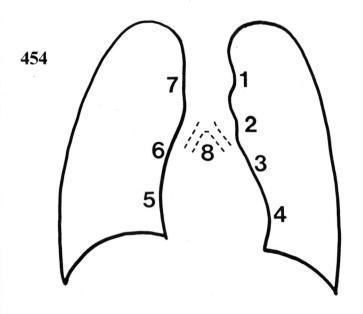

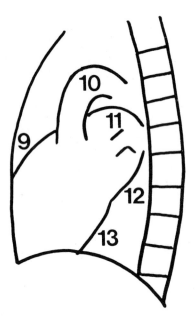

**454  Diagrams of the postero-anterior and lateral views of the cardiac silhouettes.** The position of the cardiac chambers and great vessels comprising the cardiac silhouette on the two standard views are shown. 1, aortic knuckle; 2, main pulmonary artery; 3, position of the left atrial appendage when this is visible; 4, left ventricle; 5, right atrium; 6, position in which a dilated ascending aorta will appear; 7, superior vena cava; 8, left atrium within heart shadow under main carina; 9, right ventricle (meeting sternum) ascending to main pulmonary artery; 10, aortic arch; 11, pulmonary artery bifurcation; 12, left atrium; 13, left ventricle.

**455**

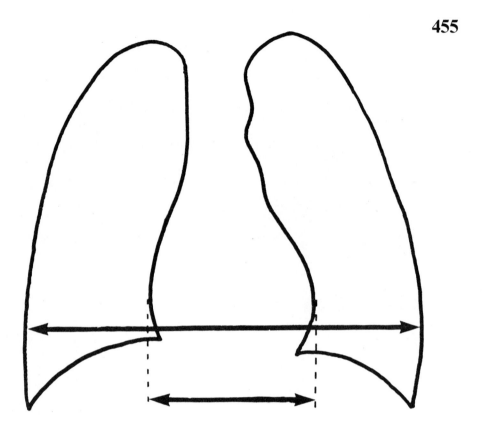

**455  Measurement of cardiothoracic ratio.** The ratio of the transverse diameter of the heart shadow to the widest transverse diameter of the thoracic cage is a crude but simple method of defining abnormal cardiac size; above 50%, cardiac enlargement is present. Since the chest is roughly symmetrical the widest thoracic diameter will be a horizontal line. Note that this diameter may not cross the heart shadow as it does in the diagram—for instance, if the lower ribs splay out. The measurement must be made from the internal or pleural borders of the ribs, *not* the external ones. The heart, of course, is not symmetrical, so an artificial transverse diameter is obtained by measuring a horizontal line joining perpendiculars dropped from the points furthest from the midline on each side, regardless of their relationship to one another—they are most unlikely to be on a level.

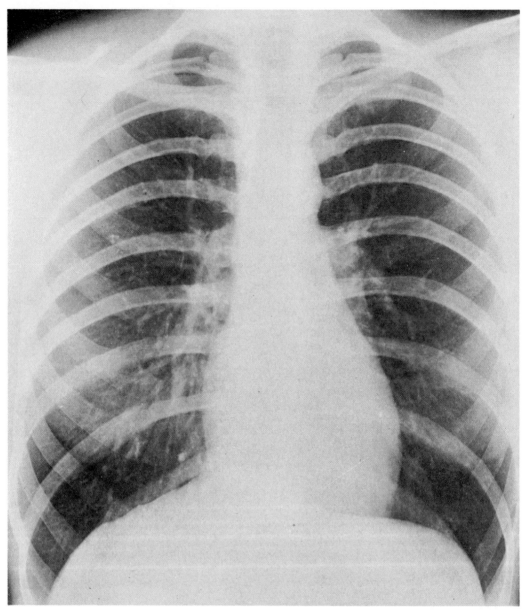

**456–458  Normal cardiac x-ray.** None of the cardiac chambers or great vessels is enlarged (cardio-thoracic ratio less than 50%), and the lung vascularity is normal. There is no intracardiac calcification. To confirm all these points both a lateral and a penetrated postero-anterior view—for carinal angle (see **502**) as well as calcium—are needed.

**457**

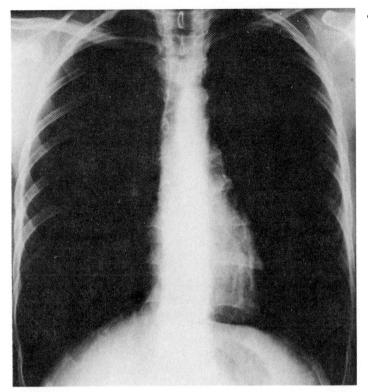

**458**

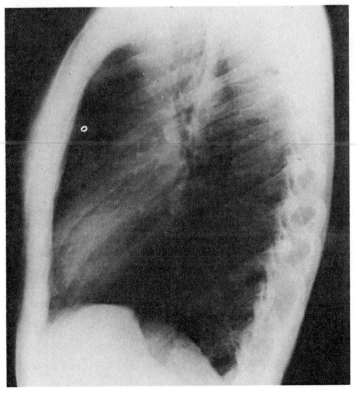

**459**

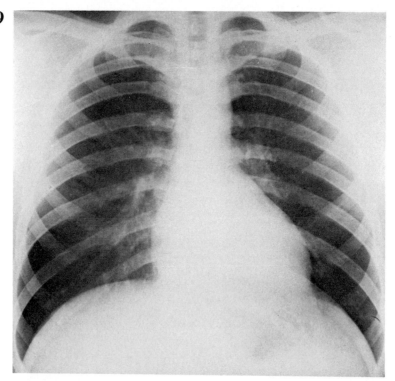

**460**

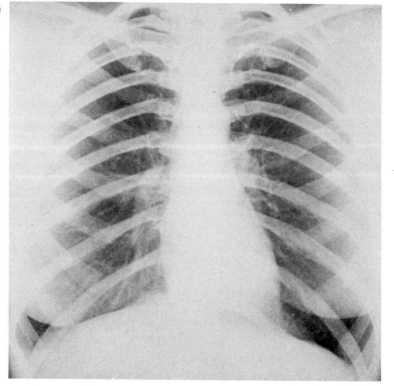

**459–462 Normal cardiac x-ray.** The range of normal appearances is too wide to attempt comprehensive illustration, but four examples are shown. Note the considerable range of shape and size even in this small sample. The slight pro-minence of the main pulmonary conus in one or two of the films is a common normal finding.

**461**

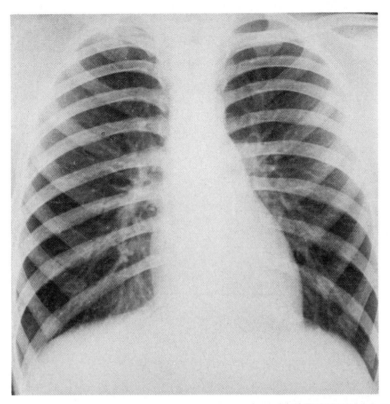

**462**

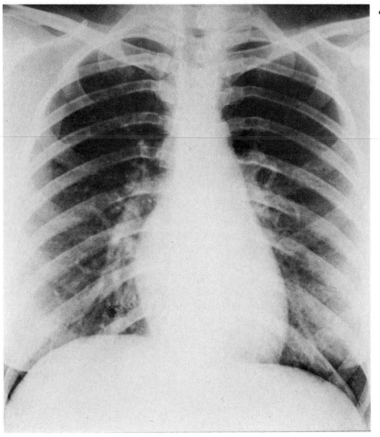

**463**

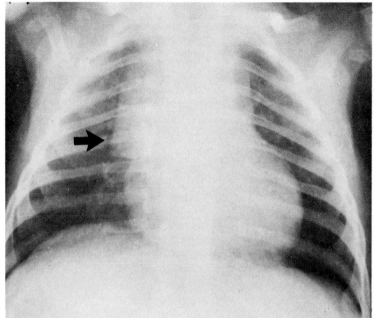

**464**

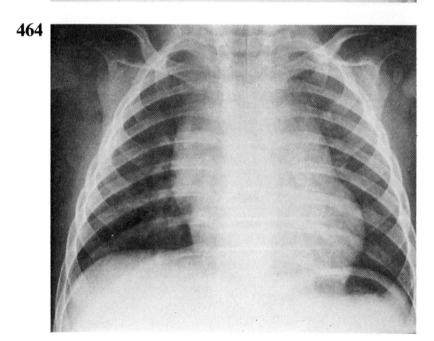

**463–466 Normal cardiac x-ray, children.** As in adults, there is considerable variation in what may safely be placed within the limits of normality. Four representative films are shown. Figure **463** illustrates the neonate. Note that the heart may well appear relatively large and yet be normal at this period, reflecting the supine position, the antero-posterior projection, and the difficulty of obtaining a truly inspiratory film. The so-called 'sail' shadow of the thymus is well seen (arrow). Figure **464** shows the situation towards the end of the first year of life.

Heart shape and size are partly obscured by the prominent thymus, especially on the right. Figure **465** illustrates middle childhood, and by late childhood (**466**), adult appearances are achieved.

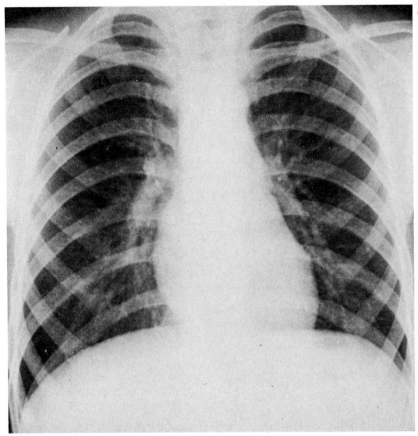

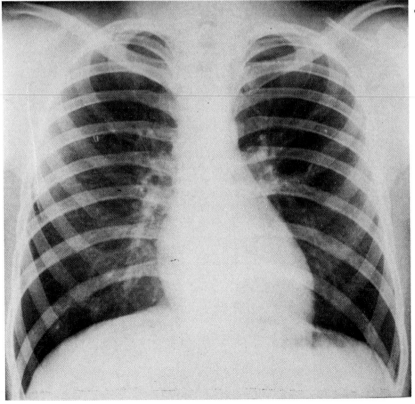

**467**

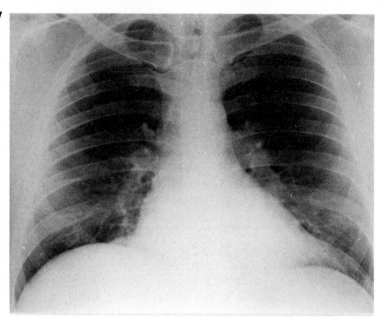

**467    Marked obesity.** Such subjects are often broad and squat with high diaphragms which may exaggerate heart size. The presence of pericardial fat also increases the apparent transverse cardiac diameter. (See **483**.)

**468    Normal cardiac x-ray, the 'suspended' heart.** This term is applied to films showing the apex of the heart well above the diaphragms in inspiration—it appears partly surrounded by lung. Subjects tend to be tall thin adolescents. A characteristic electro-cardiogram is found (see **15**).

**468**

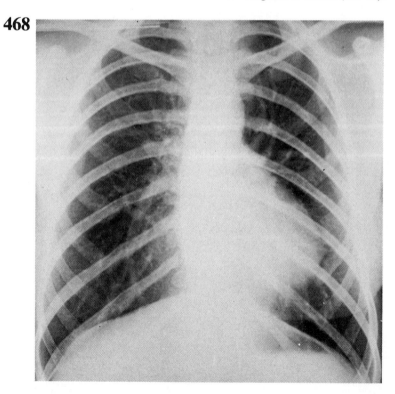

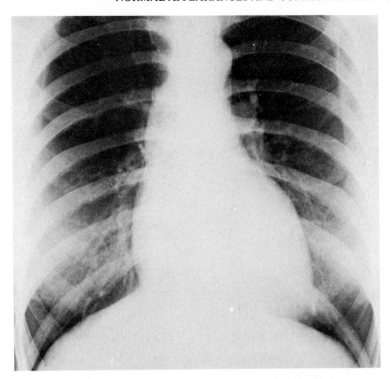

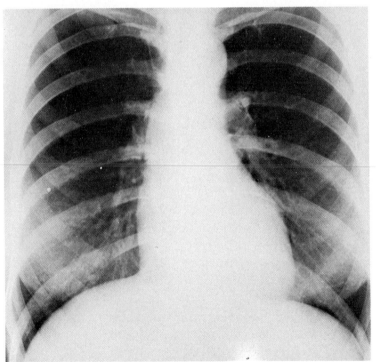

**469, 470  The effect on heart size of the antero-posterior view.** The x-ray in **469** is an antero-posterior film. The heart, being anteriorly situated in the chest, is magnified by the divergent x-ray beam, and appears just above normal in transverse diameter (cardiothoracic ratio, 51 %). The standard postero-anterior film (**470**) gives a much more accurate indication of heart size (cardiothoracic ratio, 44 %).

**471**

**472**

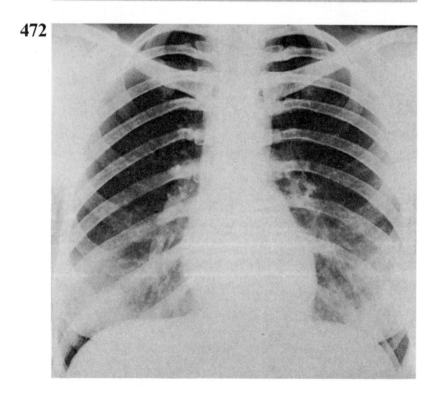

**471, 472 Apparent cardiomegaly produced by inadequate inspiration.** Figure **471** shows a heart at the upper limit of normal in size; the diaphragm is high (at the level of the anterior end of the fifth, instead of the seventh, rib). Figure **472** shows the true state of affairs—a film taken in full inspiration; the heart is small. Films in children are frequently expiratory and falsely exaggerate heart size. (See also **484, 485.**)

**473**

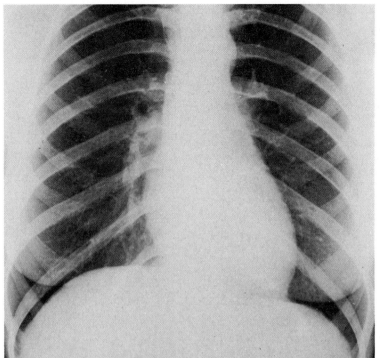

**474**

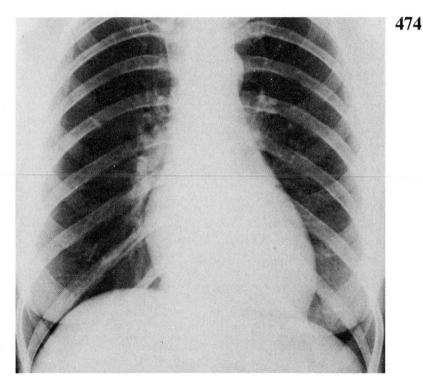

**473, 474   Effect on heart size of systolic-diastolic difference.** An alteration in heart size of 1cm of transverse diameter between two films may be attributable simply to the extremes of cardiac volume during the cardiac cycle. In this instance, the difference is as much as 1.5cm. Figure **473** was taken during systole and **474** in diastole.

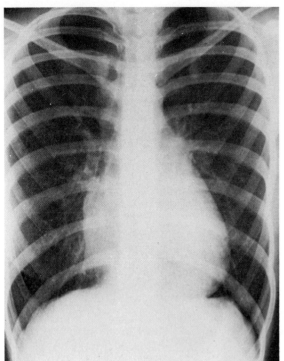 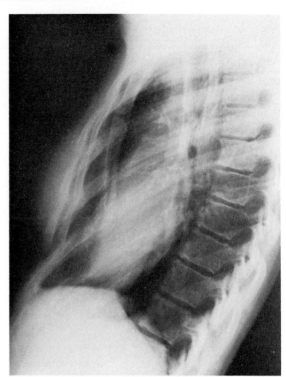

**475, 476 Apparent cardiomegaly produced by sternal depression.** In marked degrees of sternal depression the heart is compressed between the sternum and spine, as can be seen in the lateral view. Apparent cardiomegaly is produced (cardio-thoracic ratio, 57%). In the postero-anterior view the obliquity of the ribs anteriorly provides a clue.

**477, 478 Apparent cardiomegaly due to a flat chest.** The transverse cardiac diameter is increased but the cause is compression of the heart due to a greatly diminished antero-posterior dimension of the thorax as revealed in the lateral view.

**477**

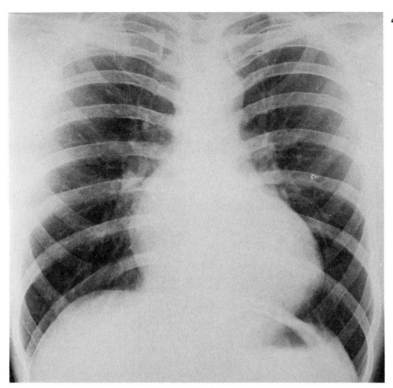

**478**

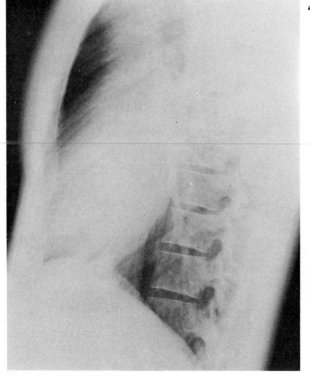

**479**

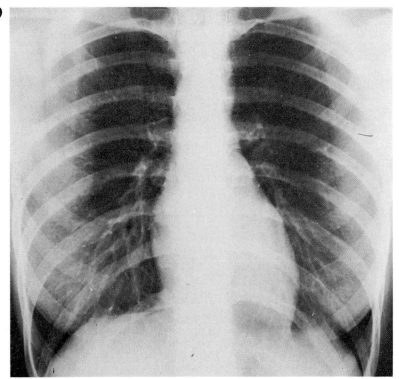

**480**

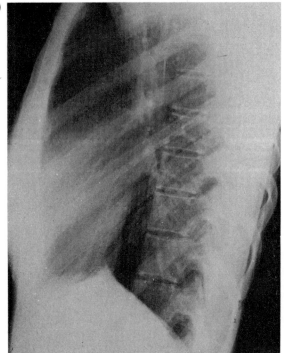

**479, 480 Straight back syndrome.** The normal dorsal curvature of the spine is absent. In some cases this can produce false cardiac enlargement due to antero-posterior compression of the heart.

**481, 482 Atrial fibrillation, effect on heart size.** The development of atrial fibrillation will cause the heart to enlarge, particularly, as in this case, when mitral valve disease is present. Figure **481** shows the appearances in sinus rhythm, and **482**, the increase in size (especially of the left atrium) after the onset of atrial fibrillation. N.B. **482** was taken after an increase in anti-failure therapy, including full digitalisation, and represents the permanent change which resulted.

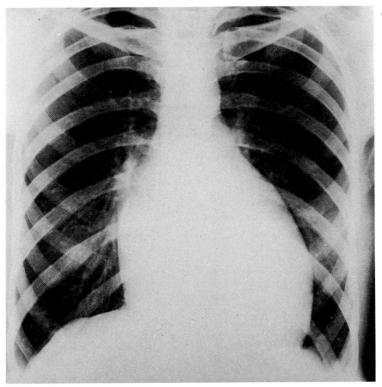

**481**

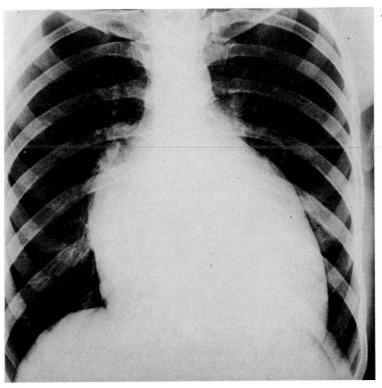

**482**

**483**

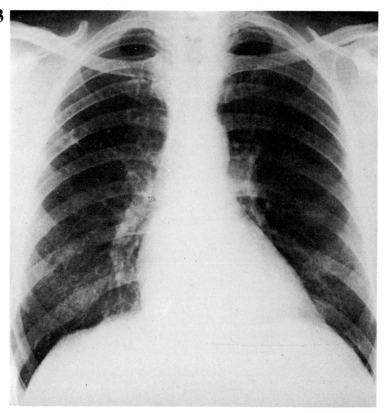

**483   Effect on heart size of apical pericardial fat pad.** The left cardiac border is prolonged in a straight line to meet the diaphragm, thus falsely exaggerating the transverse diameter of the heart. Sometimes (but not here) the actual border of the heart can be seen as a rounded shadow medial to the edge of the pad of fat. (See **467**.)

**484, 485   Effect of crying on the heart size in children.** Figure **484** was taken when the child was crying; note the wide mediastinum, high diaphragms, and apparently grossly enlarged heart. Figure **485** shows the true state of affairs: the heart is only moderately enlarged, the mediastinum is normal. Now the lungs can be seen properly.

**486   Athlete's heart.** Athletes undertaking strenuous training tend to have suspiciously large hearts. This is due mainly to the marked sinus bradycardia they develop, which gives them a large stroke volume. They do have some ventricular hypertrophy too, but this is not seen on chest x-rays unless dilatation is present.

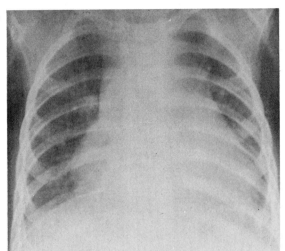

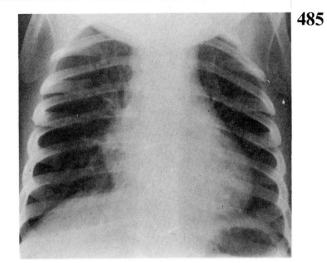

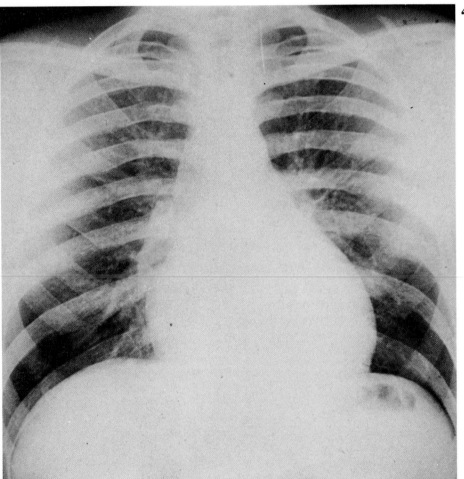

**487**

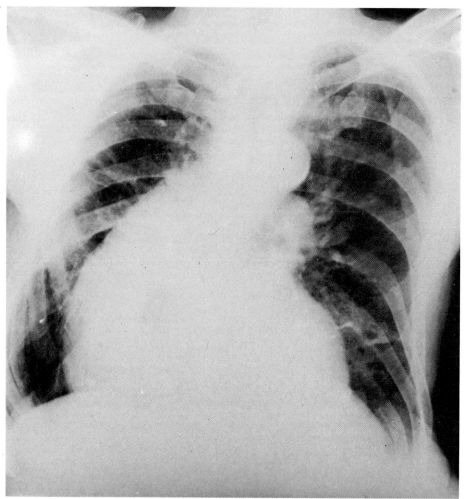

**487–489   Distortion of the cardiac shadow by severe kyphoscoliosis.** Two examples are illustrated: **487** shows an apparent enlargement of the heart to the right of the sternum which is in fact largely the spine; the degree of kyphosis can be appreciated in the lateral view (**488**). The second example (**489**) shows an apparent enlargement of the aortic arch and a curious triangular heart outline. In this film the bulge to the right of the mediastinum is, of course, the spine. Both these patients had normal hearts and great vessels. N.B. in the postero-anterior view the different obliquity of the ribs on the two sides furnishes a clue to the presence of kyphoscoliosis in less obvious cases than these.

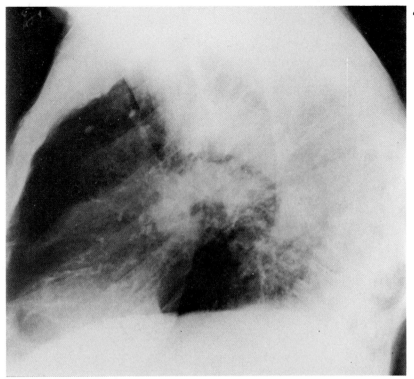

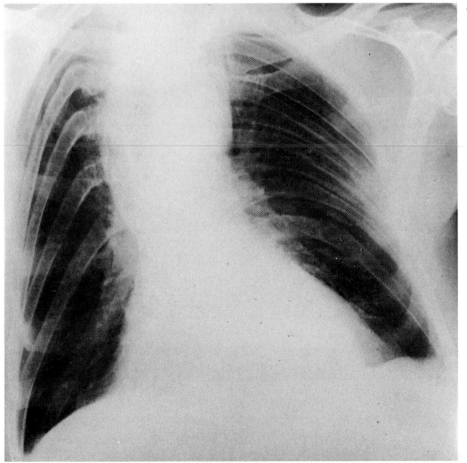

**490–493 Exaggeration of the heart size by mediastinal masses.** Obvious as it may seem, it is important to bear in mind that mediastinal masses may overlie the heart and great vessels and falsely exaggerate their real size or shape. Figure **490** shows a large air-containing structure with a fluid level within it behind the left cardiac border. This was a rolling hiatus hernia; the heart was enlarged due to a cardiomyopathy complicated by heart block. Figure **491** shows a mass protruding from the right cardiac border. It is not the left atrium, for this would tend to project from both sides of the heart when as big as this (**583**) although it is true there is slight prominence of the left atrial appendage. It is too high for the right atrium, and the superior vena is not enlarged as it should be with right atrial enlargement (**497**). A lateral view (not illustrated) showed it to be in the anterior mediastinum, probably a dermoid cyst. Close examination shows linear calcification in the wall of this structure (arrowed). Figure **492** shows apparent dilatation of the main pulmonary artery, and again, closer scrutiny reveals linear calcification in the edge. The lateral view (**493**) confirms the presence of a dermoid cyst in the anterior mediastinum.

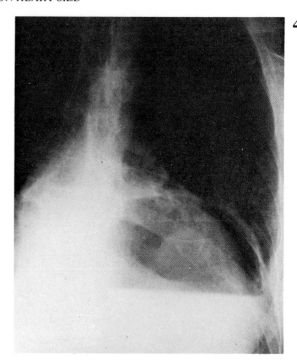

**491**

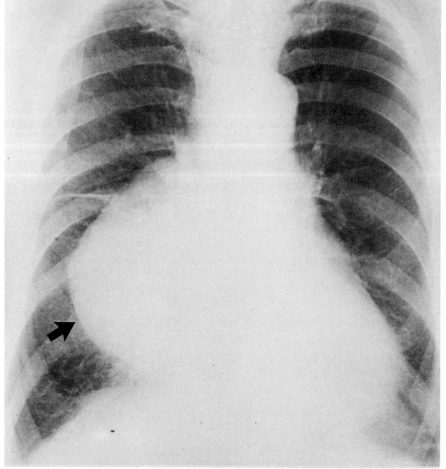

**492**

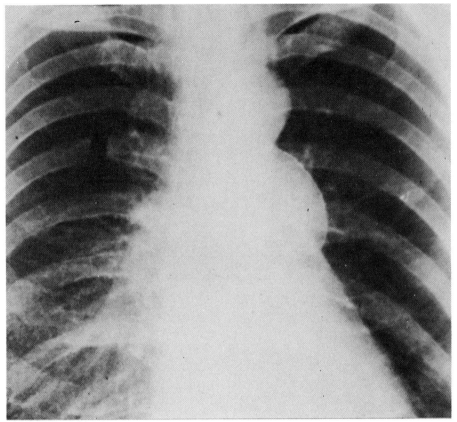

**493**

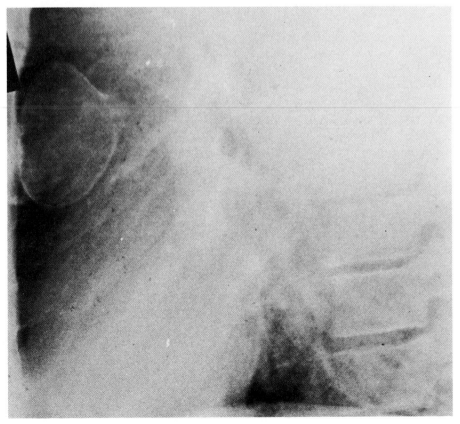

**494**

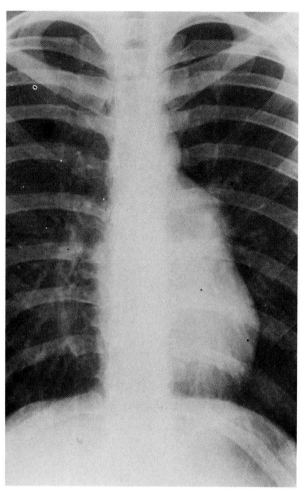

**494, 495  Large left atrial appendage mimicking dilatation of the pulmonary artery.** The true cause of the prominence in the region of the main pulmonary conus is shown in the angiogram (**495**). A catheter has been passed to the pulmonary artery from the right arm and contrast medium injected. The contrast has left the pulmonary artery and has now reached the left heart, outlining the pulmonary veins, the left atrium, the left ventricle (indistinctly), and the aorta. The abnormal shadow is a large left atrial appendage (arrow).

**496  Loss of cardiac silhouette.** The heart is normally visible because of the contrast provided by the air-containing lung around it. This is dramatically illustrated in this x-ray of a patient with a left lung destroyed by tuberculosis (note the calcified lesions on the right side too). The heart has been displaced into the left side of the thorax but cannot be seen, for it is no longer in contact with aerated lung.

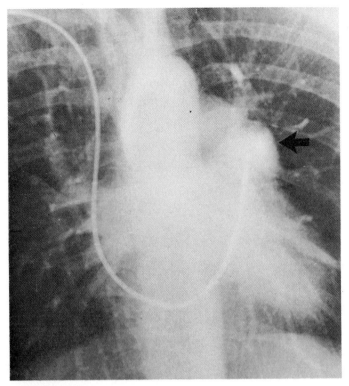

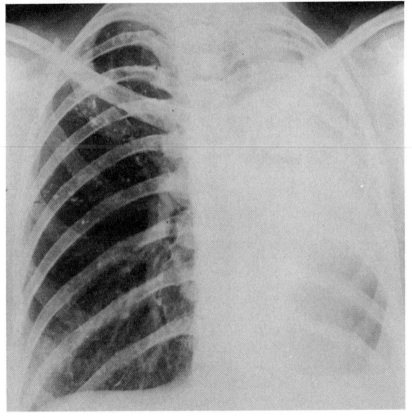

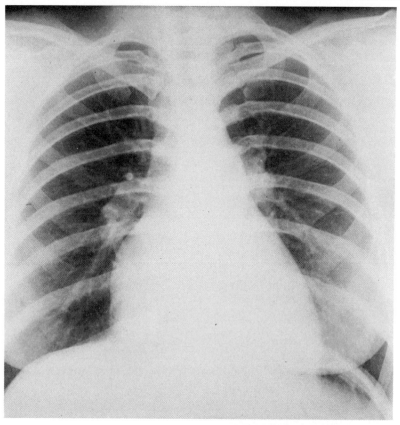

**497, 498   Right ventricular and right atrial enlargement.** Right ventricular enlargement is best recognised on the lateral view, when the upper border of the heart shadow meets the rear of the sternum at a point higher than the junction of the lower one-third with the upper two-thirds (see **454**). On the postero-anterior view, the left cardiac border may be rounded and the apex somewhat tip-tilted. Right atrial enlargement produces a rightwards projection of the right cardiac border and the superior vena caval shadow is also usually prominent (**454**). The example illustrated shows a little rotation to the right which exaggerates the superior vena cava and right atrium, but even so the right border is abnormal. Note the presence of proximal pulmonary artery enlargement due to pulmonary hypertension.

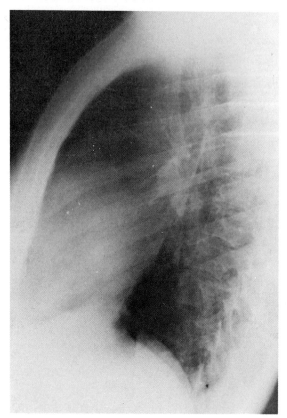

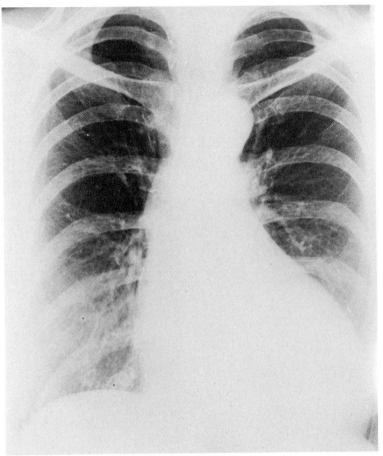

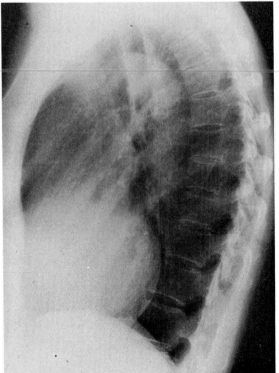

**499, 500 Left ventricular enlargement.** The transverse diameter of the heart is usually enlarged, the left cardiac border showing a gentle convexity descending to the diaphragm in the antero-posterior view, but the lateral provides more reliable information about enlargement of the left ventricle in the backwards projection of the posterior cardiac border (see **454**). Note the prominence of the ascending aorta to the right of the mediastinal shadow in this particular case—a patient with aortic regurgitation.

**500**

**501**

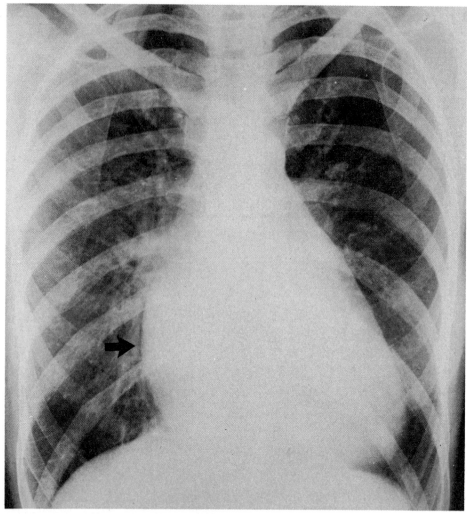

**502**

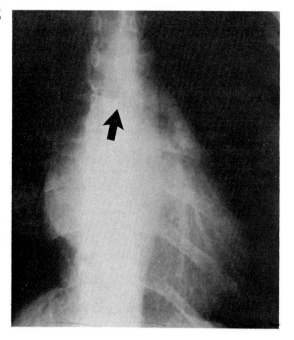

**501–504 Left atrial enlargement.** This is best illustrated by a case of mitral valve disease. On the normally penetrated postero-anterior view (**501**) left atrial enlargement is suspected by a fullness of the left cardiac border (the left atrial appendage may cause a localised bulge—see **577**) and the suspicion of a double contour at the right cardiac border (arrowed). The over-penetrated view (**502**) confirms the double shadow, which is produced by superimposition of the edges of the two atria. It also shows another sign of left atrial enlargement— elevation of the left main bronchus so that the angle formed by the main carina is 90° or more (arrow), see also **454**. On the lateral view (**503**) left atrial enlargement is seen as a backward projection close to the spine (see **454**), and this may be confirmed by barium swallow (**504**), when the oesophagus is seen to be displaced by the enlarged atrium.

**503**

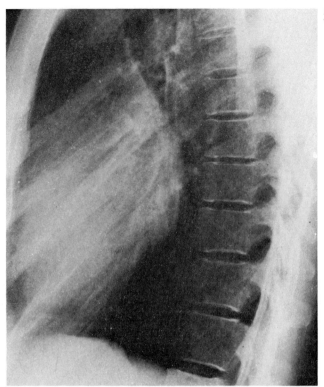

**504**

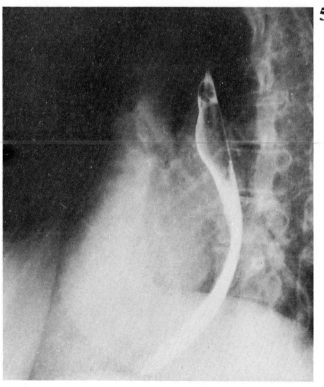

**505**

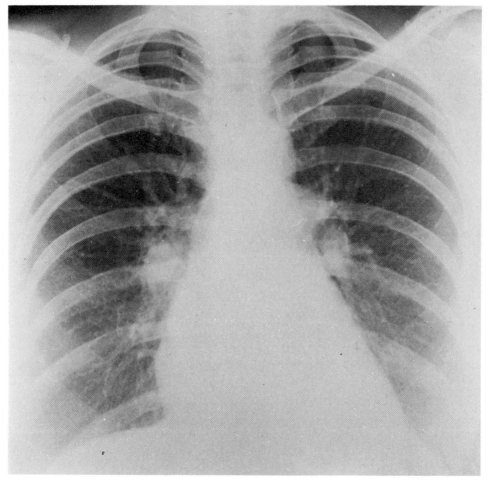

**505  Pulmonary venous congestion, reversal of normal vascular pattern.** Normally, the upper lobes of the lungs are relatively oligaemic compared to the lower lobes. When the left atrial pressure is markedly raised the upper lobe veins distend but the lower lobe veins constrict. This reversal of vascular pattern is accentuated if pulmonary arterial hypertension develops as a consequence for once again, the effect is to constrict the arteries to the lower zones only. These changes are best appreciated in patients with mitral valve disease as in the case illustrated, in whom they are prominent and long-standing.

**506, 507  Pulmonary venous congestion, upper lobe veins.** Figure **506** shows a close-up of distended upper lobe veins, **507** illustrates their reduction in size after diuretic therapy.

**508, 509  Left heart failure, Kerley's lines.** Horizontal lines of interstitial oedema are seen in the lower zones just above the diaphragm in the costo-phrenic angle (**508**). With successful treatment they disappear (**509**).

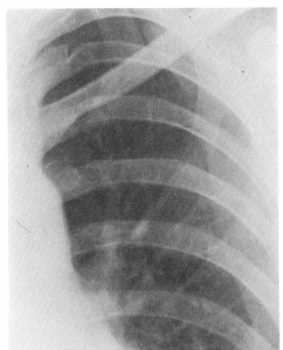

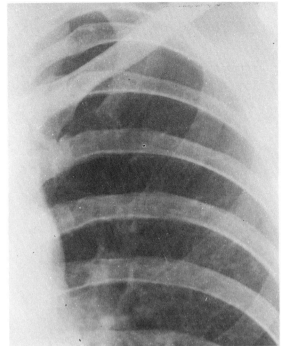

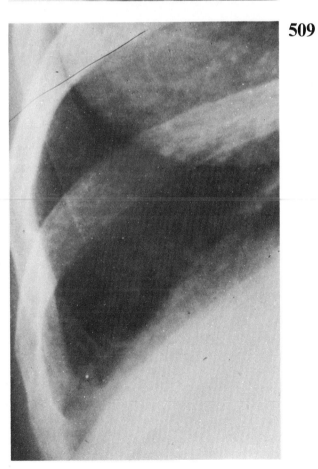

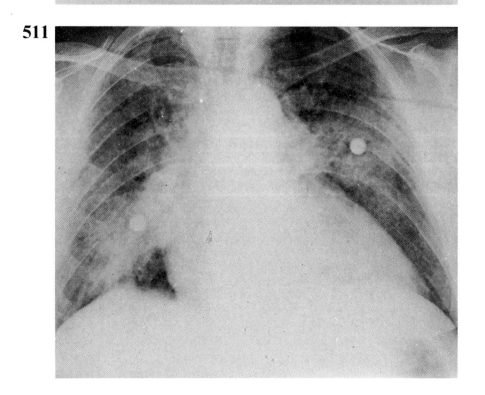

**510–513 Pulmonary oedema.** The lung fields are almost completely obscured by ill-defined fluffy shadows so that the heart silhouette can hardly be seen (**510**). Early oedema appears as a flare extending out from both hila (the so-called 'bat's wing' shadow, **511**) or as a diffuse haziness which, however, tends to be maximal centrally (**512**). Pulmonary oedema may be entirely or predominantly unilateral (**513**).

**512**

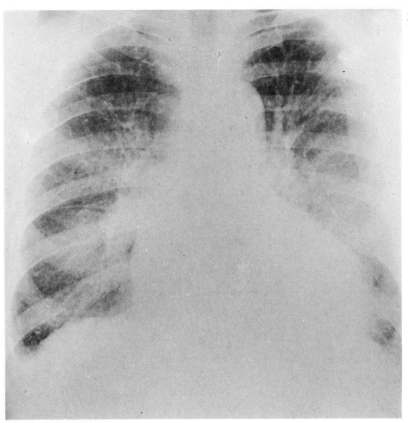

**513**

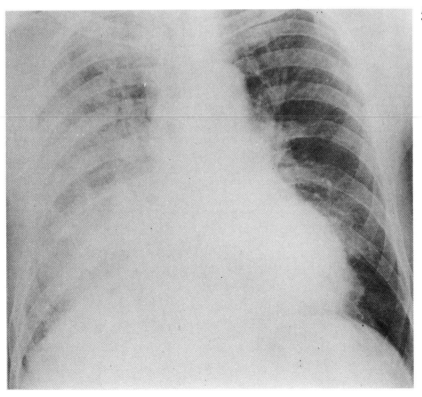

**514**

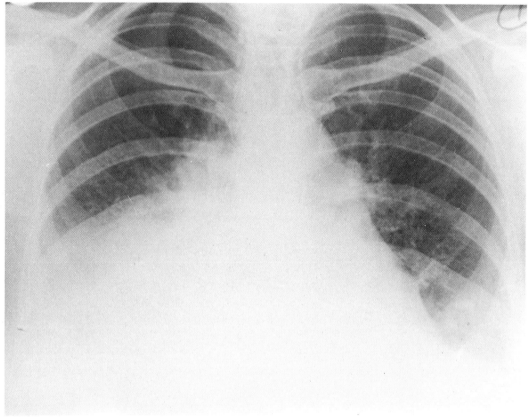

**514 Heart failure, pleural effusions.** Pleural effusions due to heart failure are often largely unilateral, although there is usually evidence of some fluid on the other side (note the blurring of the left costo-phrenic angle. This patient had mitral valve disease. It is difficult to see the pulmonary venous congestion which was present. Note how the large effusion blanking out the right lower zone obscures the right border of the heart. A combination of fluid and underlying collapse has removed any air-containing lung to silhouette the right atrium (see **496**).

**515–517 Heart failure, encysted pleural effusion, the 'vanishing tumour' of lung.** Encysted effusions in one of the pleural fissures often produce rounded shadows in the lung fields (usually on the right side). This is shown in **515**. Note the pulmonary venous congestion (compare **516**) and the haziness in the lower zone due to fluid in the general pleural cavity (which will always be present in some degree with an encysted effusion). The lateral (**517**) shows an elongated shadow (arrowed) in the rather depressed horizontal fissure, which, seen foreshortened in the postero-anterior view, is producing the round shadow. The thickened greater fissure containing fluid can be seen clearly—this is perhaps the commoner place for an encysted effusion. Figure **516** shows the appearance after anti-failure therapy. The fluid has gone.

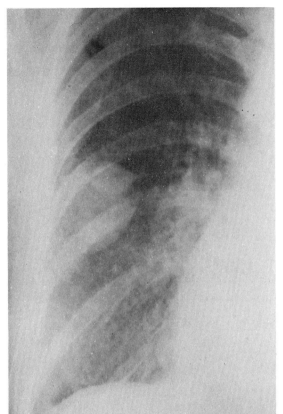

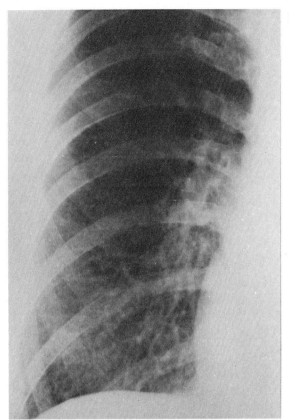

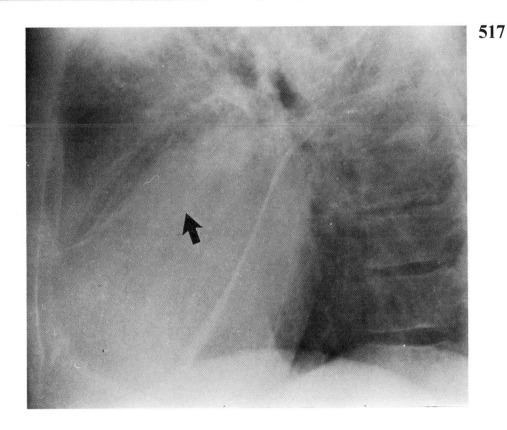

**518**

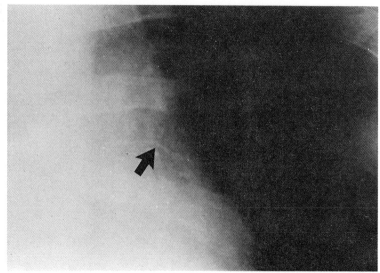

**518 Coronary heart disease, calcification in the left coronary artery.** This may be seen as linear calcification just within the cardiac border a little below the hilum, as shown in this close-up.

**519 Myocardial infarction, 'step shadow'.** An infarction involving the left border may be seen occasionally as an angular distortion—probably a small ventricular aneurysm. The cardiomegaly in this case was due to heart failure.

**519**

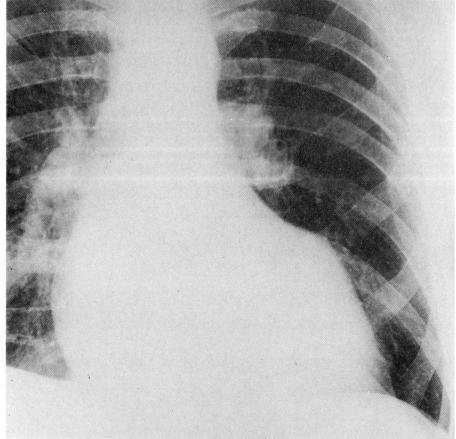

**520**

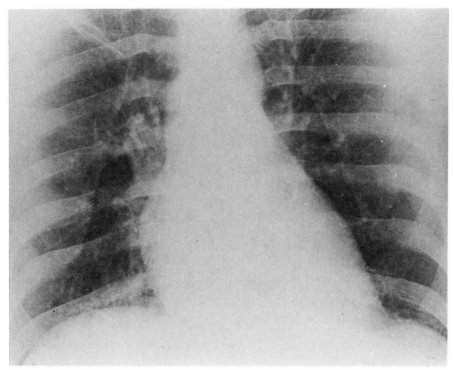

**521**

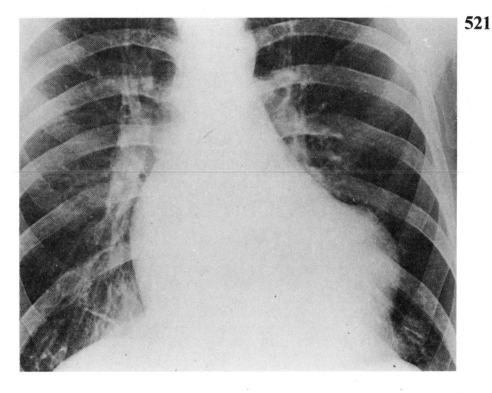

**520, 521  Acute myocardial infarction, appearance of ventricular aneurysm.** Figure **520** shows the heart outline in a patient admitted with an acute antero-lateral myocardial infarction, and **521** the same patient three weeks later. A bulge has appeared on the left cardiac border. On screening, this would be found to move paradoxically (outwards) during systole and is a ventricular aneurysm of moderate size.

**522**

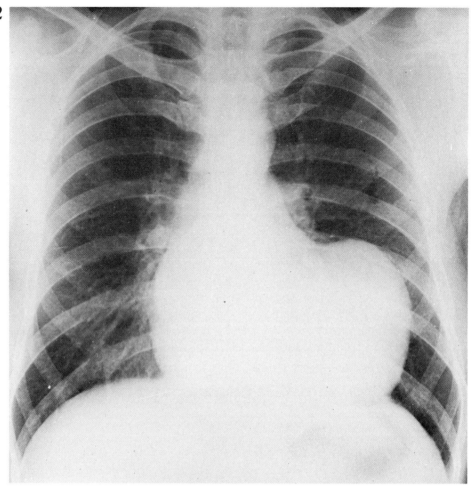

**522–524 Large ventricular aneurysm.** In **522** the
left cardiac border is distorted by a rounded
dilatation of the cardiac shadow with characteristic
tip-tilting. There is mild pulmonary venous
congestion. The lateral view (**523**) shows a curved
shadow overlying the heart (arrowed) that is the
upper margin of the aneurysm. Figure **524** was
taken after resection of the aneurysm.

**523**

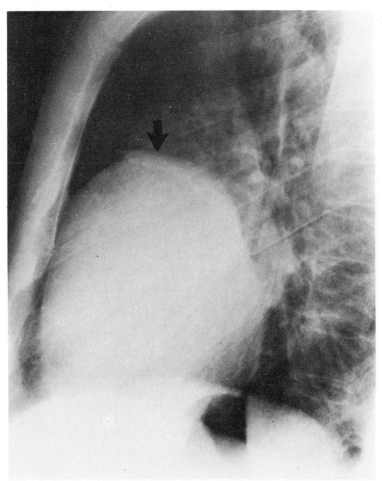

**524**

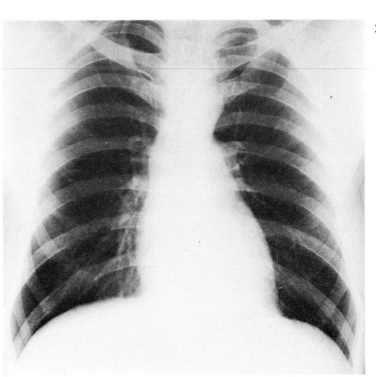

**525**

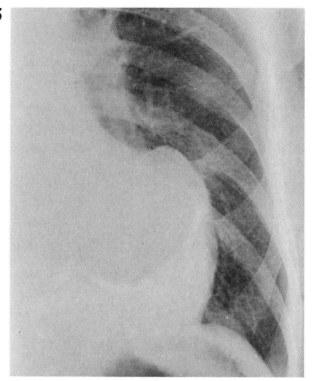

**526**

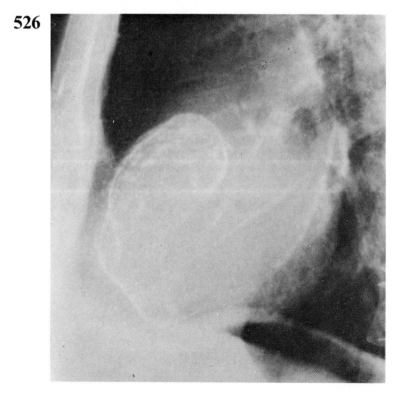

**525, 526 Calcified left ventricular aneurysm.**
Extensive calcification in a ventricular aneurysm of
long standing; some is probably in mural clot.

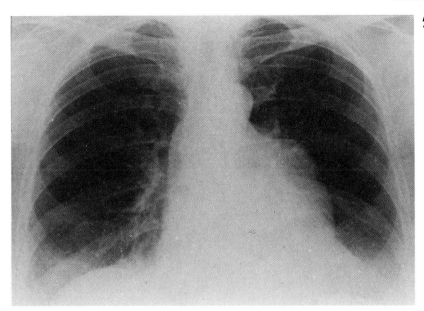

**527 Left ventricular aneurysm in an unusual site.** Most left ventricular aneurysms involve the antero-lateral region of the myocardium but they may occur inferiorly (when they cannot be seen on the plain chest x-ray) or, as in this case, the high lateral area of the myocardium, just under the aortic valve. The abnormal shadow mimics a hilar or mediastinal mass, or dilatation of the pulmonary conus.

**528 Possible left ventricular aneurysm after myocardial infarction.** While the diagnosis of left ventricular aneurysm is easy when it is in the classical site (**522**) aneurysms involving the antero-septal or inferior surface of the heart are commonly overlooked. They should be suspected when the left cardiac border has an unusually rounded, convex shape associated with cardiac enlargement. The lateral view is not helpful as it is with classically sited aneurysms (**523**). The importance of not missing occult left ventricular aneurysms is well demonstrated in **529, 530**.

**528**

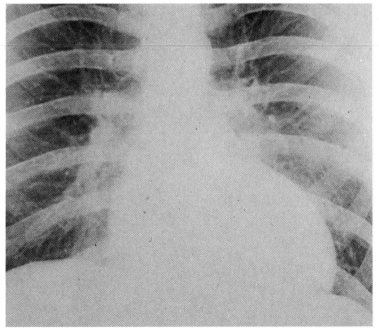

**529**

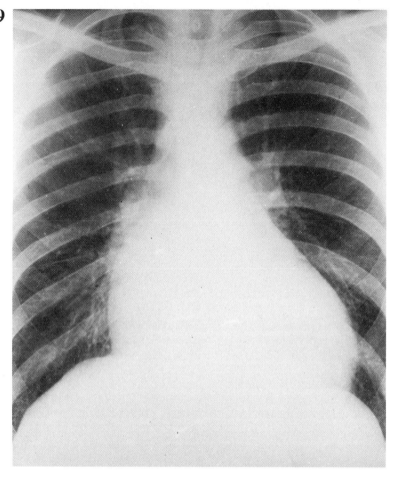

**529, 530 Heart failure after myocardial infarction.**
Figure **529** shows generalised cardiac enlargement
with pulmonary venous congestion and Kerley's
lines following a large myocardial infarction. This is
likely to mean diffuse involvement of the left
ventricle, but, despite the absence of a characteristic
bulge, a localised left ventricular aneurysm is
possible (see **528**), and this was so in this patient.
The appearances eight months after resection of the
aneurysm is seen in **530**. The shadow has returned to
normal; pulmonary venous congestion persists,
however.

**531 Myocardial infarction, acquired ventricular
septal defect.** Rupture of the interventricular
septum is suggested by the development of a loud
pansystolic murmur at the left sternal border. The
chest x-ray shows pulmonary plethora. The large
heart is partly attributable to this being a ward film
(antero-posterior view) but cardiomegaly and
congestive failure are the rule in any sizeable defect.

**530**

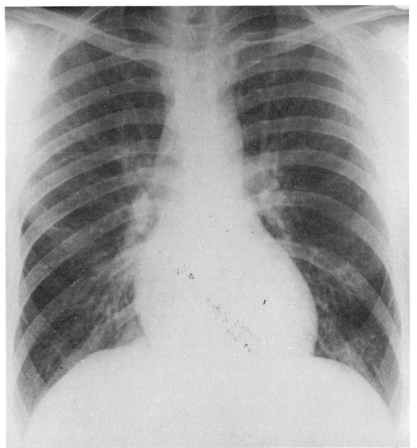

**531**

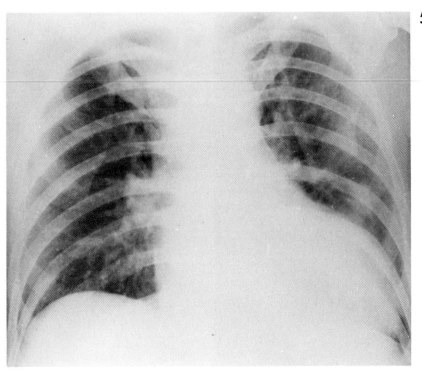

**532**

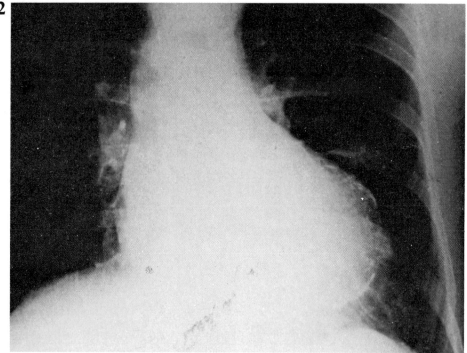

**533**

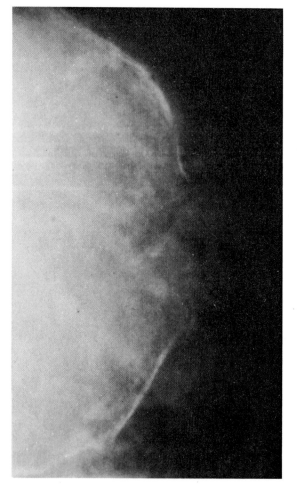

**532–534  Old myocardial infarction, calcification.**
Calcification may occur in the fibrotic wall of the ventricle or in organised mural clot. Figure **532** shows linear calcification (shown in close-up in **533**); a ventricular aneurysm may be present. Figure **534** shows irregular calcification.

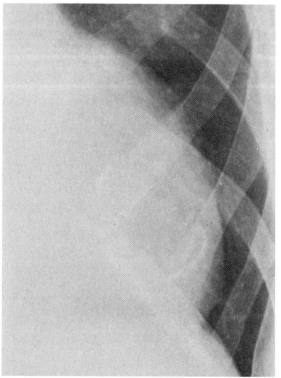

5

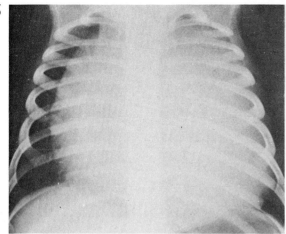 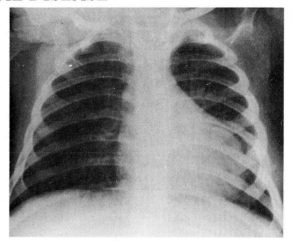

**535, 536  Large pericardial effusion.** The cardiac shadow is grossly enlarged and has a globular shape. All details of the normal cardiac silhouette are smoothed out and characteristically, the right border meets the diaphragm at an acute angle. The shadow is dense, and has a well-defined or 'stencilled' edge. Figure **536** shows the appearances after the effusion had gone. These films were obtained from a child with purulent pericarditis. See **417, 418** for electrocardiographic changes.

**537, 538  Small pericardial effusion.** Small pericardial effusions are difficult to detect radiologically. Figure **537** shows an apparently normal sized heart shadow in a patient with pericarditis. Nevertheless, pericardial fluid was present. The film in **538** shows the true heart size. Even allowing for a deeper inspiration in the latter, the difference in cardiac silhouette is striking.

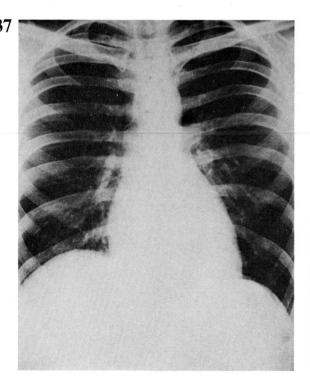 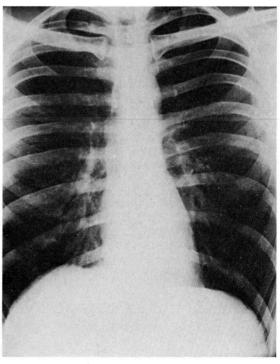

**539**

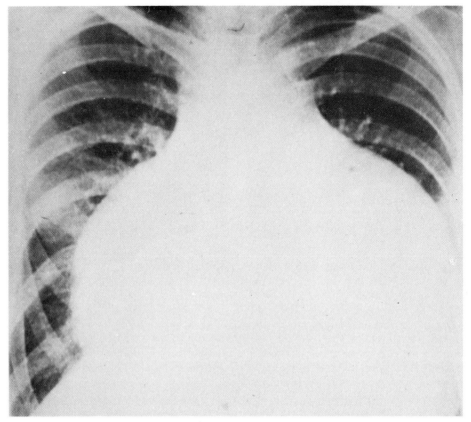

**540**

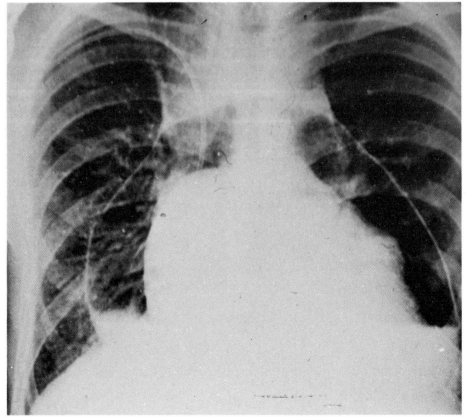

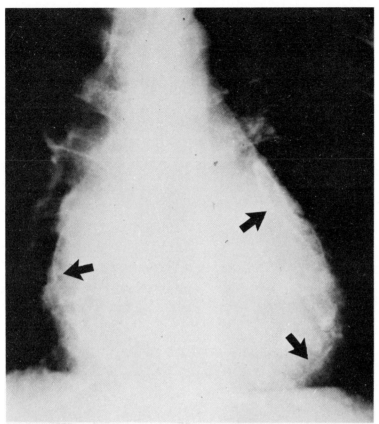

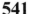

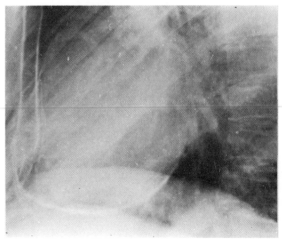

**539, 540 Aspiration of pericardial effusion.** In this patient the large pericardial effusion (**539**) was aspirated and the fluid transiently replaced by carbon dioxide (**540**). The thin pericardium, the small underlying heart, and fluid levels can be seen.

**541, 542 Calcific constrictive pericarditis.** The extensive irregular calcium encasing the heart is best seen on penetrated postero-anterior views and on the lateral. The heart is normal in size; its shape is sometimes rather angular. Calcification in the superficial layers of the myocardium may also occur after an infarction (**532**) or in a ventricular aneurysm (**525**). Fibrous constriction may occur without calcification. See **416** for the characteristic electrocardiogram.

**543**

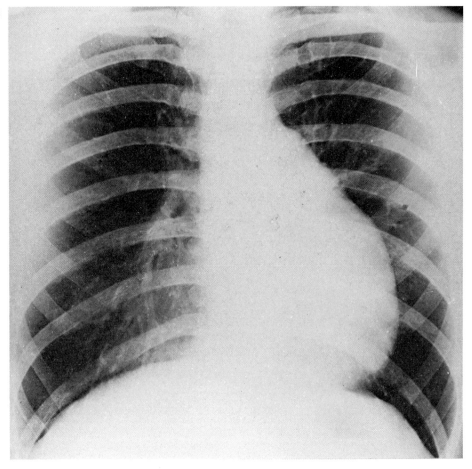

**544**

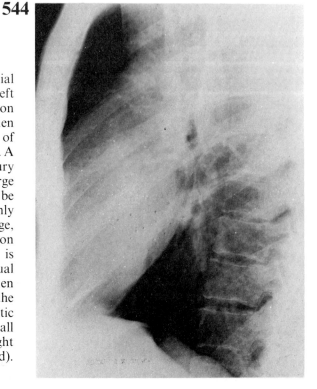

**543–546  Absent pericardium.** Congenital partial absence of the pericardium usually occurs on the left side. Although rare, it may be readily recognised on the plain x-ray, and, because it may lead to sudden death by herniation, torsion and strangulation of the heart, it is an important anomaly to recognise. A similar situation is seen after pericardial injury during pneumonectomy. The defect may be a large one, as in **543**, permitting the entire heart to be displaced into the left chest, or localised, when only a part of the heart, usually the left atrial appendage, forms an unusual bulge. Marked sternal depression or flat chest as the cause of this displacement is excluded by the lateral (**544**), while the unusual mobility of the heart is confirmed by films taken lying on one side (**545** was taken left side up, yet the heart remains within the left chest). Diagnostic proof is afforded by the induction of a small pneumothorax (**546**) when air appears in the right (but of course, not the left) pericardium (arrowed). N.B. the lung edge cannot be seen in this film.

**545**

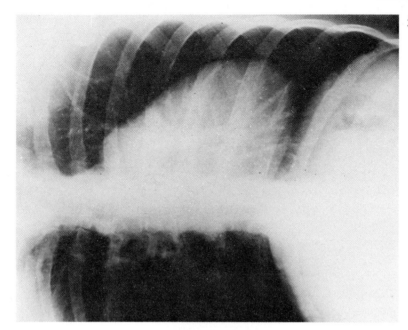

**546**

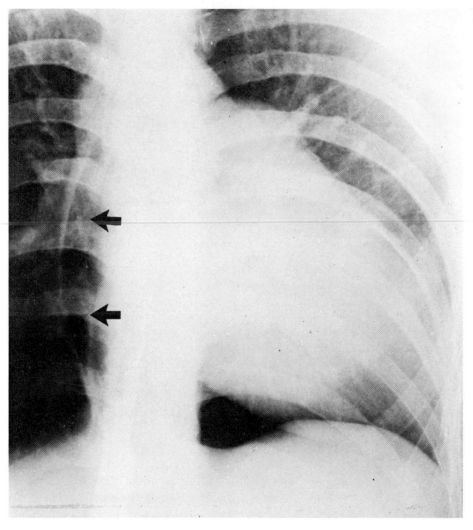

**547**

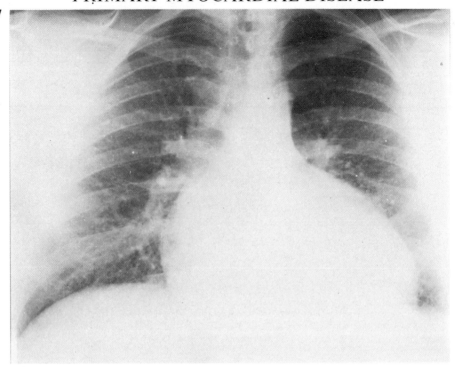

**548**

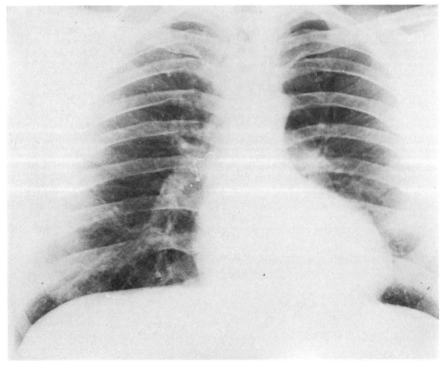

**547, 548 Acute myocarditis.** Marked cardiac enlargement affecting all chambers is seen in **547**; there is pulmonary venous congestion. This film was taken in a young man with acute viral myopericarditis and congestive cardiac failure (there was no evidence of pericardial effusion). Full recovery occurred and the film four months later (**548**) shows a normal heart size. The slight irregularity of the left cardiac border may be due to pericardial-pleural adhesions.

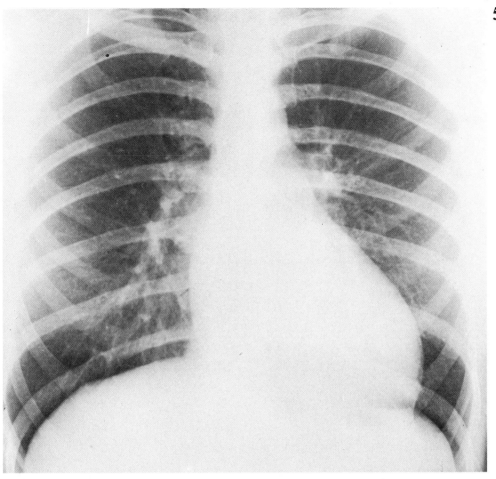

**549, 550   Hypertrophic cardiomyopathy.** The heart size and shape in this disease are very variable and may be virtually normal. Typically, as in this example, left ventricular enlargement is suggested by the left cardiac border in the postero-anterior view and by slight backward projection of the posterior cardiac border in the lateral (**454**).

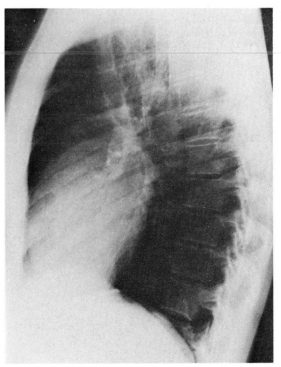

**551**

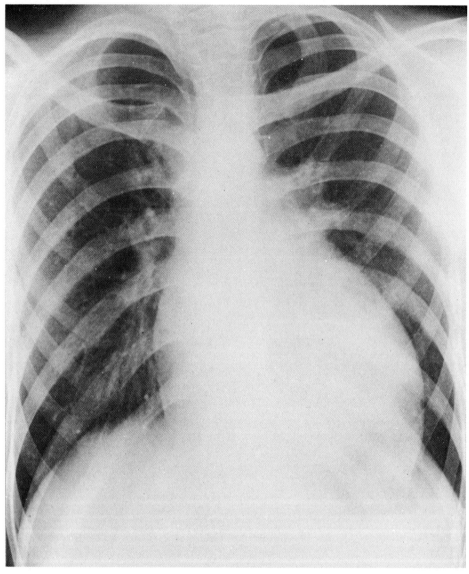

**551  Cardiac involvement in muscular dystrophy.**
This boy with a known muscular dystrophy
presented in congestive cardiac failure. The left
ventricle was huge and poorly contractile.

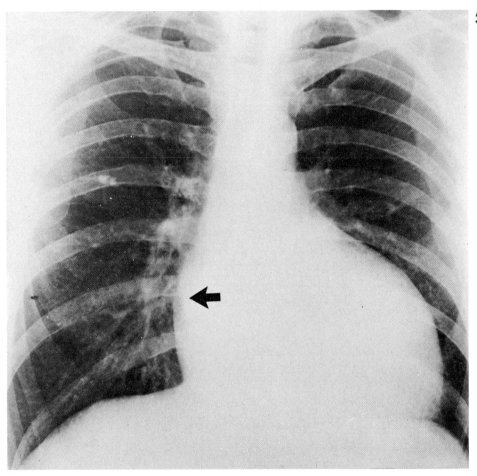

**552, 553  Congestive cardiomyopathy.** The heart is generally enlarged but the chamber principally affected is the left ventricle. Despite the frequent presence of mitral regurgitation and pulmonary hypertension the left atrium is only modestly enlarged (note the double shadow at the right cardiac border) and the main pulmonary arteries are normal. No valvar calcium can be seen; the ascending aorta is normal. These appearances are not by themselves diagnostic but taken with the physical signs and electrocardiogram provide a very good lead to the correct aetiology. Similar appearances are seen in acute myocarditis (**547**) but the main problem in differential diagnosis is how to exclude one of the mechanical complications of myocardial infarction— a ventricular aneurysm or inert segment (see **529**). N.B. this example shows no evidence of pulmonary venous congestion which, of course, is usually to be seen. The films were taken after intensive antifailure treatment prior to catheterisation.

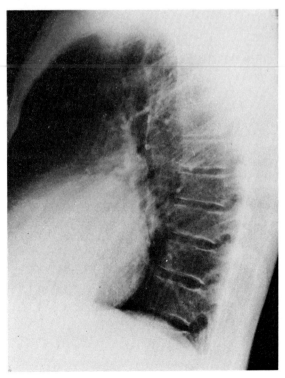

**554**

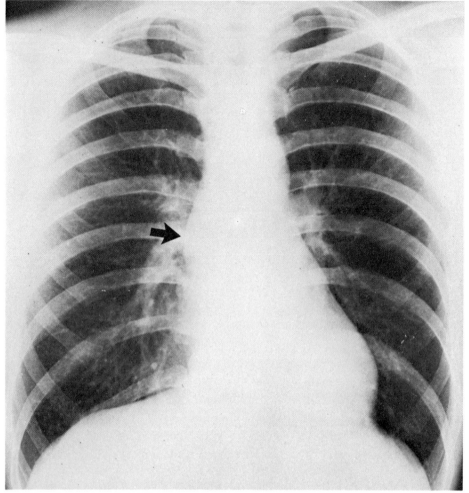

**554–556 Aortic stenosis.** In uncomplicated cases of aortic stenosis the heart shadow is not enlarged (**554**). In many instances post-stenotic dilatation of the ascending aorta (arrowed) is the only clue in the postero-anterior view although the lateral may show aortic valve calcification and left ventricular enlargement as illustrated in **569**. In other patients with severe aortic stenosis, and in cases of fixed sub-aortic stenosis, even this sign may be absent or inconspicuous and the chest x-ray passes for normal (**555**). When left ventricular failure occurs the heart will enlarge (**556**)—note the Kerley's lines.

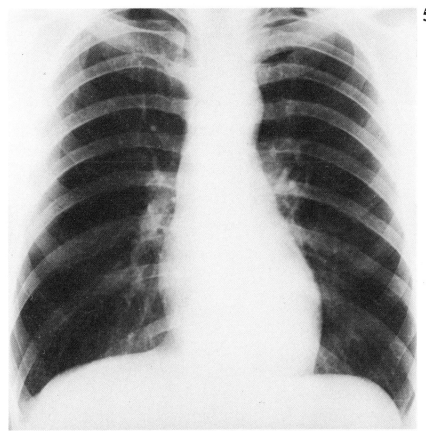

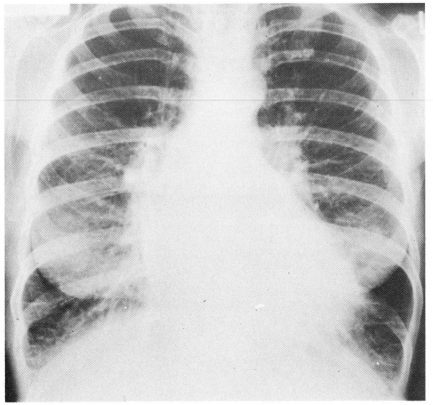

**557**

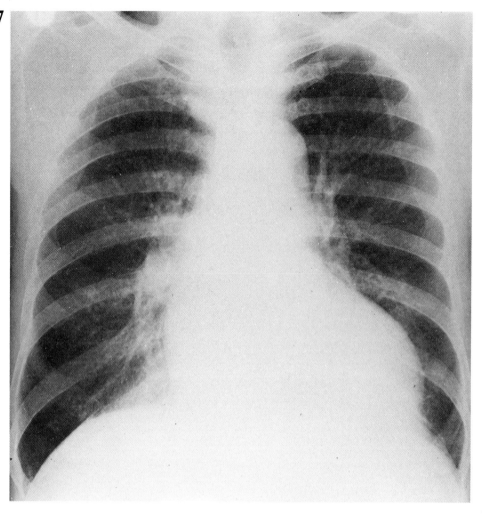

**557 Aortic regurgitation.** Although with mild aortic regurgitation the heart may not be enlarged, moderate, and certainly severe, regurgitation produces cardiomegaly due to left ventricular dilatation in addition to hypertrophy (but see **558**). Figure **557** shows a typical silhouette of such a case. Note the slight prominence of the ascending aorta. This may be marked, depending on the cause of the lesion (**559, 709, 711**). Pulmonary venous congestion is prominent. This patient later developed left ventricular failure (**512**). See also **559**.

**558 Aortic regurgitation.** Although most patients with aortic regurgitation of significance will show cardiomegaly it is important to be aware that this is not always the case, as in the example illustrated. This man had very severe aortic regurgitation of long standing and required aortic valve replacement because of left ventricular failure.

**558**

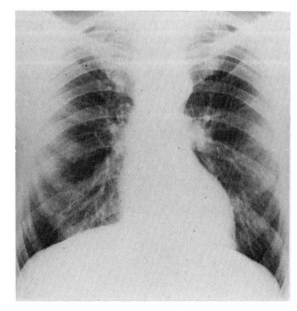

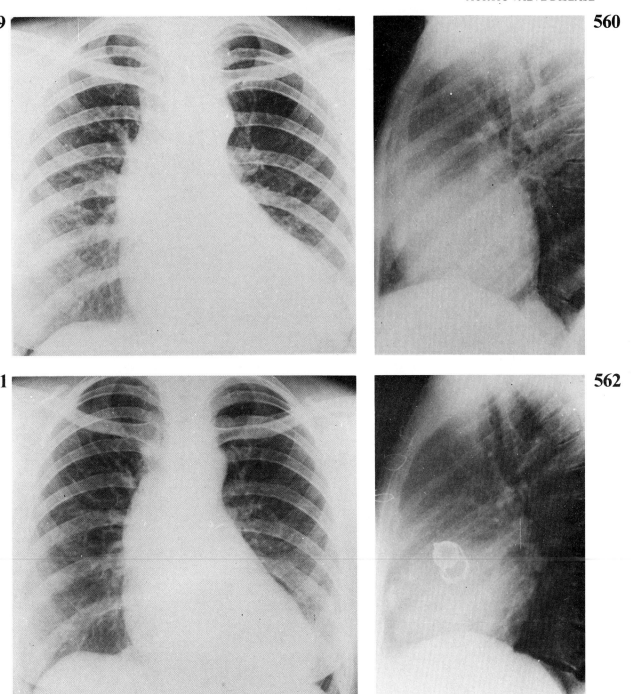

**559–562 Severe aortic regurgitation, results of surgery.** Figures **559**, **560** show the pre-operative appearances in a young woman with severe aortic regurgitation. There is considerable prominence of the ascending aorta to the right of the mediastinum, and massive left ventricular enlargement (the lateral is particularly impressive). Figures **561**, **562** were taken after successful aortic valve replacement. The reduction in left ventricular size is noteworthy (especially in the lateral view) reflecting principally the diminution in stroke volume.

**563**

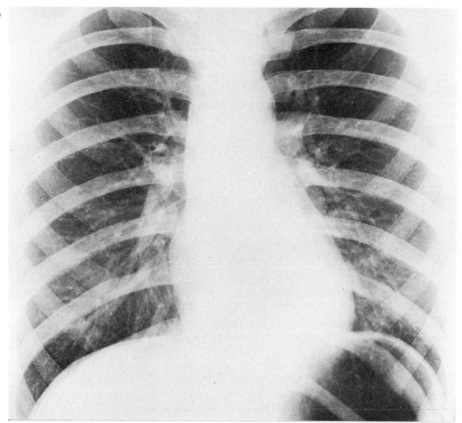

**564**

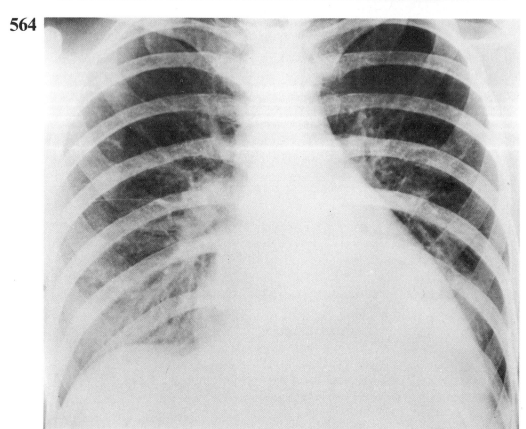

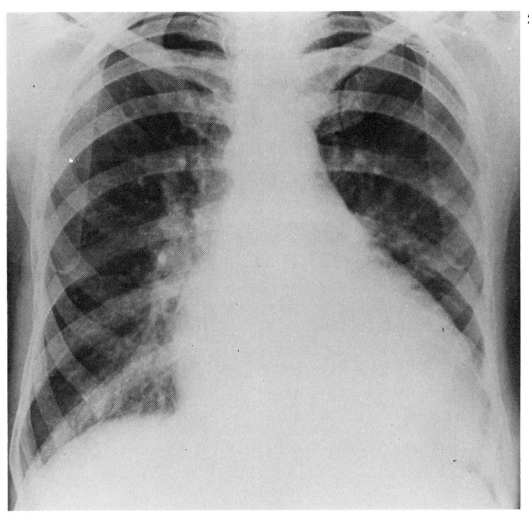

**563, 564 Acute aortic regurgitation following bacterial endocarditis.** Figure **563** was taken when a trivial congenital aortic valve lesion was diagnosed. A year or so later bacterial endocarditis followed dental fillings undertaken without antibiotic cover and severe aortic regurgitation was produced. The dramatic increase in heart size which resulted is seen in **564**. There is pulmonary venous congestion. Aortic valve replacement was necessary to control heart failure before endocarditis could be cured; afterwards, the heart size returned to normal.

**565 Sinus of Valsalva aneurysm, rupture into the right heart.** Aneurysms may develop in any of the three sinuses of Valsalva but are commonest in the right. Rupture into the right heart (usually the ventricle) is the classical termination. The result is the combination of sudden aortic regurgitation (with a continuous murmur) and acute pulmonary plethora. The heart is enlarged. Congestive failure is inevitable if the communication is of any size.

**566**

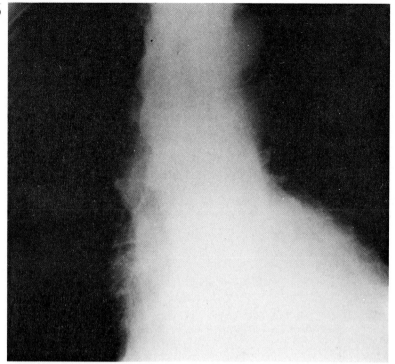

**567**

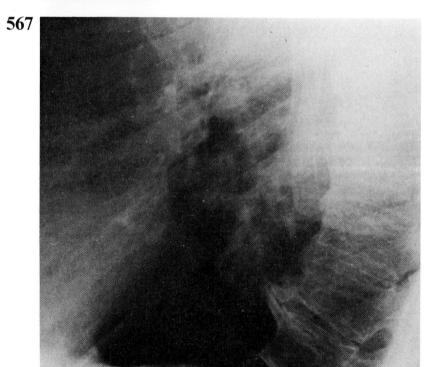

**566, 567 Aortic regurgitation in ankylosing spondylitis.** Sometimes the chest x-ray furnishes clues to the aetiology of aortic regurgitation—in syphilis, Marfan's syndrome, or dissecting aneurysm for instance (see **691–712** for examples), and ankylosing spondylitis is another cause which may be obvious. These films show the abnormal spine clearly. There is also some osteoarthritic lipping.

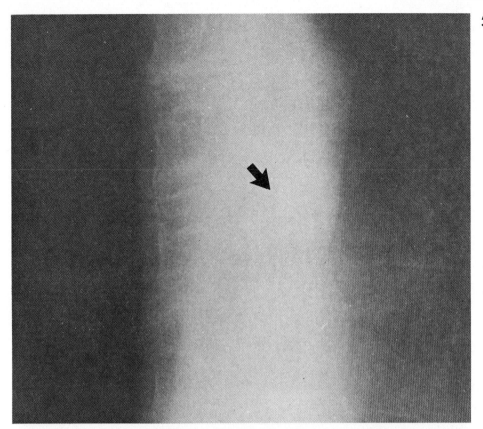

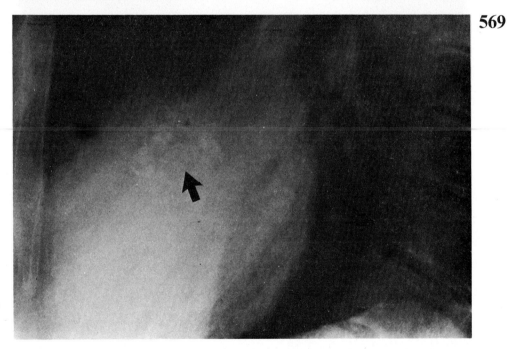

**568, 569   Aortic valve calcification.** Even in the penetrated antero-posterior view (**568**) aortic valve calcification is difficult to see for it overlaps the spine. It is arrowed in the illustration. The lateral view (**569**) however shows it clearly. Note the backward projection of the posterior surface of the heart shadow indicating left ventricular enlargement. (See also **570, 571, 609**.)

**570**

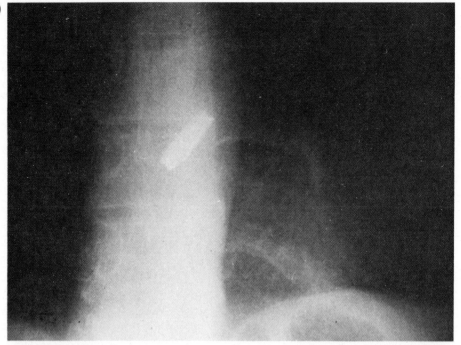

**571**

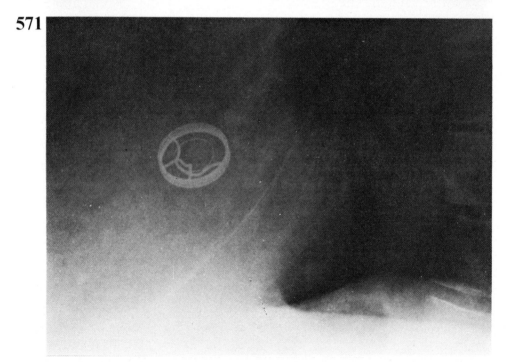

**570, 571 Aortic valve replacement.** The aortic valve has been replaced by a tilting disc prosthesis. The position of the aortic valve within the heart is thus well demonstrated (see also **613–617**). The attitude of the prosthesis remains reasonably constant from film to film, allowing for slight discrepancies of posture and x-ray technique, and this point can be of diagnostic importance (see **572, 573**). Note the very fine ring crossing the valve struts in the lateral view—this is a radio-opaque ring within the disc of this particular model of prosthesis which is helpful in demonstrating the range of movement of the disc if this is in doubt.

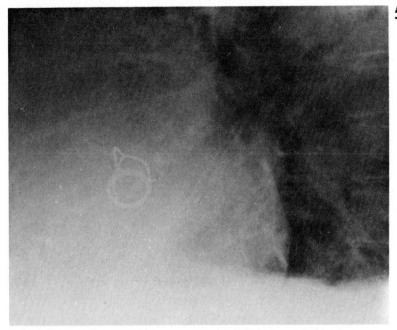

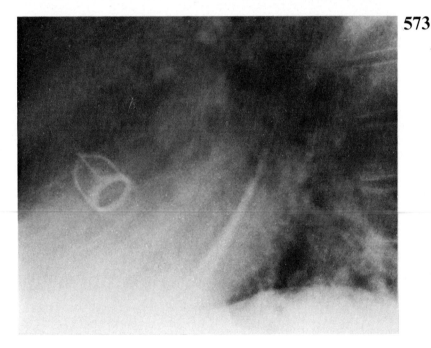

**572, 573 Dehiscence of aortic valve prosthesis.**
Figure **572** shows a close-up lateral view of a ball-in-cage aortic valve prosthesis shortly after insertion. Owing to the development of bacterial endocarditis, separation of the sewing ring of the prosthesis occurred later producing severe para-valve aortic regurgitation. Figure **573** shows that the valve has altered its attitude within the heart—it has tilted forwards and somewhat vertically. Such a con- siderable change in position of a prosthesis means detachment of the sewing ring over about two-thirds of its circumference; lesser degrees of dehiscence are not so easily detected. Screening reveals an abrupt rocking of the prosthesis. N.B. the consequences of this and any other acutely developing severe valvar regurgitation is an abrupt descent into heart failure (see **593, 605**)—note the fluid in the greater fissure in **573**.

**574**

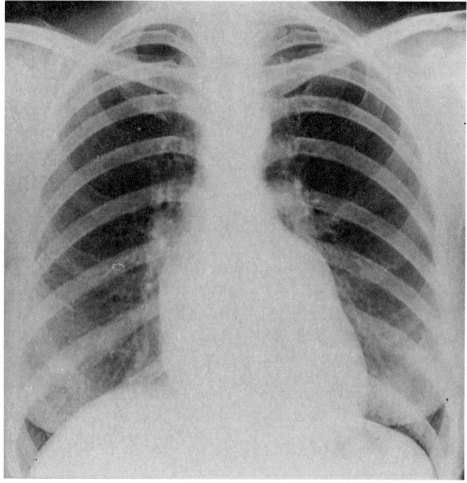

**574  Mitral stenosis.** The characteristic change in the cardiac silhouette in dominantly stenotic or purely stenotic mitral valve disease is enlargement of the left atrium and left atrial appendage. In the absence of pulmonary hypertension or any other valve lesion the heart is not enlarged. Although pulmonary venous congestion is typical, it is not uncommon to see little evidence of it when diuretics have been given, as in the case illustrated. Mitral valve calcification may be present. (See **586–589**.)

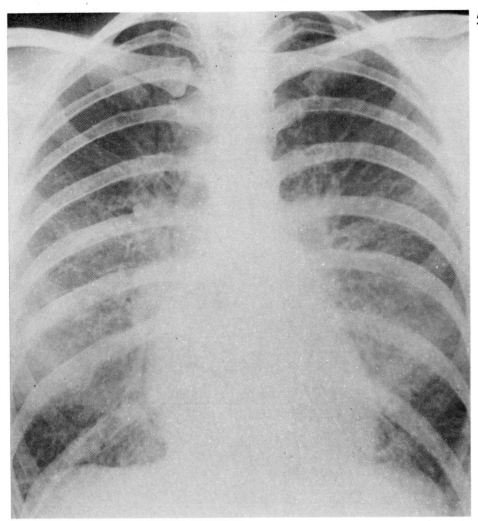

**575 Mitral stenosis without left atrial enlargement.**
Although left atrial enlargement is usual in mitral
stenosis, its degree is not always well correlated with
the severity of the stenosis. In some instances tight
stenosis is unaccompanied by detectable left atrial
enlargement, particularly in patients presenting
acutely with incipient or actual pulmonary oedema.
The illustration shows just such a case. The heart
silhouette is normal but there is marked pulmonary
venous congestion, Kerley's lines, and soft
shadowing around both hila indicating early
pulmonary oedema.

**576**

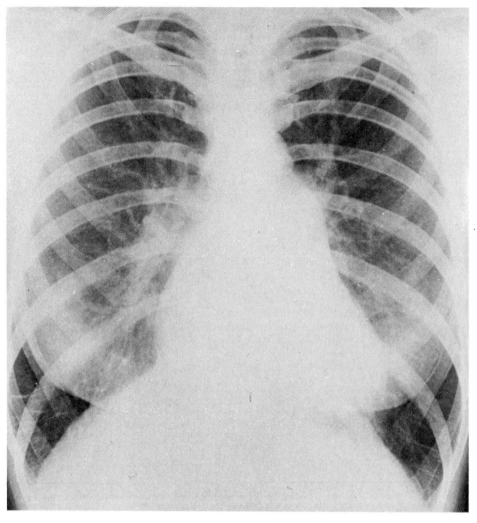

**576 Mitral stenosis, pulmonary hypertension.** In this film the left atrium is not prominent as is sometimes the case in severe mitral stenosis but the severity of left atrial hypertension is shown by the presence of pulmonary venous congestion, and Kerley's lines at the bases. Pulmonary arterial hypertension is suggested by the enlargement of the main pulmonary conus but the absence of marked constriction of the more peripheral pulmonary arteries suggests that the pulmonary vascular resistance has not risen to extreme levels. In such a case, it is likely that pulmonary hypertension will be at least part passive. The right atrial shadow is prominent due to functional tricuspid regurgitation.

**577, 578 Mitral stenosis, successful mitral valvotomy.** Figure **577** shows the pre-operative state. The heart is not enlarged but the left atrium is just above normal in size and has a prominent appendage (arrowed). The lungs do not show pulmonary venous congestion because of intensive diuretic therapy. After valvotomy (**578**) the reduction in left atrial size is evident, mainly due to amputation of the appendage. The heart has not increased in size overall, indicating that significant mitral regurgitation has not been induced (see **595–600**). Note the re-uniting rib at the site of the left thoracotomy.

**577**

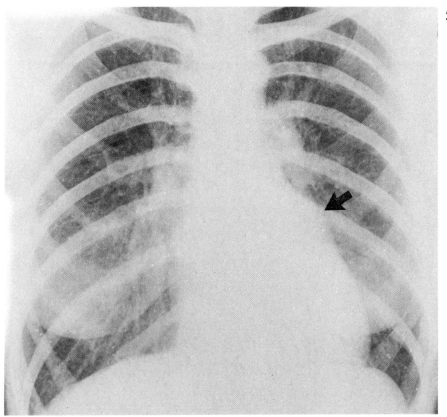

**578**

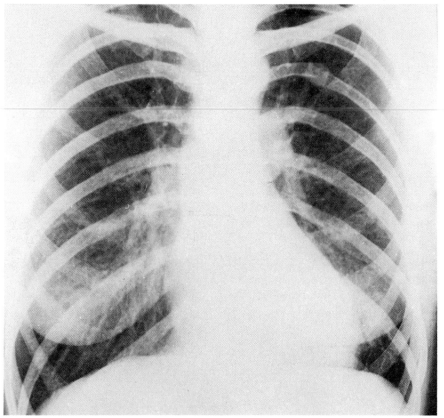

**579**

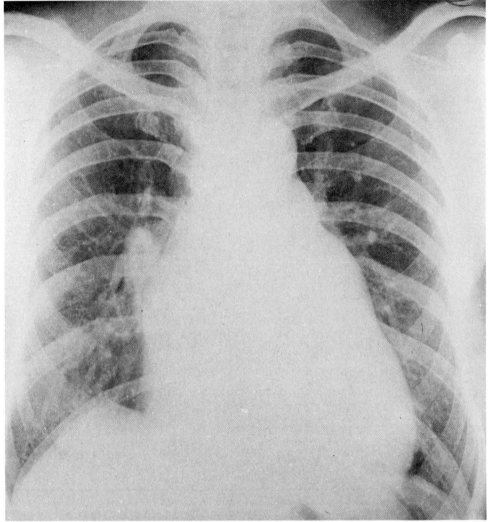

**579, 580   Mitral regurgitation.** In mitral regurgitation, or in cases of mixed mitral valve disease in which regurgitation is significant, left ventricular enlargement is present as well as left atrial enlargement, pulmonary venous congestion and all the other features of mitral valve disease. Figure **579** is an example. Note the long projection of the left ventricle, confirmed on the lateral view (**580**). There is some right ventricular enlargement too, judging by the high take-off of the cardiac shadow behind the sternum (**498, 499**), but the pulmonary hypertension which caused it is not reflected in florid radiological changes (see **576, 620**).

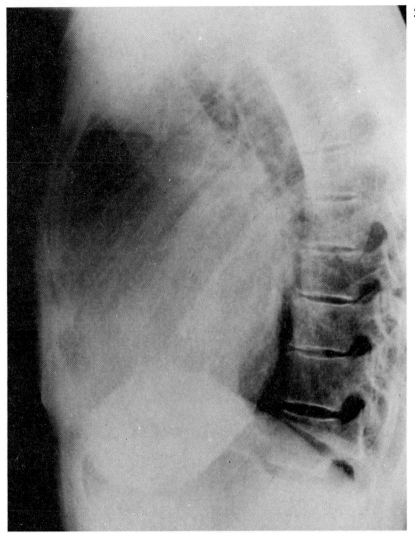

**581**

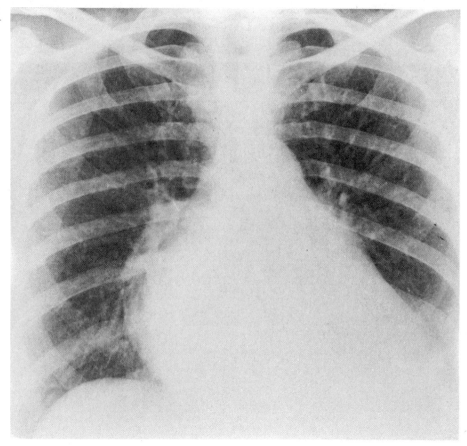

**581, 582 Disproportionate cardiac enlargement in mitral valve disease, cardiomyopathic disease.** If a mitral lesion appears to be modest (whether stenotic, regurgitant, or both) disproportionate cardiomegaly suggests myocardial disease, in the absence of severe pulmonary hypertension or other valve lesions. In a rheumatic case this implies extensive myopathic involvement in the rheumatic carditis (and patients with giant left atria are examples—see **583**), but in others it is likely that the mitral lesion (always then regurgitation, of course) is secondary to the myocardial disease. Figure **581** shows such a film. Note the very large left atrium on the penetrated view in this instance (**582**); atypically, it constitutes the entire right border of the heart and meets the diaphragm, overlying the right atrium, which, judging by the superior vena caval shadow, is not markedly enlarged (**497**).

**583 Mitral valve disease, giant left atrium.** In some patients with rheumatic mitral disease, gross enlargement of the left atrium occurs due to rheumatic myopathic involvement. Invariably they have mitral regurgitation. In severe cases, as illustrated, the left atrium may extend to the chest wall and produce an enormous cardiac shadow. Right atrial enlargement may also be gross. The ventricles are often quite small.

**582**

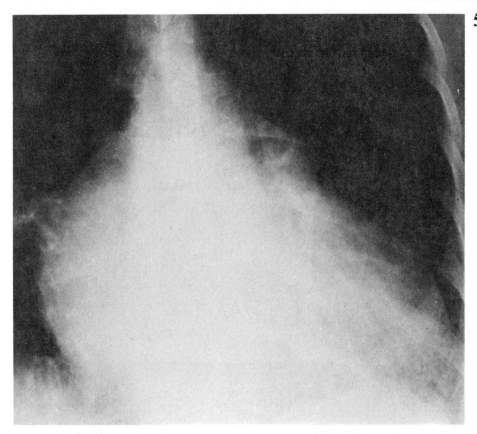

**583**

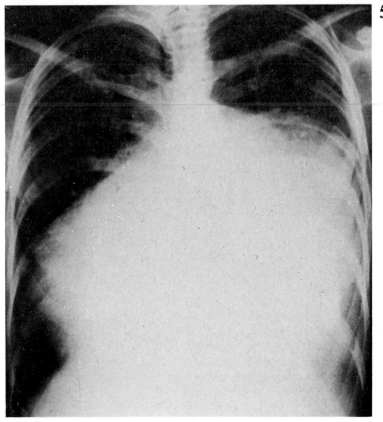

**584**

**585**

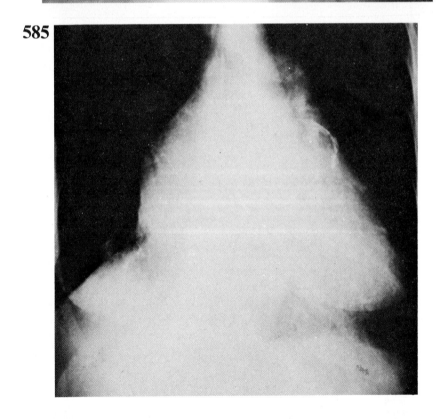

**584, 585 Calcification of the left atrium in rheumatic mitral valve disease.** Calcification may occur extensively in the left atrial wall (**584**) or be largely confined to the appendage (**585**). The calcium is largely laid down in mural thrombus.

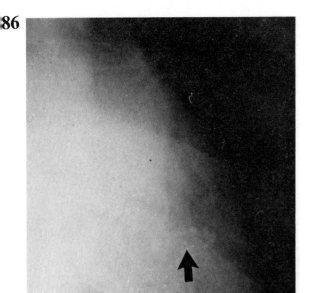

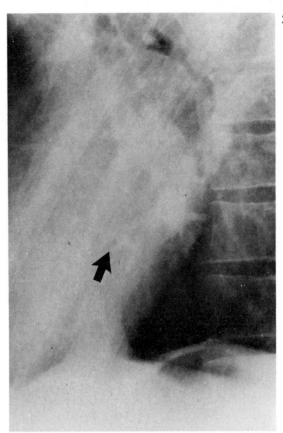

**586, 587  Mitral valve calcification.** This can be seen faintly alongside the spine in penetrated postero-anterior films but, like aortic calcium, is best appreciated in lateral views. In both **586** and **587** the arrow points to the calcification. Note the enlarged left atrium.

**588**

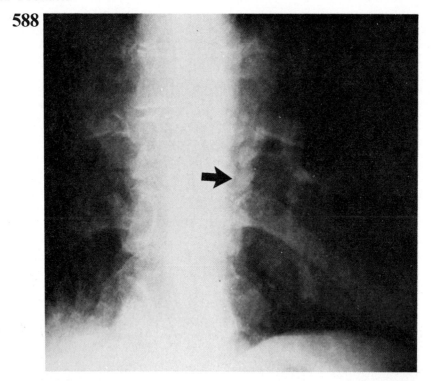

**589**

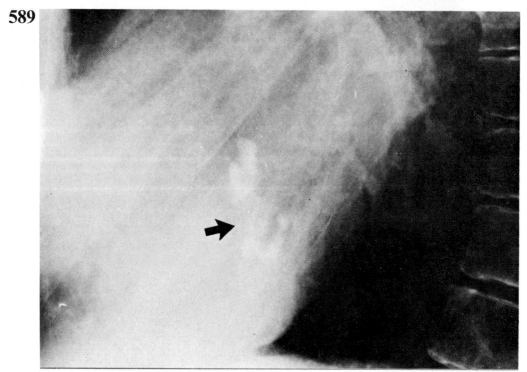

**588, 589 Heavy mitral valve calcification.** In **588** the overpenetrated film shows a thick bar of calcium close to the spinal shadow (arrow). The lateral (**589**) confirms this finding. On screening, the mitral valve was totally immobile.

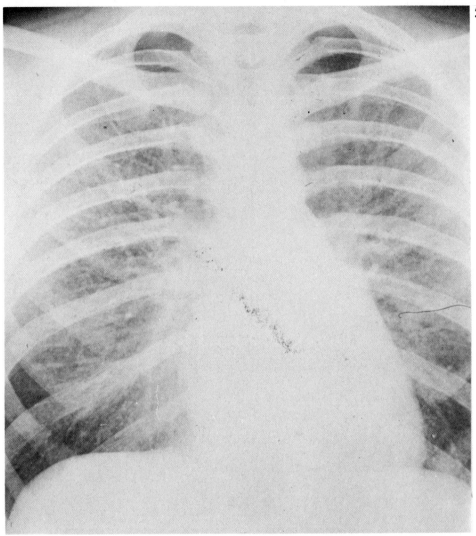

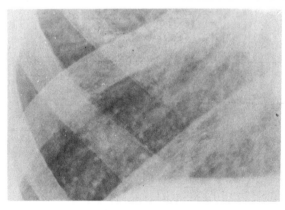

**590, 591   Mitral valve disease, pulmonary haemosiderosis.** Nodular deposits of haemosiderin are seen in some patients with chronic pulmonary venous congestion due to mitral valve disease. Classically, it is seen in longstanding, unrelieved mitral stenosis as in the x-ray of the patient illustrated. The close-up shows the fine nodular shadows in one zone.

**592**

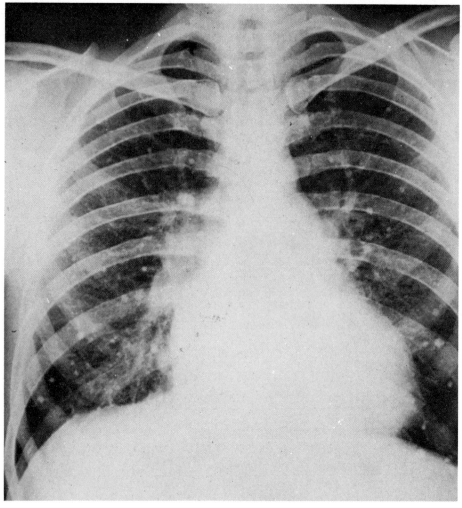

**592 Mitral valve disease, pulmonary haemosiderosis with secondary ossification.** Occasionally in a case of pulmonary haemosiderosis due to chronic unrelieved pulmonary venous congestion, bone formation may occur in some of the nodules as in the film illustrated.

**593, 594 Acute mitral regurgitation due to chordal rupture of the mitral valve.** If regurgitation is anything more than trivial such patients present very soon after the event with symptoms of left heart failure, often well before the heart has had time to enlarge significantly. The lungs, however, show pulmonary venous congestion and even oedema. The contrast is striking and, together with the history and electrocardiogram (**306**) bring the diagnosis readily to mind. Figure **593** shows moderate left atrial enlargement, but chordal rupture had occurred some months earlier. Note the congested lungs. Figure **594** shows the post-operative appearances six weeks later. Note how readily the heart, relieved of the acute insult and relatively undamaged still, returns to its normal dimensions.

**593**

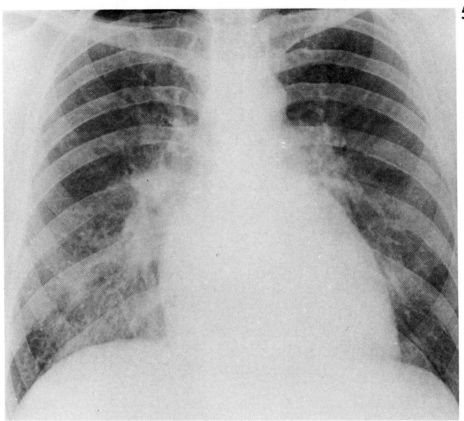

**594**

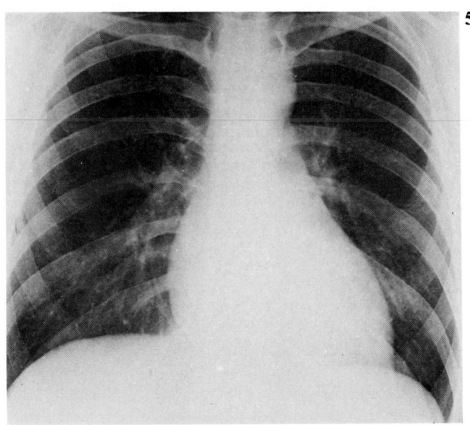

**595–600 Surgically induced mitral regurgitation.** This series of x-rays is valuable in charting the progress of a relatively acutely produced mitral regurgitation, demonstrating the effects on the right heart in particular. The initial film (**595**) shows a normal sized heart with left atrial enlargement showing characteristically as a bulge on both sides of the heart shadow. Mitral valvotomy reduces the size of the heart and especially of the left atrium; the appendage has been amputated (**596**). However, improvement is short-lived and the next film (**597**), taken a year later, shows an increase in heart size. The left atrium is bigger and there is some dilatation of the main pulmonary artery shadows and right atrium. Pulmonary venous engorgement (never previously marked) has appeared. The last three films (**598–600**) show progressive deterioration, with the appearance of severe pulmonary venous congestion, Kerley's lines, and enormous dilatation of the heart and pulmonary arteries as pulmonary hypertension, tricuspid regurgitation and biventricular failure supervened. The time scale from start to finish was seven years.

**595**

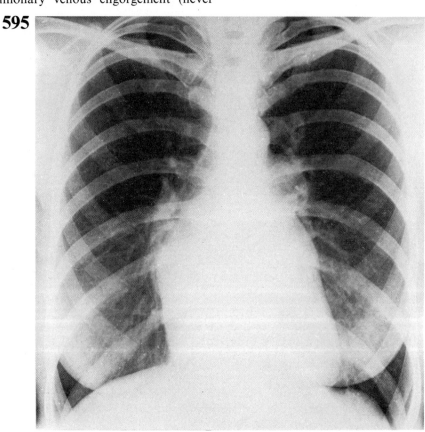

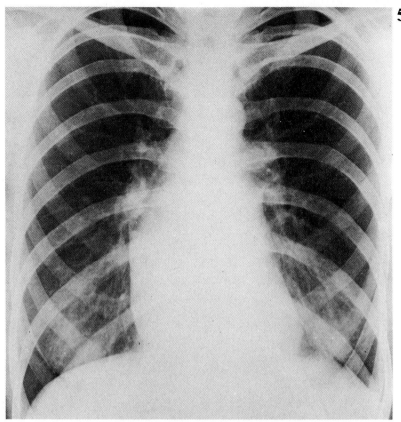

**596**

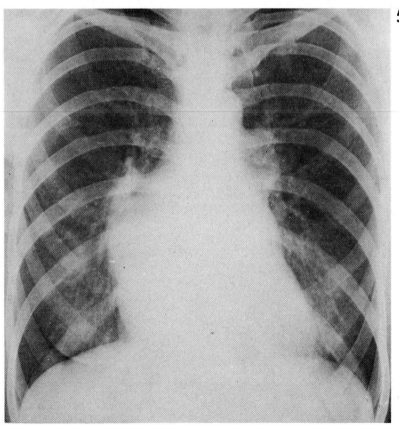

**597**

**598**

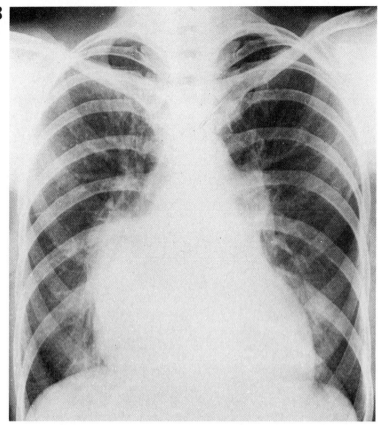

**599**

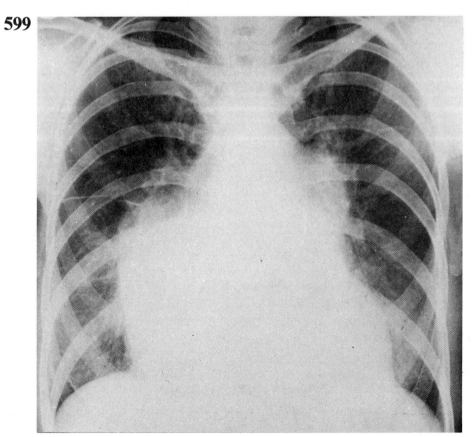

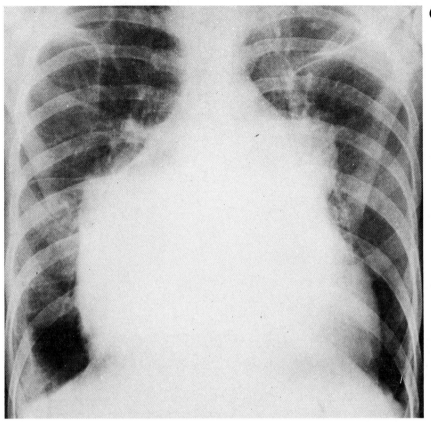

The caption to pictures **598–600** is on the previous
page.

**601**

**602**

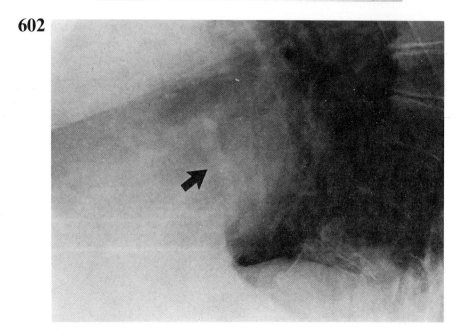

**601, 602 Senile mitral valve ring calcification.**
Heavy calcification in the mitral valve ring in the
elderly leads to mitral regurgitation. The heart is
enlarged, the left ventricle and left atrium being
prominent. The calcium can be seen on the antero-
posterior view and easily on the lateral (arrowed in
both). In normally penetrated films pulmonary
venous congestion was present.

**603, 604 Successful mitral valve replacement.**
Figure **603** shows the pre-operative state. The heart
is enlarged with considerable dilatation of the left
atrium, and there is a prominent main pulmonary
conus due to pulmonary hypertension, pulmonary
venous congestion, and Kerley's lines. The film in
**604** shows the post-operative result. The heart is
much smaller; the left atrium is invisible; and
pulmonary venous congestion has gone.

**603**

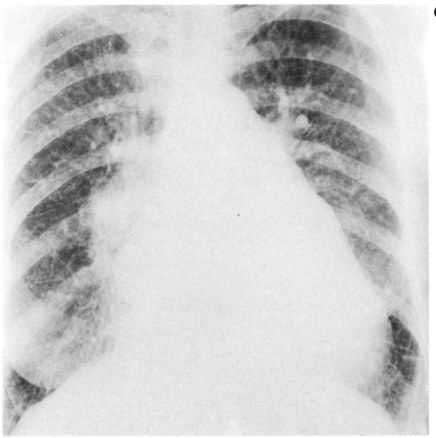

**604**

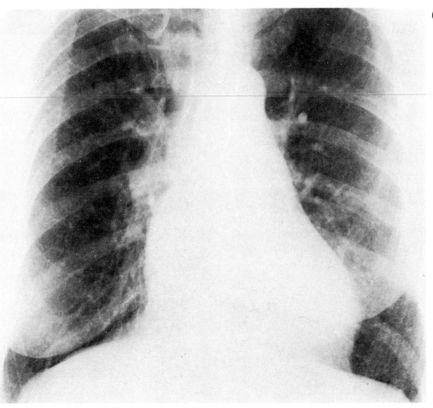

**605**

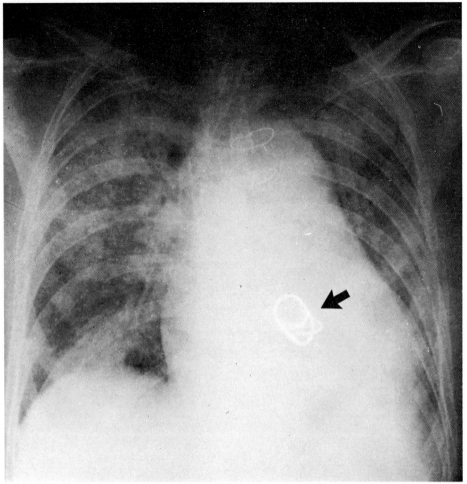

**605 Dehiscence of prosthetic mitral valve.** When a prosthetic valve becomes detached from its seating (usually due to infection) the acute regurgitation which results has catastrophic consequences. Here, the sudden severe mitral regurgitation around the edge of the sewing ring has produced pulmonary oedema. A similar appearance would be produced with a dehisced aortic prosthesis. Comparison with previous films may be helpful in demonstrating an alteration in the attitude of the prosthesis within the heart (see **572, 573**). In the illustration various intravenous catheters and the endotracheal tube can be seen.

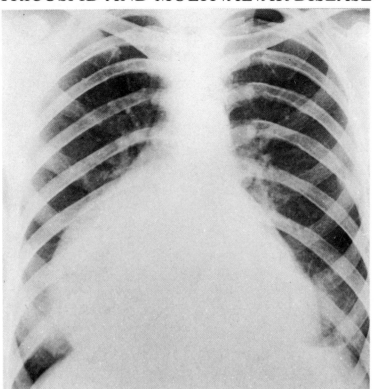

**606 Severe tricuspid valve disease.** Organic rheumatic tricuspid valve disease is usually associated with mitral and aortic lesions. Rarely, as in this case, it dominates the clinical picture. The film shows gross dilatation of the right atrium. A previous mitral valvotomy accounts for rib abnormalities and diaphragmatic tenting on the left. Other examples of right atrial enlargement suggesting either organic or functional tricuspid disease are shown elsewhere, e.g. in **576, 595–600, 607**.

**607  Mitral and tricuspid valve disease.** Severe tricuspid valve disease produces considerable right atrial (and right ventricular) enlargement (**606**). Lesser lesions should also be suspected when the right atrium is unusually prominent. Figure **607** shows clear left atrial enlargement with a double shadow half way down the right border, but the right atrium is prominent too. In the presence of pulmonary hypertension, this could indicate functional tricuspid regurgitation; otherwise it suggests organic tricuspid disease. The proximal pulmonary arteries *are* a little prominent in **607** but in fact pulmonary hypertension was modest and tricuspid stenosis was present.

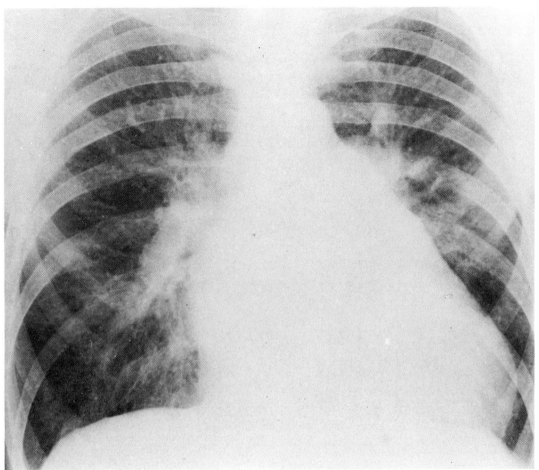

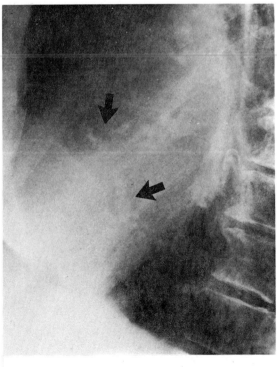

**609**

**608 Aortic and mitral valve disease.** In a case of aortic valve disease a minor degree of mitral valve involvement cannot be identified on the chest x-ray, and vice versa, but significant lesions of both valves coexisting in the same patient may be suspected from a study of the size of the cardiac chambers. If **608** showed the film of a patient with obvious aortic valve disease, the size of the left atrium would suggest an additional mitral lesion, for it is too large for straightforward aortic disease. Alternatively, if mitral valve disease were present, the size of the left ventricle might indicate additional aortic valve disease, although with mitral lesions, other factors may cause cardiac enlargement (see **581**).

**609 Calcification in both aortic and mitral valves.** The upper arrow points to aortic and the lower to mitral calcium in this case of rheumatic heart disease. The relationship of the two valves is well shown. (See also **569, 589, 613–617**.)

**610**

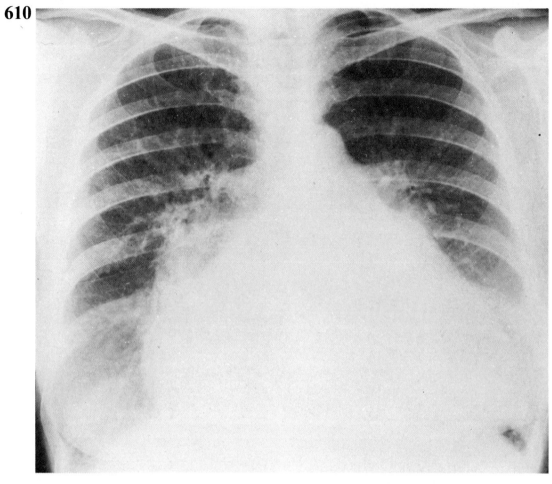

**611**

**612**

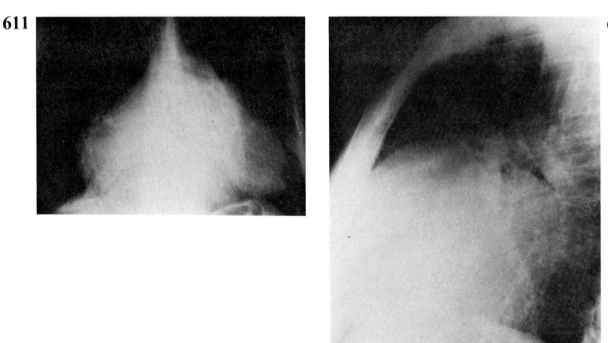

**610–612   Rheumatic valve disease, involvement of aortic, mitral, and tricuspid valves.** The heart is enormously enlarged, all four chambers being affected. The huge left atrium is best appreciated on the penetrated postero-anterior view; the right atrium projects beyond it. The lateral view shows the enlarged right ventricle behind the sternum and the dilated left ventricle filling in the gap in front of the spine. There is pulmonary venous congestion. Note the dilated pulmonary conus due to pulmonary hypertension, and also linear atheromatous calcification in the descending aorta.

**613–615   Aortic and mitral valve replacement.** The proximity of the aortic and mitral valves within the heart is well demonstrated. The type of prosthesis used has a metal ball which makes timing of the phase of the cardiac cycle easy. Two lateral views are illustrated. Figure **614** shows a systolic film with the ball at the end of the cage of the aortic valve and seated at the base of the mitral one. Figure **615** shows the opposite situation—a diastolic film, therefore.

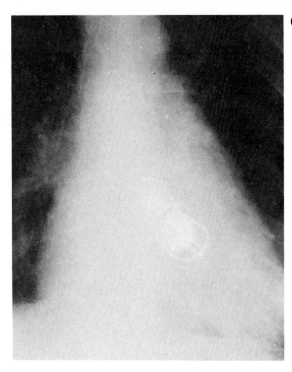

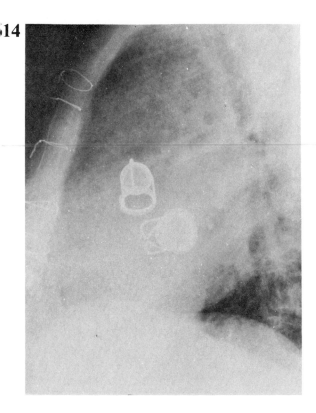

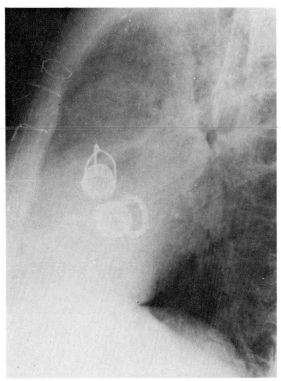

**14**

**615**

**616**

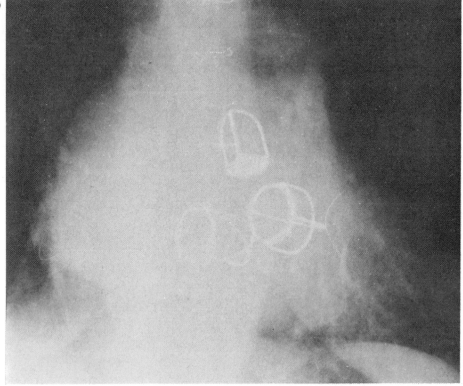

**617**

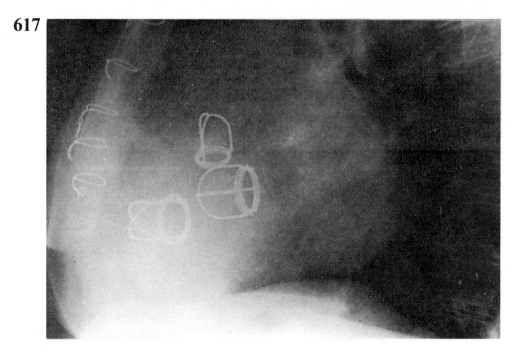

**616, 617  Triple valve replacement.** The mitral, tricuspid, and aortic valves have been replaced. In this variety of prosthesis the ball is non radio-opaque. The relative position of the three valves is well shown, the anterior situation of the tricuspid valve in the lateral view being noteworthy.

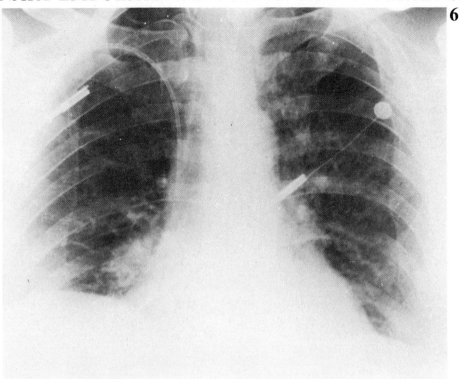

**618 Acute massive pulmonary embolism.** The cardinal features are an area or areas of diminished vascularity (here, the right lung) often associated with a loss of volume. The heart is not greatly enlarged. Note the presence of a cardiac catheter passed from an antecubital vein on the right through the right atrium and ventricle to the pulmonary artery in preparation for a pulmonary angiogram. Electrocardiogram monitoring wires and electrodes are also shown (N.B. see **419**). This is an antero-posterior film. Note the absence of pulmonary infarction which does not occur at this early stage.

**619**

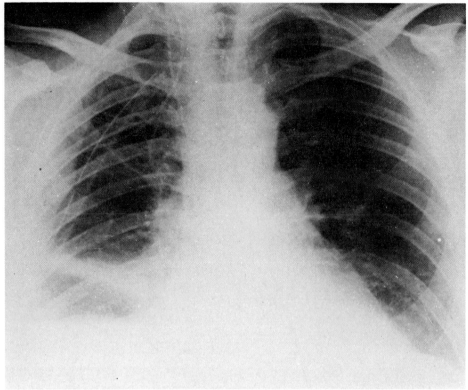

**619 Pulmonary embolism, pulmonary infarction.** An area of collapse and consolidation is present in the right lower zone. This followed fragmentation of a large embolus temporarily lodged in the right pulmonary artery. The heart shadow (allowing for the portable film) is not enlarged. A central venous pressure line is in situ.

**620, 621 Thrombo-embolic pulmonary hypertension.** The main pulmonary conus is enlarged and this dilatation extends to the proximal branches. Thereafter, there is an abrupt diminution in the calibre of the pulmonary arteries and the peripheral lung fields are underfilled. There is right ventricular hypertrophy and enlargement best appreciated in the lateral view where the anterior surface of the heart meets the sternum at a higher point than normal (i.e. above the junction of the lower one-third with the upper two-thirds, **497**). Evidence of infarction is unusual (for these are micro-emboli) unless secondary pulmonary arterial thrombosis-in-situ has occurred.

**620**

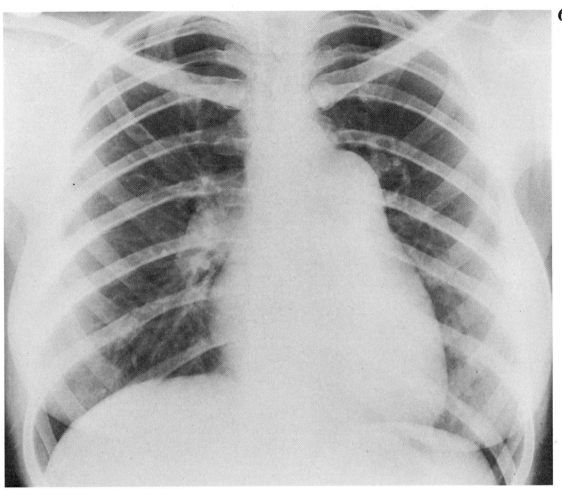

**621**

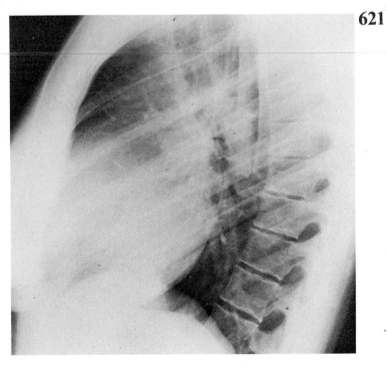

**622**

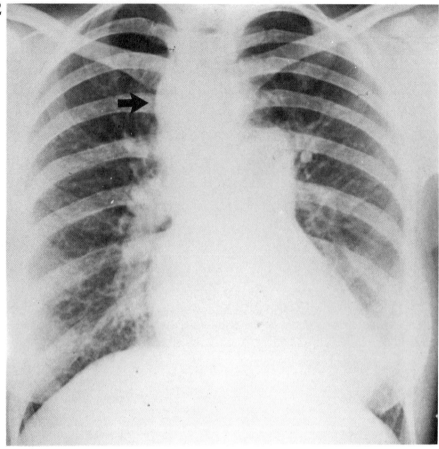

**624**

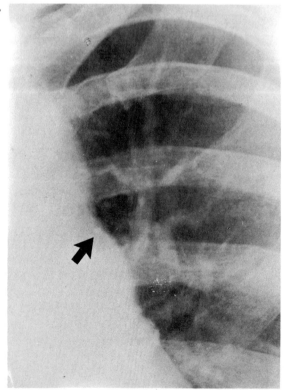

**622–624 Eisenmenger's syndrome.** Essentially, the appearances are those of long-standing pulmonary hypertension and have been summarised under 'thrombo-embolic hypertension'. However, often there are radiological clues to the presence of Eisenmenger's syndrome, e.g. a right sided aortic arch (**622**), which is an anomaly associated with ventricular septal defect, unusually large proximal pulmonary arteries (**623**), which suggests an atrial septal defect, or calcification in a persistent ductus arteriosus (**624**).

**625 Severe pulmonary hypertension, thrombosis-in-situ.** Massive thrombosis in a pulmonary artery secondary to pulmonary hypertension and associated with pulmonary artery atheroma is a complication of any variety of severe long-standing pulmonary hypertension. The shadow of the pulmonary artery (here the right) becomes bulky and very dense. Peripherally, oligaemia is present.

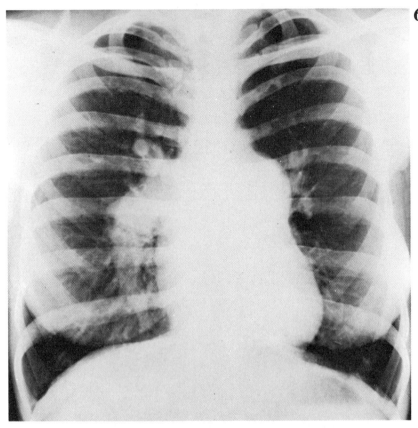

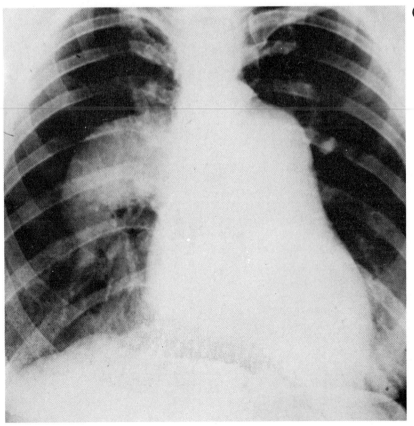

**626   Left superior vena cava.** This is shown by the presence of a linear shadow to the left of the aortic knuckle. It usually drains to the right atrium via the coronary sinus. A right superior vena cava is also present. In this example the abnormal shadow is more obvious than in most.

**627   Idiopathic dilatation of the pulmonary artery.** The main pulmonary conus is enlarged but the pulmonary vascularity is normal and the heart is not enlarged. On chest x-ray mild pulmonary valve stenosis produces identical appearances.

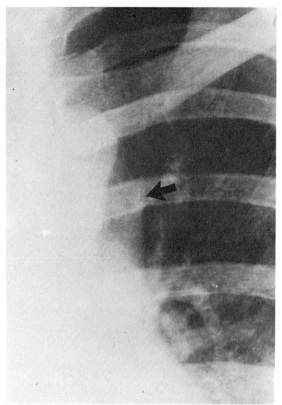

**627**

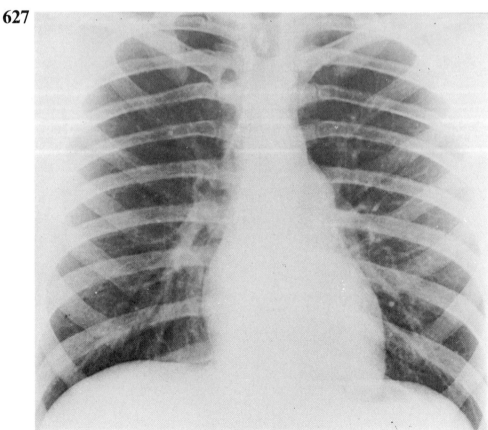

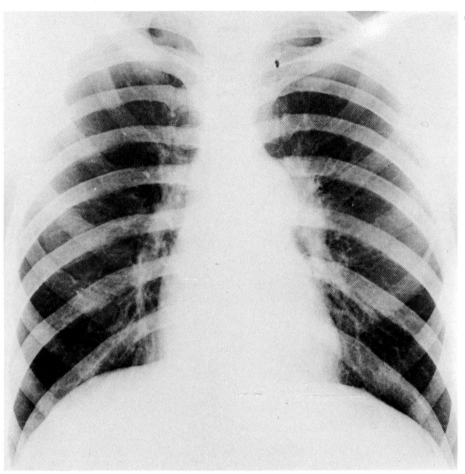

**628  Moderately severe pulmonary valve stenosis.**
The heart is not enlarged though the right ventricle
is prominent on the lateral view (not illustrated).
The main pulmonary conus shows post-stenotic
dilatation which may extend (as in this example)
into the main proximal branches. The peripheral
lung vascularity is diminished but not strikingly so
and in many cases it will be normal. See **631**.

**629**

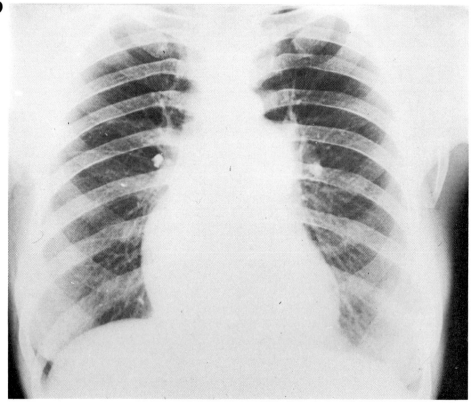

**630**

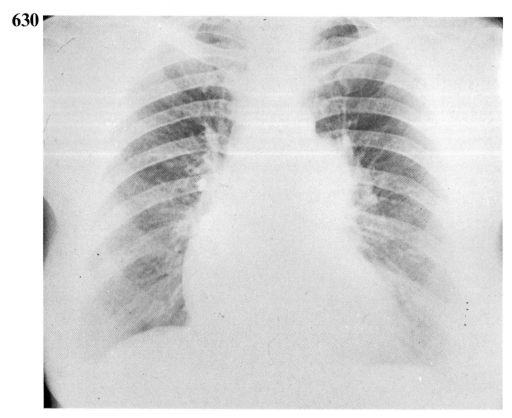

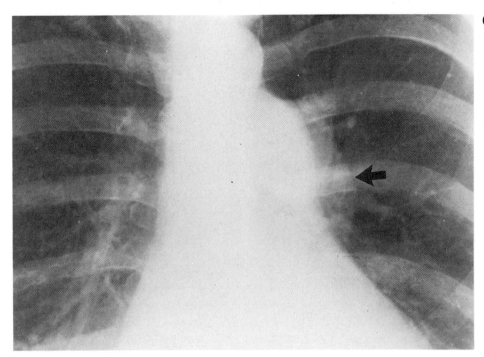

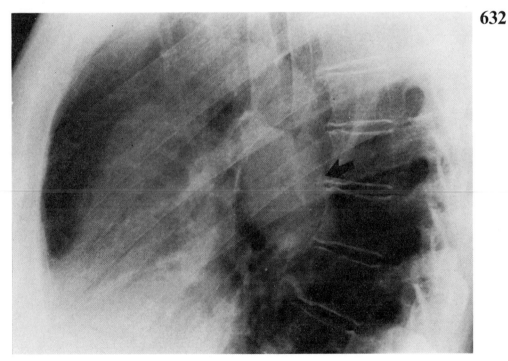

**629, 630   Very severe pulmonary valve stenosis.** The cardiac silhouette is described above (**628**). When stenosis is very severe the lungs are definitely underfilled. Figure **630** shows the results of operation; lung vascularity has improved but the heart is a little larger because of pulmonary regurgitation induced at surgery.

**631, 632   Post-stenotic dilatation of the pulmonary artery extending into the left branch.** Involvement of the left pulmonary artery in post-stenotic dilatation can be seen in the postero-anterior view as a shadow beside the dilated main pulmonary conus and in the lateral view as a wide shadow beneath the aortic arch.

**633**

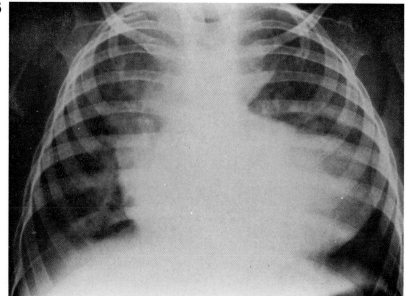

**634**

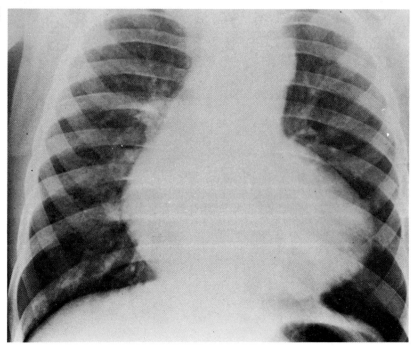

**633–636  Fallot's tetralogy.** The classical appearances are a tip-tilted apex due to right ventricular hypertrophy (the so-called *coeur-en-sabot*), an absent pulmonary conus producing a 'bay' or indentation in the left cardiac border, and under-filled lung fields. In a quarter of cases the aortic arch is right-sided. The four cases illustrated show how greatly the reality may differ from this typical appearance. All have severe Fallot's tetralogy. All show a pulmonary bay but this may not be present if stenosis is valvar rather than infundibular. Figures 633, 634 show the *coeur-en-sabot*; 635 has a somewhat rounded apex, but 636 shows a silhouette that would pass for normal. It is difficult to assess 635 which is overpenetrated but the lungs *are* underfilled; the vascularity of the others is unremarkable. The reason for this is the presence of systemic arteries supplying the lungs. Note the characteristic reticular pattern sometimes seen when this is so (636). Note too how readily the chest x-ray could pass for normal.

**635**

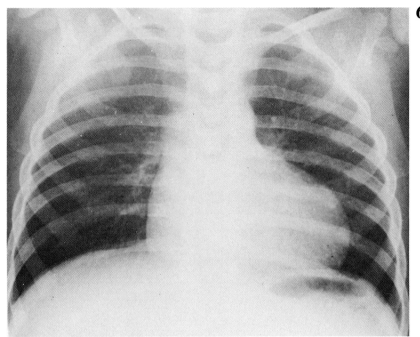

**636**

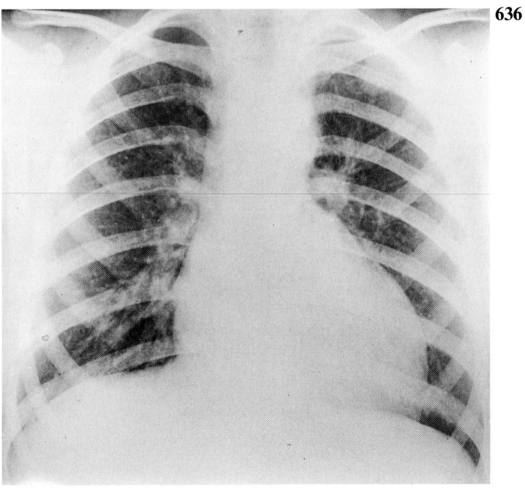

**637**

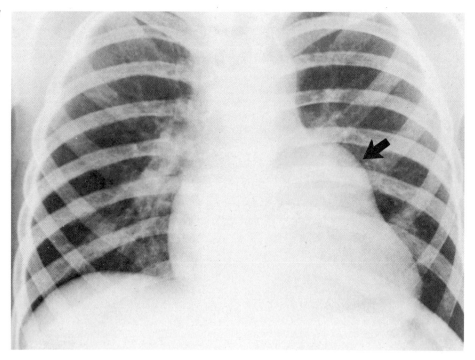

**637 Fallot's tetralogy, aneurysm of right ventricular outflow tract following repair.** Following resection of infundibular stenosis in the total correction of Fallot's tetralogy, with or without the insertion of a patch, aneurysm formation may occur and will produce a bulge on the left cardiac border.

**638, 639 Pulmonary atresia.** This usually presents in early infancy (**638**). The heart is normal in size, with a characteristic projection to the right of the upper mediastinum which could be thymus but which is in fact the large aorta. The lungs are markedly underfilled. If the child survives, many systemic arteries proliferate and attempt to supply the gravely ischaemic lungs producing a reticulated pattern well seen in **639**. The same pattern is also seen in severe Fallot's tetralogy of which this condition is essentially an extreme form (**636**).

**638**

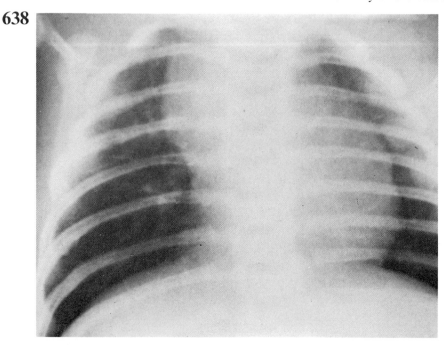

**639**

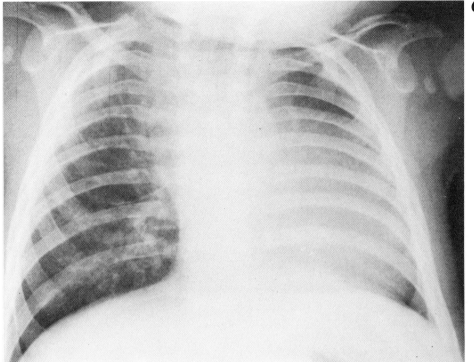

**640**

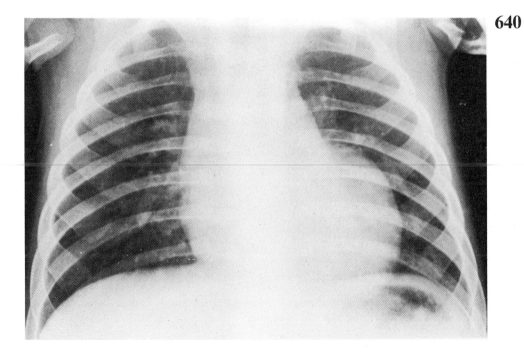

**640 Tricuspid atresia.** This usually presents in infancy. Transposition of the great arteries is a frequent association but the commonest form has additional pulmonary valve and subvalve stenosis and presents as illustrated with a normal-sized heart with underfilled lungs and a tip-tilted apex reminiscent of Fallot's tetralogy. See **449** for the characteristic electrocardiogram.

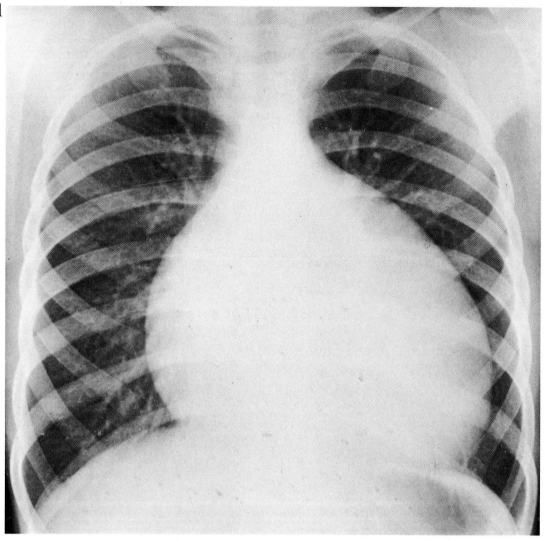

**641  Ebstein's disease of the tricuspid valve.** This uncommon congenital anomaly of the tricuspid valve in which it is displaced into the right ventricle results in a greatly dilated right atrium which becomes the largest chamber in the heart. The globular cardiac shadow with its well-defined margins mimics that of a pericardial effusion. The lungs are underfilled and neither great vessel is prominent. See **447** for the characteristic electro-cardiogram.

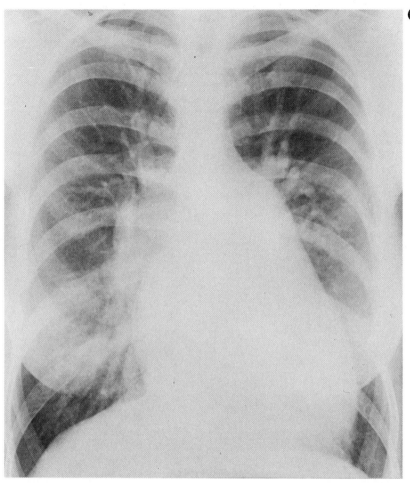

**642, 643  Atrial septal defect, large left to right shunt.** The heart is enlarged. The aortic knuckle is inconspicuous and its small size is emphasised by the dilated main pulmonary conus immediately below. A fullness of the right cardiac border indicates enlargement of the right atrium, but the left atrium is not enlarged unless additional mitral stenosis ('Lutembacher's syndrome'—**648**) is present. On the lateral view the right ventricle is seen to be enlarged. The proximal pulmonary arteries are large and they extend into the periphery of the lung fields—pulmonary plethora. (See **645, 646**.) Ostium secundum and ostium primum defects cannot be distinguished on chest x-ray appearances, though, of course, their respective electrocardiograms are very different (see **329, 340**). For the Eisenmenger syndrome and atrial septal defect see **623**.

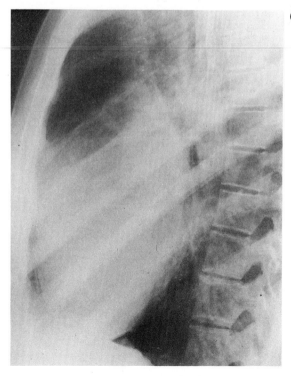

**644**

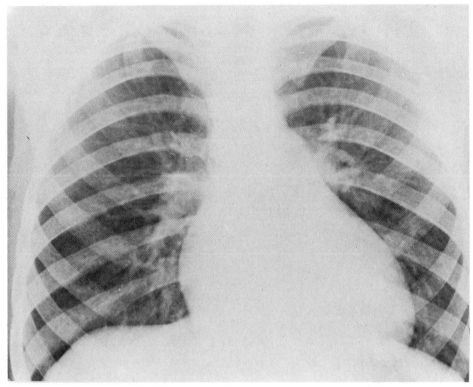

**644   Atrial septal defect, small or moderate left to right shunt.** This can be difficult to diagnose on x-ray. The heart is not definitely enlarged. Some prominence of the main pulmonary conus is seen in normal subjects; pulmonary plethora is not seen (allowing for the increased vascularity of the expiratory film in the case illustrated, this is so).

**645, 646   Atrial septal defect, effect of closure.** The film in **645** shows all the features of atrial septal defect listed in **642** except that the main pulmonary conus is not very large. The defect was closed and **646** shows the post-operative result—an obvious reduction in heart size and plethora.

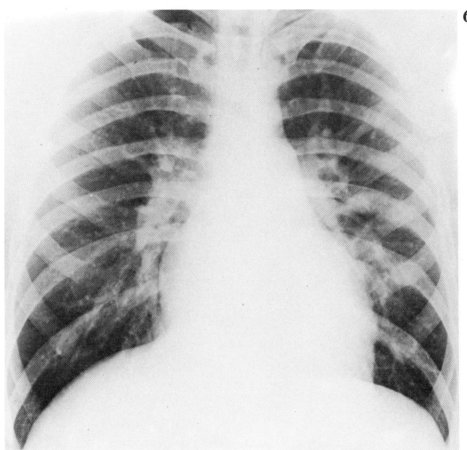

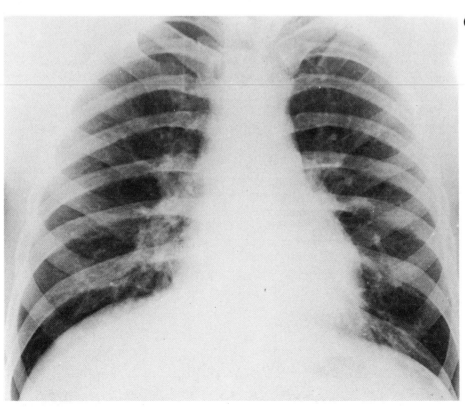

**647**

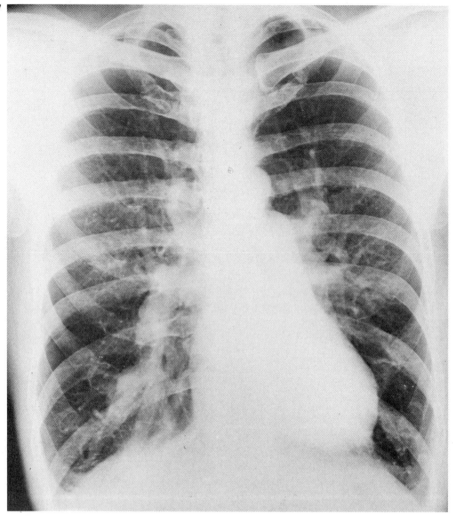

**647 Atrial septal defect, grossly dilated pulmonary arteries.** Since patients with large atrial septal defects survive well into adult life, time may produce considerable dilatation of the proximal pulmonary arteries (**642**) especially if pulmonary hypertension develops (**623**). The patient in **647**, however, showed dilatation extending well down into the vessels to the right lower zone. Angiography showed no other lesion in the region; this was simply pulmonary artery dilatation associated with a heavy left to right shunt.

**648, 649 Lutembacher's syndrome.** The combination of mitral stenosis and an atrial septal defect is suspected on the plain chest x-ray by unusual enlargement of the left atrium (note widening of the carinal angle just visible on the postero-anterior view, and the posterior prominence on the lateral), and by mitral valve calcium (not present in this case). Pulmonary venous congestion is not seen, because of the open septum, but the heart may be unusually large. The electrocardiogram may help in diagnosis—see **453**.

**648**

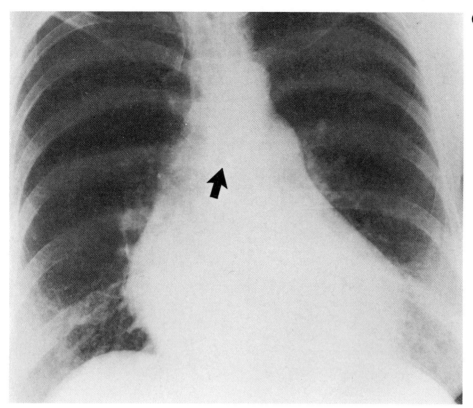

**649**

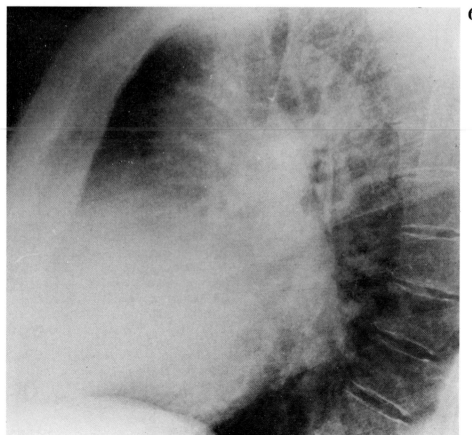

**650**

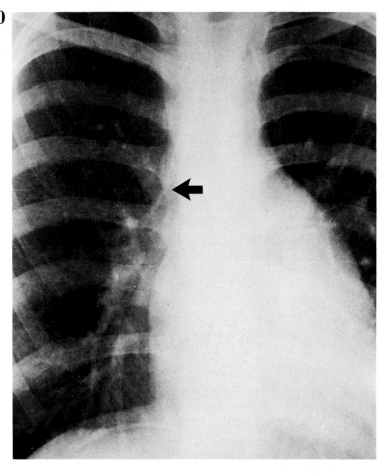

**651**

**650, 651 Partial anomalous pulmonary venous drainage.** Either one or more pulmonary veins drain abnormally into the right atrium or a vena cava. This is commoner on the right. An associated atrial septal defect is almost always present and tends to dominate the chest x-ray appearances, though of course, the anomalous veins also produce a left to right shunt and contribute to any pulmonary plethora that may be present. When the anomalous vein joins the lower part of the superior vena cava or the caval-right atrial junction it may occasionally be suspected on the x-ray as an ill-defined vascular shadow (arrowed in **650**) and there may be a bulge in the caval outline at this point. Figure **651** shows the position of such a vein in another patient by the presence of a catheter within it.

See also the scimitar syndrome (**652**).

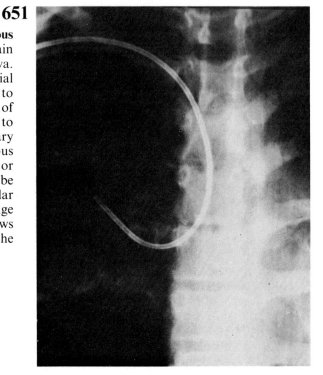

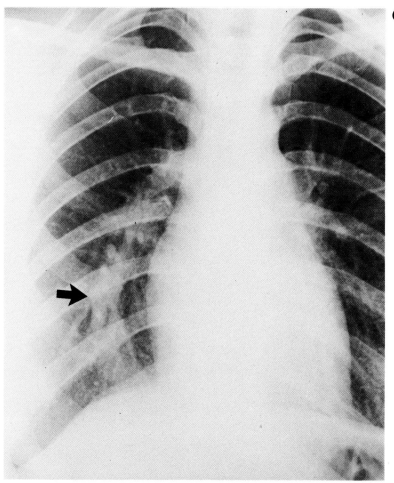

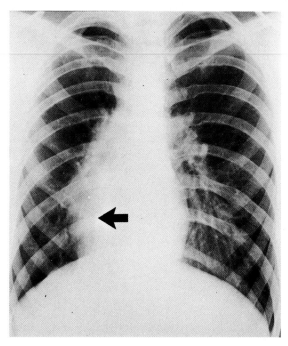

**652, 653   The 'scimitar' syndrome.** This name is given to a particular variety of partial anomalous pulmonary venous drainage in which the aberrant vein drains beneath the diaphragm (to portal, hepatic, or caval veins), and is visible as a crescentic shadow on the right of the heart (hence the name). Figure **652** shows the abnormal vessel as an ill-defined shadow (arrowed) overlapping the pulmonary arteries and descending to the diaphragm. Figure **653** shows another example of the syndrome illustrating another typical feature—displacement of the heart to the right because of associated hypoplasia and loss of volume of the right lower lobe. In this instance the abnormal vessel is behind the heart and can only just be seen (arrow).

**654**

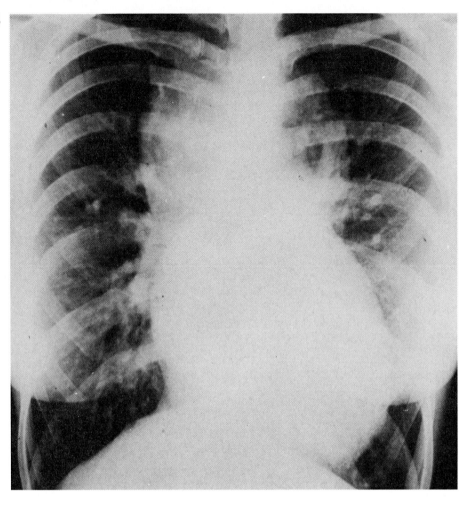

**654, 655 Total anomalous pulmonary venous drainage.** There are several types of this anomaly, most of which present in infancy (see **656**), but one of them often survives into adult life and is readily recognised on the chest x-ray. This is the supra-cardiac variety, in which the pulmonary veins meet behind the heart and join a persistent left superior vena cava which runs upward to join the left innominate vein. The result is a somewhat ill-defined shadow above the heart, producing the so-called 'cottage loaf' or 'figure of eight' appearance (**654**). The lungs are plethoric from the left to right shunt. Figure **655** shows a catheter passed from the right arm into the abnormal vessel.

**656 Infradiaphragmatic total anomalous pulmonary venous drainage.** In this variety of anomalous pulmonary venous drainage the constriction of the common pulmonary vein so characteristic of this condition tends to be more severe than in other types, and further obstruction may be produced by enforced passage of the blood through the portal system. The result is a distinctive radiological picture with a haziness throughout the lung fields. It is, however, impossible to guess the anatomy from the chest x-ray and many variations are possible. These cases present in early infancy.

**655**

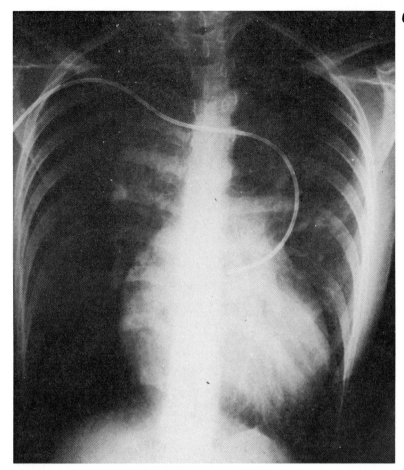

**656**

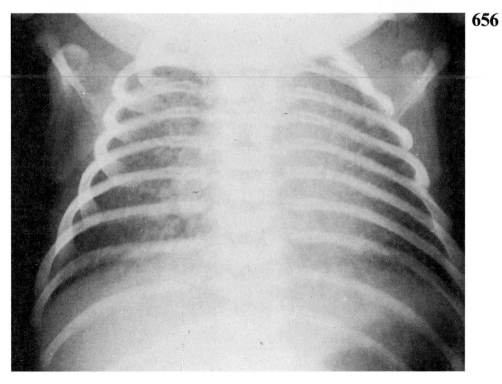

**657**

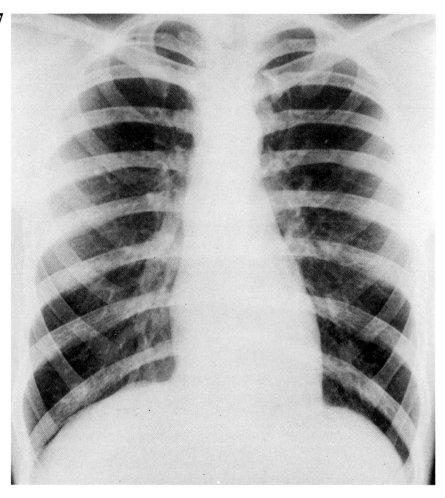

**657 Maladie de Roger.** The small ventricular septal defect to which this term is applied shows no abnormality of the chest x-ray. Heart size and shape, and lung vascularity are normal.

**658, 659 Ventricular septal defect.** Defects of moderate size carrying shunts of intermediate proportions show slight cardiomegaly and, as in the film illustrated, doubtful plethora (**658**). The main pulmonary conus, though a little prominent, is within normal limits. Nevertheless, closure of the defect produced a dramatic reduction in heart size (**659**), even allowing for the deeper inspiration of the second film.

**658**

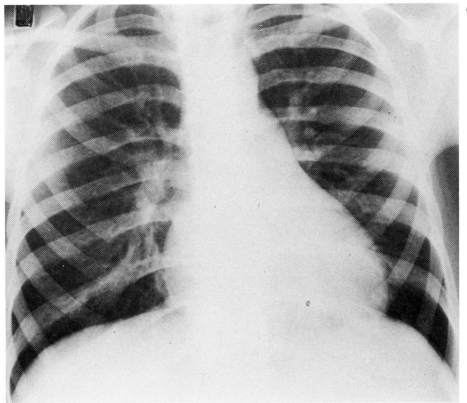

**659**

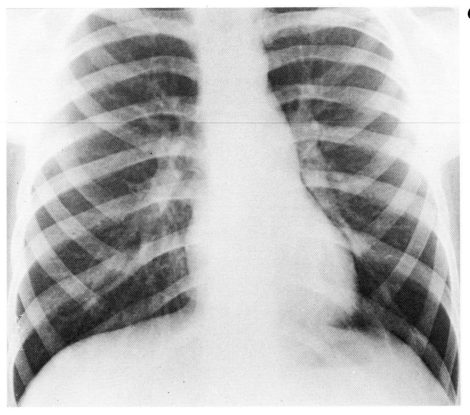

**660**

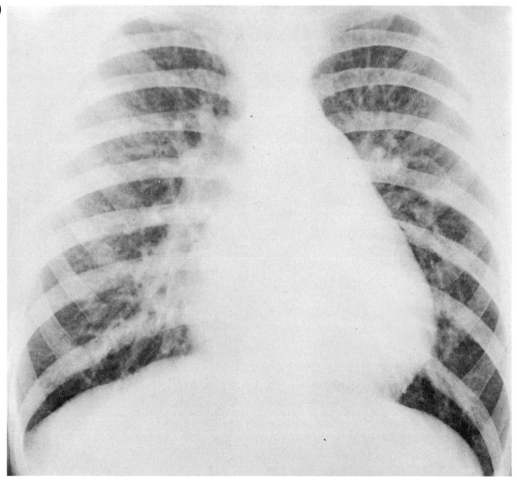

**661**

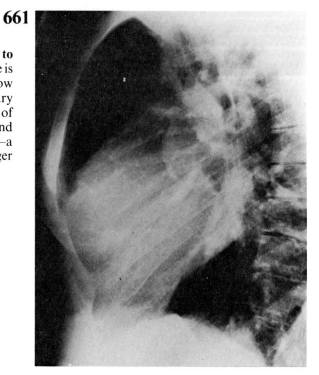

**660, 661 Ventricular septal defect with heavy left to right shunt.** Both ventricles are enlarged, and there is often mild left atrial dilatation (see double shadow in **660**). There is prominence of the main pulmonary conus and pulmonary plethora. Forward bowing of the sternum is seen in patients with large shunts and hyperkinetic pulmonary hypertension (**661**—a different patient). See **622** for the Eisenmenger syndrome and ventricular septal defect.

**662**

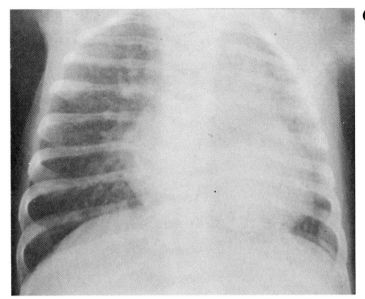

**663**

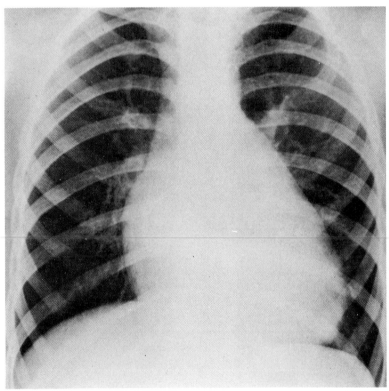

**662, 663 'Banded' ventricular septal defect.** The operation of banding was used to limit the large left to right shunt in infants with ventricular septal defects who went into intractable heart failure in the early months of life. Nowadays it is less and less often performed, primary closure of the defect being preferred. The main pulmonary artery is constricted and the shunt relieved, the distal lung vessels being protected from its consequences (possible develop-ment of pulmonary hypertension) at the price of right ventricular systolic overload. Figure **662** shows an infant with such a shunt, and **663** the appearances at the age of five immediately before projected closure of the defect and removal of the band. There is no plethora.

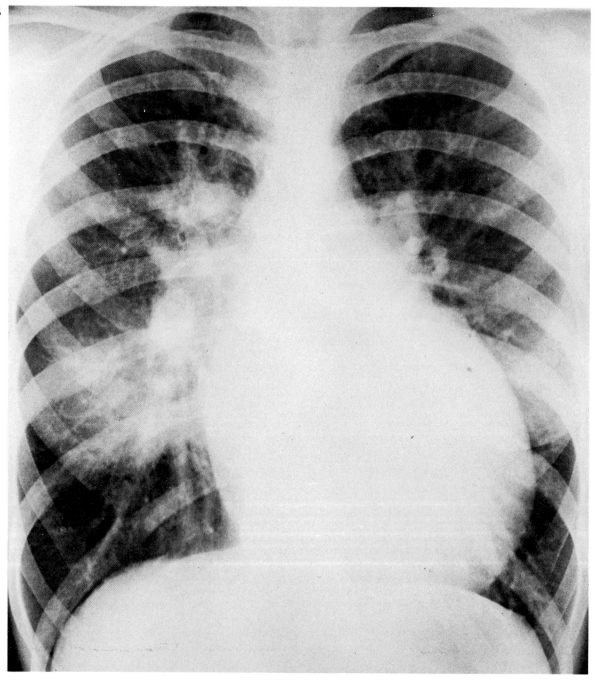

**664 Ventricular septal defect with corrected transposition.** In a case of ventricular septal defect the presence of corrected transposition may be suspected by the absence of a prominent pulmonary conus, the convex left upper cardiac border being formed by the aorta, and the narrow vascular pedicle. Note the gross pulmonary plethora in this film. The shunt was a large one and there was hyperkinetic pulmonary hypertension. See **673**. The electrocardiogram may assist the diagnosis of corrected transposition (**450**).

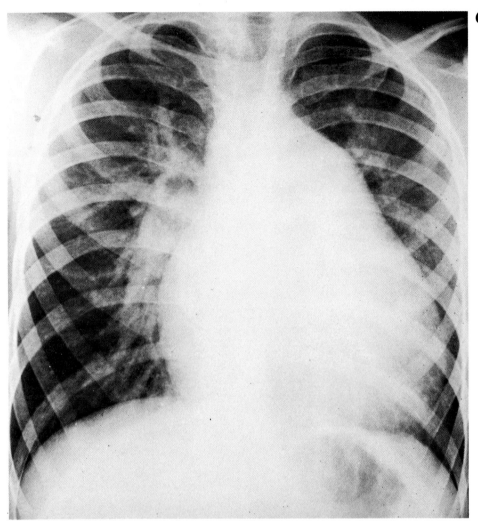

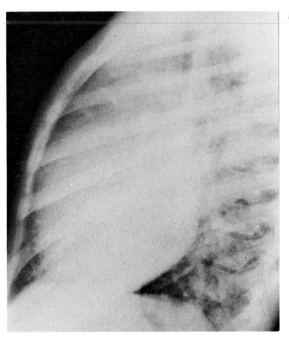

**665, 666  Atrioventricular canal with heavy left to right shunt.** With shunting at both atrial and ventricular levels and with associated mitral regurgitation, all four chambers of the heart are enlarged (the left atrium cannot be easily seen on these films). There is gross pulmonary plethora and dilatation of the main pulmonary conus (note the filling of the anterior mediastinal window on the lateral view by the huge pulmonary artery). The aorta is inconspicuous. There is anterior bowing of the sternum (see **661**). For the electrocardiographic findings in endocardial cushion defects see **340**.

**667**

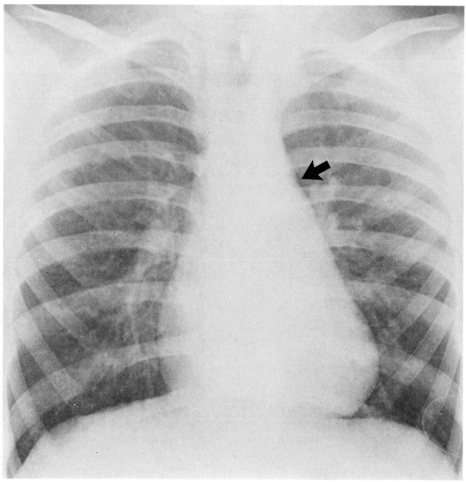

**667–669   Patent ductus arteriosus with left to right shunt.** In mild or moderate defects (**667**) the x-ray may pass for normal. Sometimes the aorta is a little conspicuous and the main pulmonary conus mildly dilated (though this is not uncommon in normal films). There is filling in of the gap between the aortic knuckle and pulmonary artery (arrow). Pulmonary plethora is absent. When heavy shunting is taking place through a large ductus (**668**) there is obvious plethora, and more prominence of the main pulmonary conus; the left ventricle enlarges and there may be visible left atrial dilatation (not on this infant's film). The position of the ductus is well shown by a catheter passed through it from the pulmonary artery and directed down the descending aorta (**669**). See also the Eisenmenger syndrome, **624**, for ductal calcification.

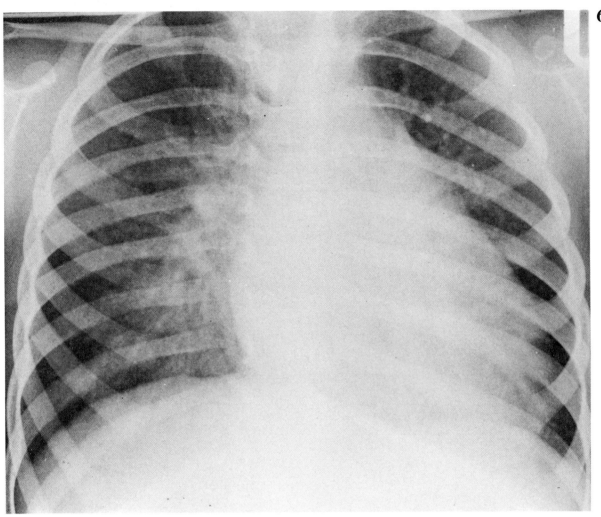

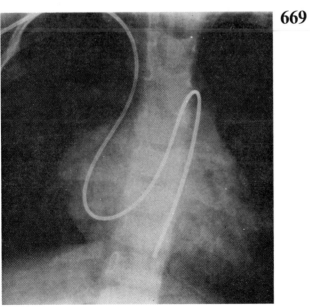

669

**670**

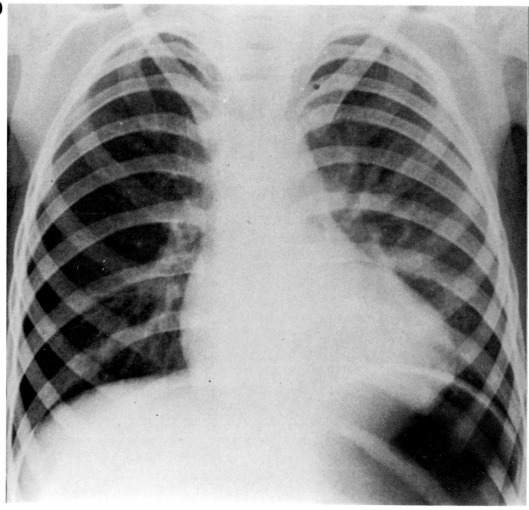

**670, 671  Unilateral pulmonary plethora.** Straight-forward left to right shunts sometimes show unilateral pulmonary plethora (**670** shows left sided plethora in a case of moderate ventricular septal defect) but the commonest cause, as in **671**, is a surgical shunt (Waterston's operation) between the ascending aorta and the right pulmonary artery performed for Fallot's tetralogy. Blood is directed with remarkable selectivity into the right lung only; indeed, unilateral pulmonary vascular disease may occur. In **671**, the left lung would pass for normal.

**672  Dextrocardia with situs inversus.** The heart and the viscera are inverted. This variety of dextrocardia is frequently unaccompanied by any congenital heart lesion, as in the case illustrated. Note the stomach bubble on the right and the higher diaphragm on the left. See **28** and **29** for the electrocardiogram.

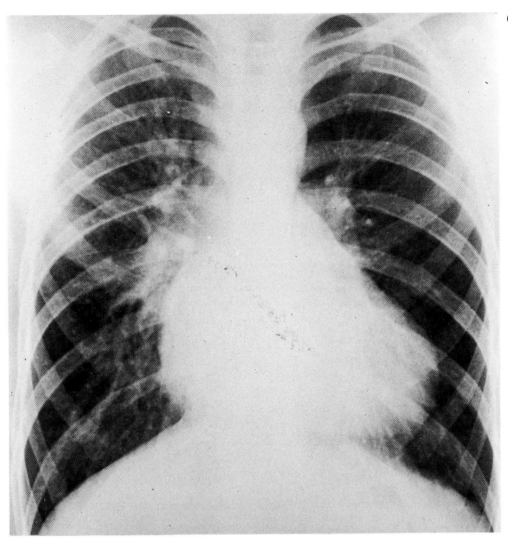

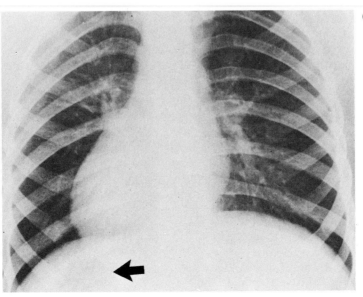

**673**

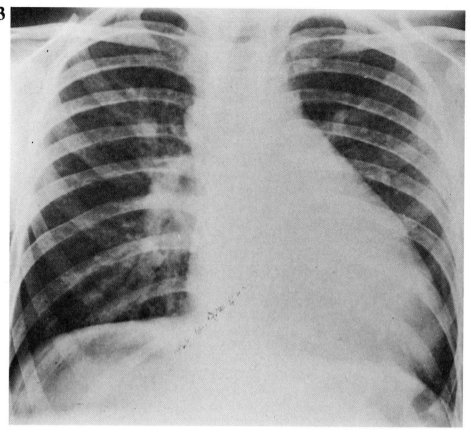

**673 Isolated laevocardia, corrected transposition.** In isolated laevocardia, the heart is normally sited but the other viscera are reversed—note the stomach bubble on the right and the hepatic flexure of the colon on the left. Isolated dextrocardia is essentially the same condition in mirror image. Most patients with isolated dextrocardia or laevocardia have a congenital heart defect and a common one is transposition of the great arteries with ventricular inversion and a ventricular septal defect as in the case illustrated (though other lesions, such as anomalous pulmonary venous drainage, occur as well). This form of transposition is the only common variety of 'corrected' transposition—i.e. *physiologically* corrected, the right atrium communicating with the pulmonary artery via an anatomically 'left' ventricle, and the left atrium with the aorta via a 'right' ventricle. The heart has a characteristic shape with a gentle convexity to the left cardiac border because of the position of the aorta there. The pulmonary artery is abnormally situated centrally in the heart shadow. The other features of a ventricular septal defect can be seen. (See **450** for the electrocardiogram in corrected transposition.)

**674 Isolated dextrocardia.** This is the mirror image of isolated laevocardia (**673**). Note the stomach bubble on the left, indicating situs solitus. As with isolated laevocardia, most of these patients have a congenital heart defect. In this case it was coarctation—rib notching is just visible. See **713–717**.

**675 Mesocardia.** This is a purely descriptive term indicating that the heart is in the midline. The position of the cardiac chambers, their relation to the viscera, and whether or not dextrocardia is present cannot be diagnosed with confidence from such a film, and cardiac catheterisation is necessary to establish these points. For instance, in the example illustrated the high left diaphragm suggests situs inversus but a faint stomach bubble is present on the left side, and despite the cardiac shape, the left ventricle was on the left.

**674**

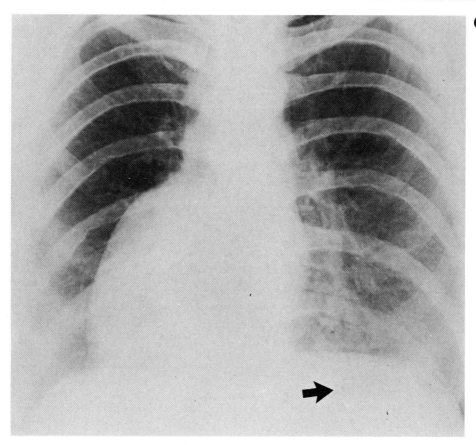

**675**

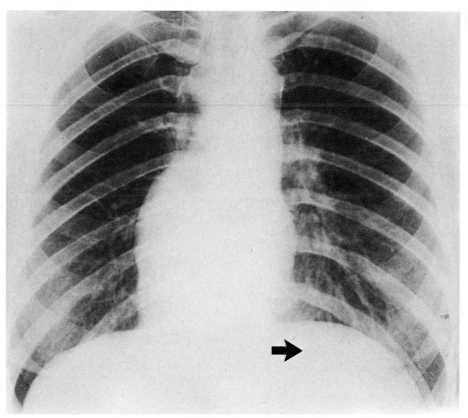

**676**

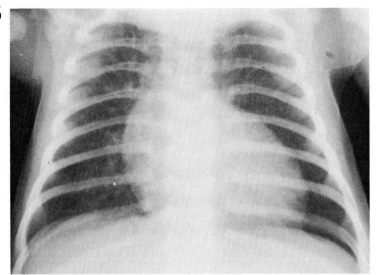

**677**

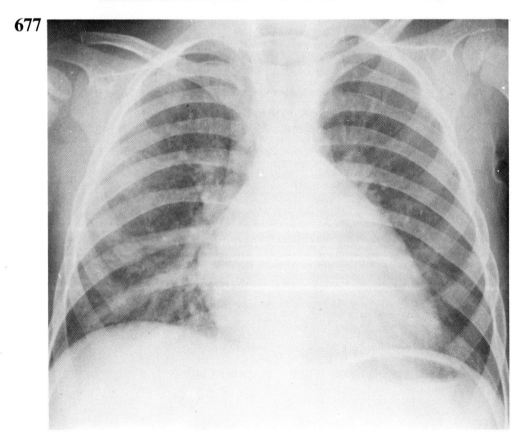

**676, 677 Transposition of the great arteries.** The majority of cases present in the first days of life (**676**) but nowadays, with balloon septostomy many survive into early childhood (**677**) and come to corrective surgery. The appearances can vary considerably, depending on associated lesions and the presence of heart failure, but the classical findings are modest cardiac enlargement, a narrow vascular pedicle (because of the position of the great artery roots behind one another), an 'egg-shaped' cardiac silhouette, and pulmonary plethora (unless pulmonary stenosis is present, when the lungs are underfilled and the appearances may be mistaken for Fallot's tetralogy).

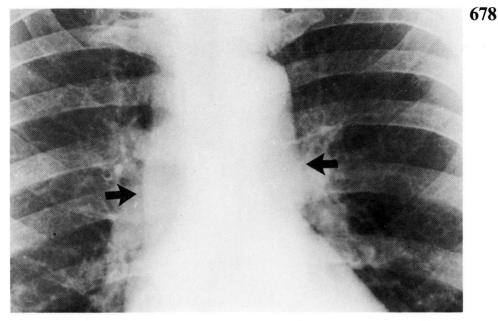

**678  Unfolded aorta.** A normal finding in older subjects. There is prominence of the ascending aorta to the right of the mediastinum, and the descending aorta is displaced to the left as it passes behind the heart, producing a linear shadow.

**679, 680  Marked aortic unfolding and kyphosis.** The combination of marked aortic unfolding and kyphosis can produce alarming prominence of the aortic shadow, as in this subject. The lateral view reveals the calibre of the descending aorta at least, to be normal. There is cardiac enlargement which is partly due to left ventricular hypertrophy and partly attributable to the chest shape. Some of the prominence of the ascending aorta is due to post-stenotic dilatation.

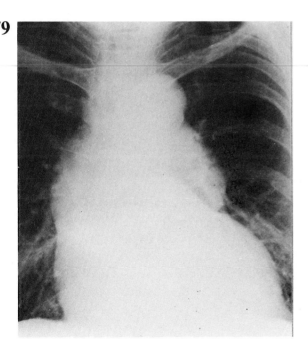

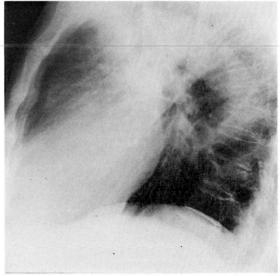

**681**

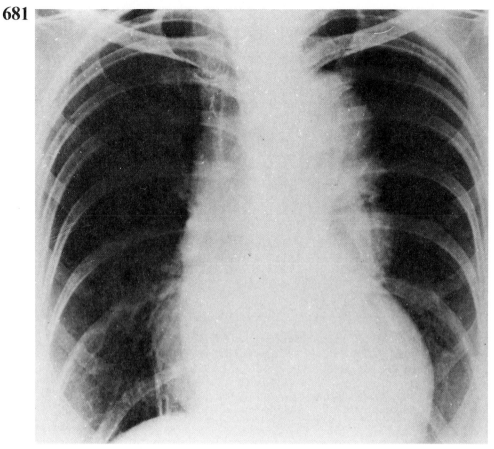

**681–683 Tortuosity of the thoracic aorta.** On the normally exposed postero-anterior view (**681**) the aorta appears to be unfolded but there is a shadow to the right of the heart above the diaphragm. The penetrated film (**682**) and lateral delineate marked tortuosity and kinking of the aorta causing it to cross the midline. This occurs in the elderly.

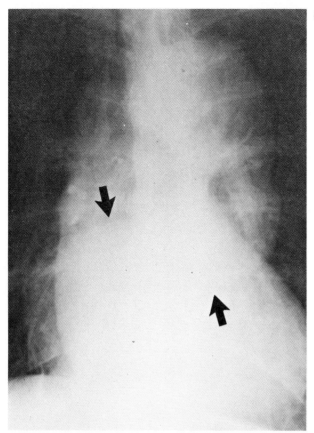

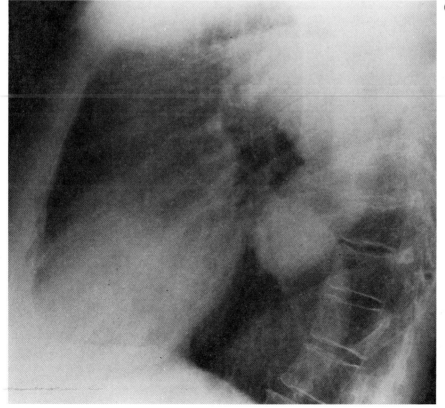

**684**

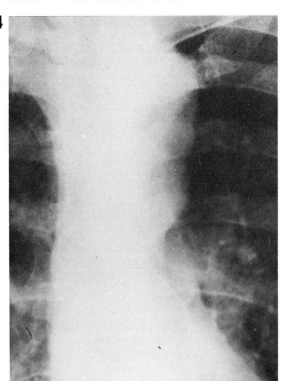

**68**

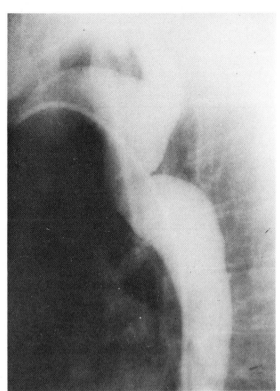

**686**

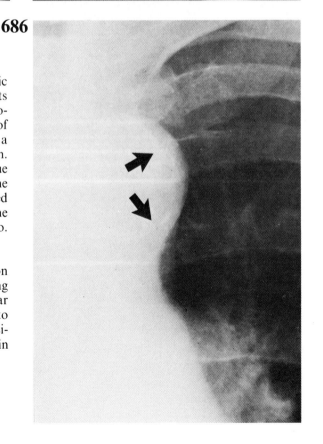

**684, 685    Kinked aortic arch.** Kinking of the aortic arch produces an abnormal aortic knuckle. Subjects are usually past middle age and the frequent co-existence of hypertension may raise the suspicion of coarctation (despite the absence of rib notching or a dilated left subclavian artery) or of aortic aneurysm. The lateral angiocardiogram (**685**) reveals the true state of affairs. The aorta is kinked just beyond the origin of the left subclavian artery but not narrowed (note the helpful position of the catheter against the aortic wall). The plain film may well show this too.

**686    Calcified aortic knuckle.** Mural calcification in the aortic arch is a common and harmless finding in older subjects. It is well seen in this particular place because the direction of the arch in relation to the plane of the film, which produces superimposition of shadows (cf. the perimeter calcification in constrictive pericarditis).

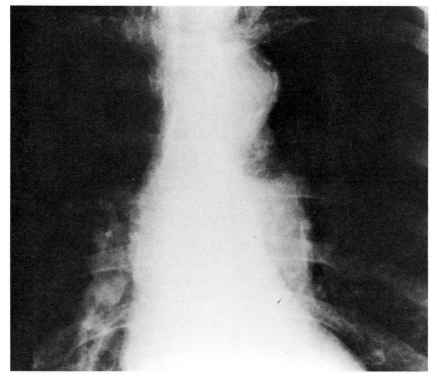

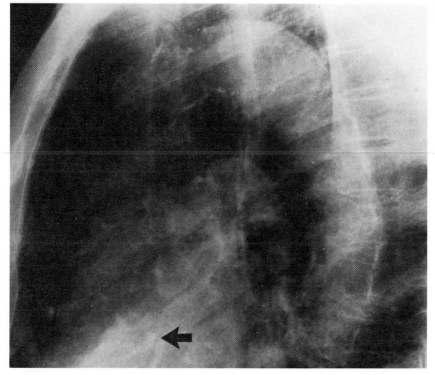

**687, 688  Aortic atheroma, extensive calcification.** Calcification in atheromatous plaques may mimic the linear calcification of syphilitic aortitis when it is as extensive as in this patient but the absence of calcification in the ascending aorta is the clue. Aortic valve calcification is present due to aortic stenosis (lateral view).

**689**

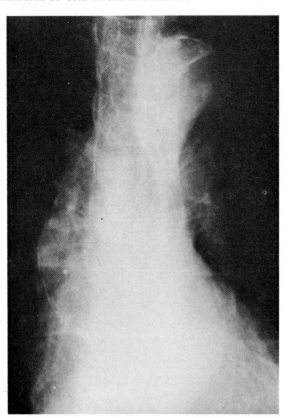

**689, 690 Syphilitic aortitis.** Linear calcification appears in the aortic wall, particularly, and classically, in the ascending aorta. This is best seen in the lateral view and in penetrated postero-anterior films. The aortic wall is a little irregular but no aneurysm is present. Syphilitic aortic valve disease is not accompanied by calcification however, and the calcium in this patient's aortic valve was associated with aortic stenosis of congenital origin—a rare association. The only other condition likely to produce calcification in the ascending aorta is old dissection (see **699, 700**).

**691, 692 Aneurysm of the ascending aorta.** This is caused by syphilis. In the postero-anterior view the bulging saccular aneurysm projects to the right; in the lateral view, it is seen projecting forwards, filling in the 'anterior window' of the mediastinum and touching the anterior chest wall. The arch and descending aorta appear dilated and this is probably due to the generalised fusiform aortic dilatation seen in syphilitic aortitis.

**690**

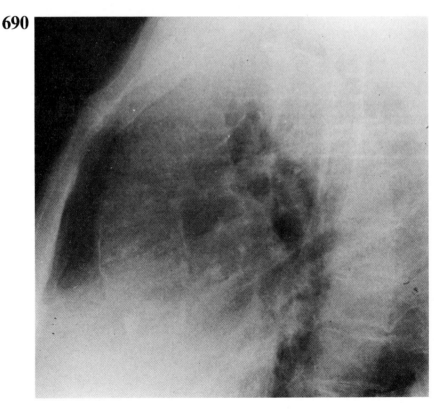

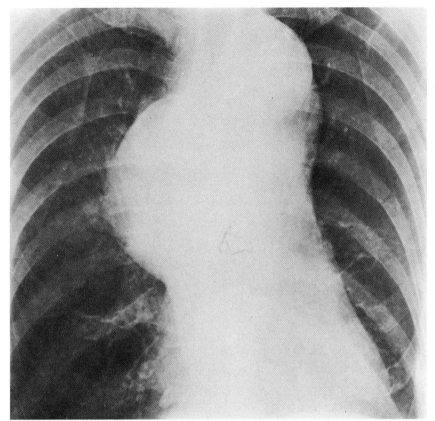

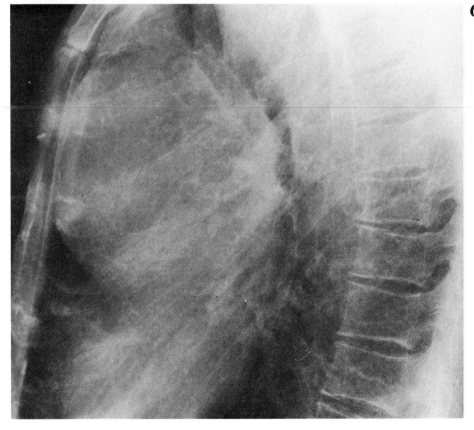

**693**

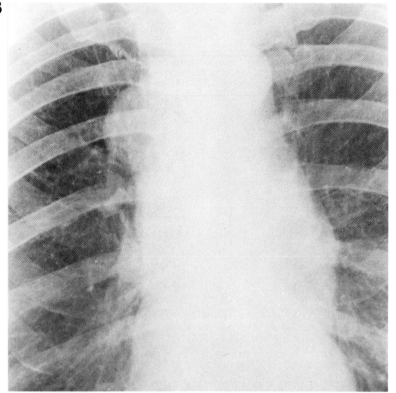

**694**

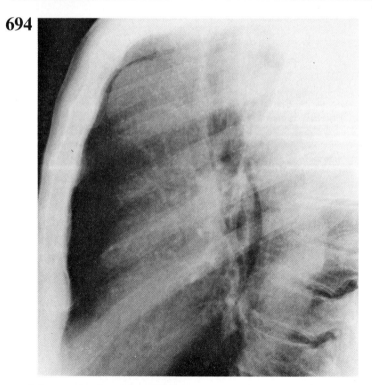

**693, 694   Aneurysm of the proximal aortic arch.** In the postero-anterior view a rounded shadow is seen projecting to the right from the mediastinum. The lateral view identifies it as a forward projection of the aortic arch shadow nearly touching the sternum.

**695**

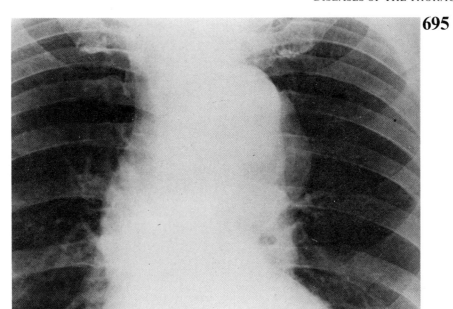

**696**

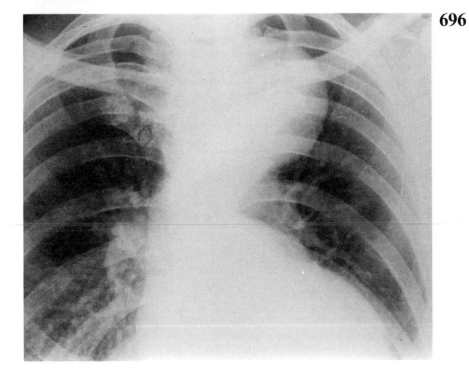

**695, 696 Aneurysm of the aortic arch.** Two examples are shown. Note how the aortic knuckle is distorted.

**697**

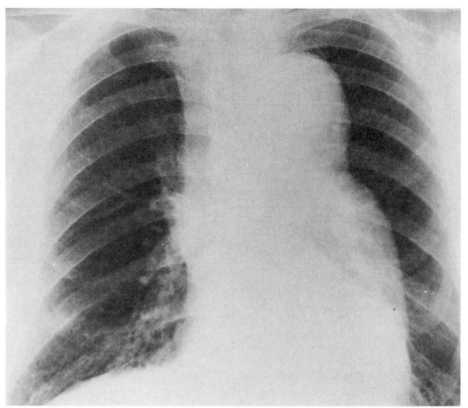

**698**

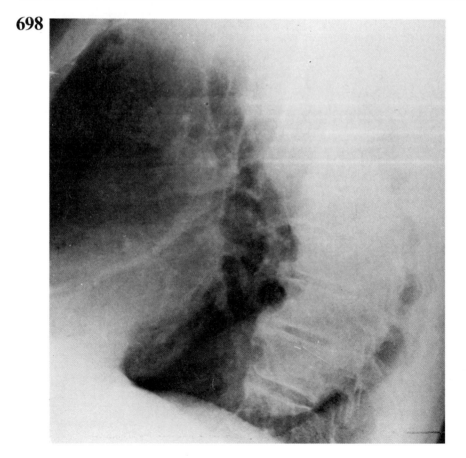

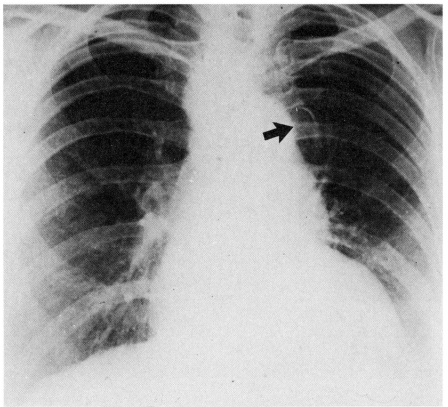

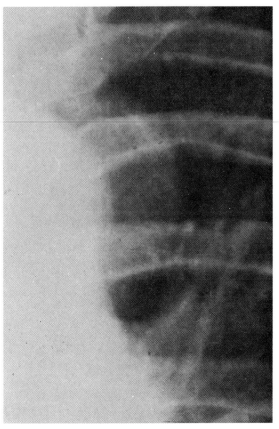

**697, 698  Dissecting aneurysm of the aorta.** The aortic shadow is markedly dilated and irregular in contour. In this instance the dissection has started in the ascending aorta and has spread over the arch to involve the descending aorta.

**699, 700  Old dissecting aortic aneurysm.** The full size film shows a shadow beyond the aortic knuckle with calcification at the edge. This is the false lumen, the calcification occurring after some years in old deposits of clot. The close-up shows the 'double' aortic knuckle at an earlier stage before such extensive calcification had occurred.

**701**

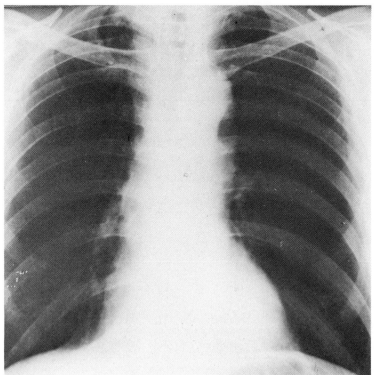

**702**

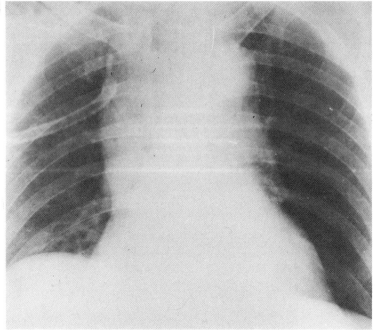

**701–704 Incorrect diagnosis of dissecting aneurysm.** Antero-posterior ward films taken from ill patients who cannot be correctly postured are a notorious trap for the unwary. With an earlier film available for comparison (**701**) the diagnosis of dissecting aneurysm seemed secure when the chest x-ray of this patient with severe chest pain was first seen (**702**). However, as his condition improved, and he was more able to co-operate, subsequent films (**703**, **704**) showed less and less abnormality of the mediastinal shadow, and allowing for the antero-posterior projection, the last of these reveals little difference on pre-admission appearances of the aorta.

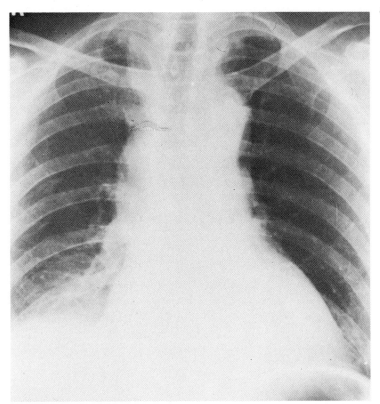

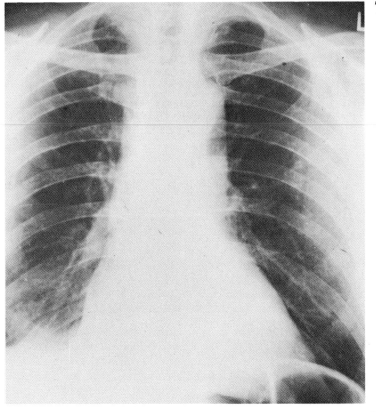

**705**

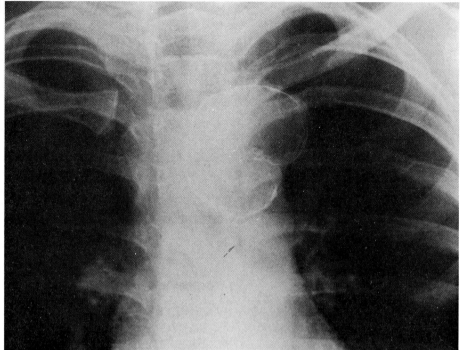

**706**

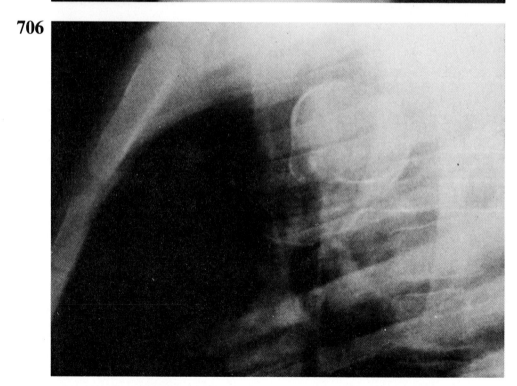

**705, 706  Traumatic aneurysm of the aorta.** A rounded, bilocular shadow is present near the aortic arch. Extensive mural calcification is present. This followed an unsuccessful repair of an aortic coarctation.

**707, 708  Aortic rupture.** The common sites are just below the origin of the left subclavian artery and in the ascending aorta. The injury may be surprisingly silent if the false aneurysm formed is temporarily contained by the adventitia, and is then discovered on routine films to exclude rib fracture. The aortic shadow is enlarged and distorted (but see **701–704**). A pleural effusion may indicate actual rupture (not present in these two examples).

**707**

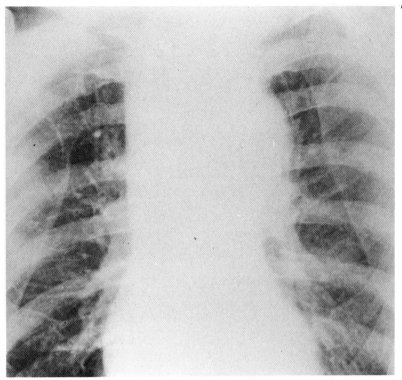

**708**

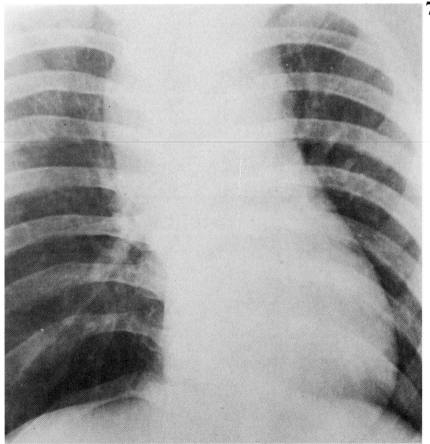

**709**

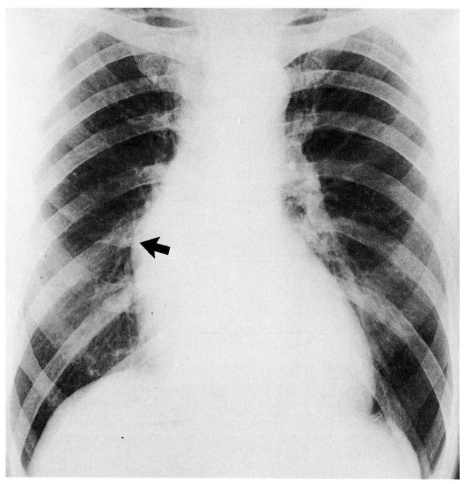

**710**

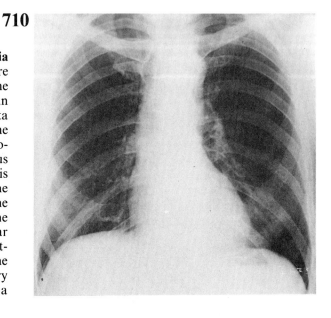

**709, 710   Marfan's syndrome with aortic hypoplasia and severe aortic regurgitation.** In this case of severe aortic regurgitation there is a prominence to the right of the mediastinum which is a little lower than the usual position of the dilated ascending aorta seen in aortic valve disease. Indeed, above it, the ascending aortic shadow is not especially prominent. This is the clue to the presence of enormous dilatation of the aortic root, the extent of which is difficult to appreciate without angiography. The dilatation tends to be confined to the first part of the aorta, which is so much larger than the rest that the angiographic appearances are likened to a pear standing upright. This is emphasised in the post-operative film (**710**) taken after replacement of the ascending aorta with a dacron graft (coronary arteries re-implanted) and the aortic valve with a ball-valve prosthesis.

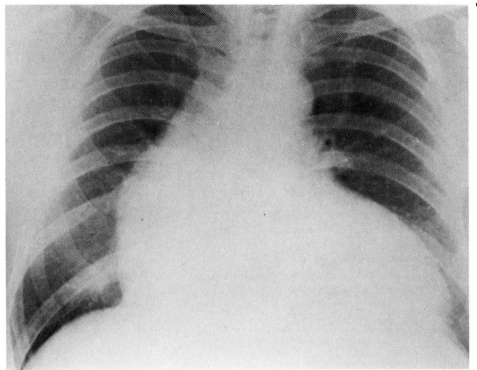

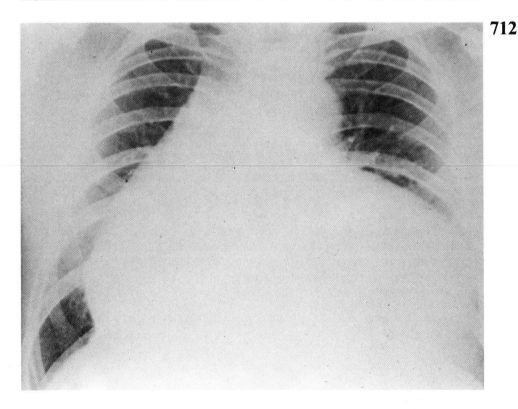

**711, 712 Marfan's syndrome with gross aortic hypoplasia.** See **709**. The two films (which are both postero-anterior views and show true heart size) illustrate the progression of untreated aortic root dilatation in patients with hypoplasia of the Marfan type. The size of the aorta in **712** is astonishing; the huge heart was produced by heart failure.

**713**

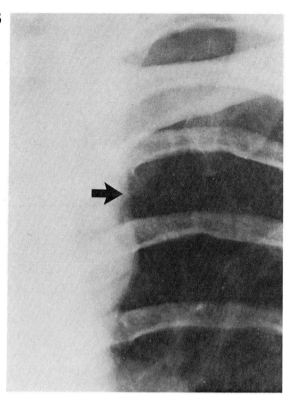

**713–717 Coarctation of the aorta.** The aortic knuckle is abnormal, being elongated into the shadow of the dilated left subclavian artery (**713**). The heart itself may be normal size (**714**), but will enlarge if aortic valve disease is present or heart failure has occurred (**715**). Rib notching (**716**) due to erosion of bone by dilated tortuous intercostal arteries is present in the upper ribs on both sides unless the left subclavian artery is involved in the coarctation itself, when it will be unilateral. The penetrated postero-anterior view (**717**) is useful in demonstrating post-stenotic dilatation beyond the site of constriction (arrowed) or aneurysms of the aorta or intercostals, which are an associated feature in some patients.

**714**

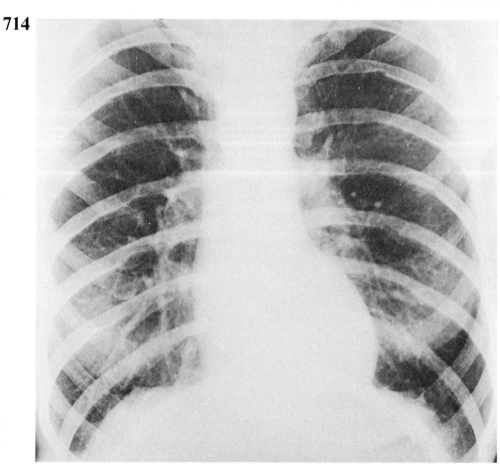

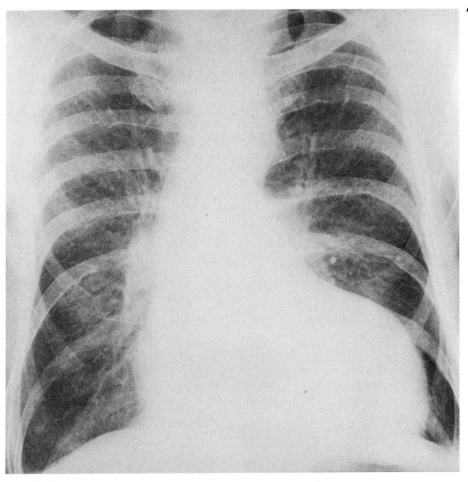

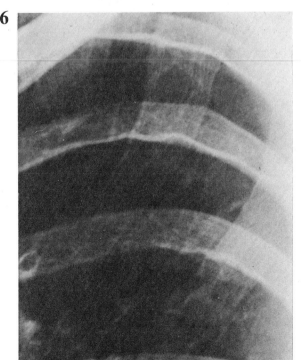

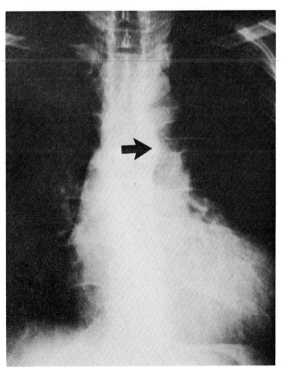

**718**

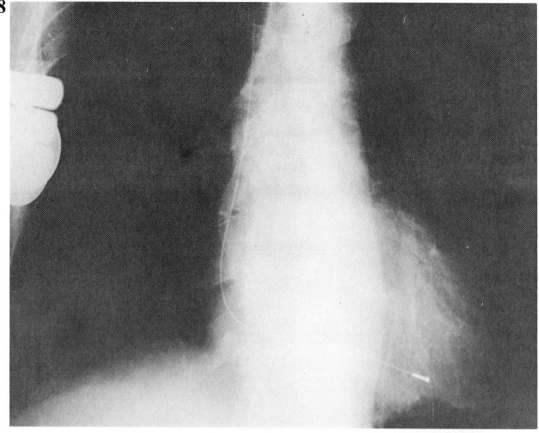

**719**

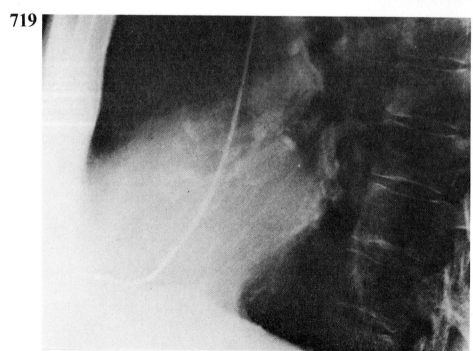

**718, 719   Endocardial pacing, acceptable electrode position.** The tip of the electrode is well out from the midline and points a little downwards. In the lateral view it points forwards. It is lodged in the apex of the right ventricle and is therefore unlikely to move. The size of the loop of catheter left in the right atrium is crucial; it is enough to preserve the position of the tip but insufficient to permit twisting, which would draw the tip backwards. Note the aortic valve calcium.

**720   Endocardial pacing, unsatisfactory electrode position.** The electrode tip is only just beyond the tricuspid valve and there is hardly any loop in the right atrium. While the tip *may* anchor in such a poor position it is unfortunately all too likely to move. The cause of this fault is usually traction on the electrode at the vein entrance but in addition, failure to leave an adequate loop in the atrium at the initial positioning of the electrode may contribute— the lower diaphragm in the upright posture must be allowed for when the catheter is secured.

**721, 722   Endocardial pacing, unsatisfactory electrode position.** Two faults are present. The electrode tip is too high in the right ventricle (well seen on the lateral view) and is likely to be displaced into the pulmonary artery; too great a loop has been left in the right atrium with the risk that this will twist on itself and draw the electrode tip backwards.

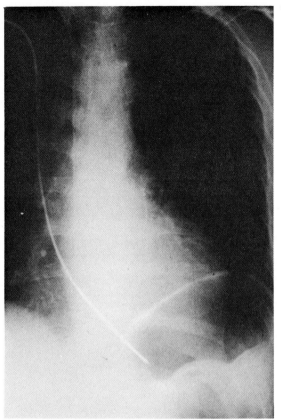

**720**

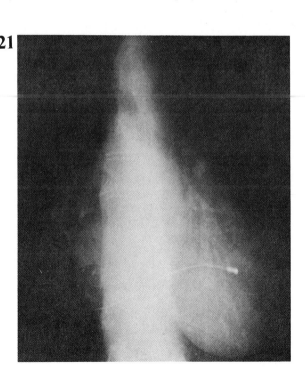

**721**

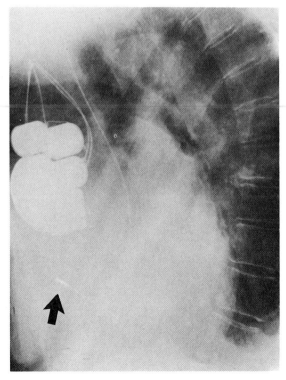

**722**

**723**

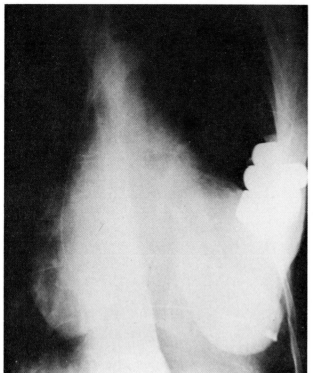

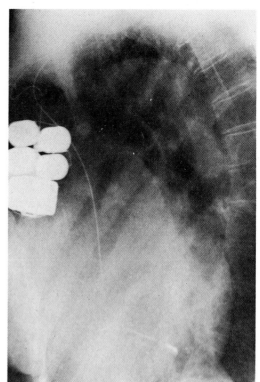

**72**

**725**

**723, 724 Endocardial pacing, inadvertent positioning of the electrode in the coronary sinus.** The postero-anterior view shows the electrode tip apparently well out in the right ventricle, pointing correctly a little downwards. A position so far from the midline is unusual but sometimes seen. The lateral view however shows that the electrode points posteriorly. It has entered the coronary sinus and been passed into the middle cardiac vein which drains the apex of the heart.

**725 Accidental perforation of the heart with a pacing catheter.**

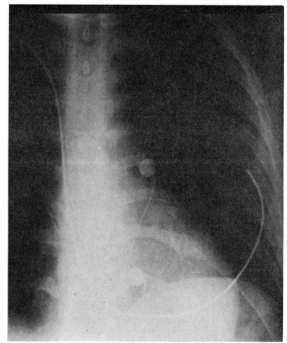

**726   Endocardial pacing catheter looped within the heart.** This remarkable position was achieved by blind insertion of a pacing catheter into the heart without fluoroscopic control. By good fortune a knot in the catheter has been avoided and the tip lodged just inside the tricuspid valve, but such manoeuvres with a semi-stiff catheter have a low success rate and are likely to cause more arrhythmias than they cure; furthermore, accidental perforation of the heart (**725**) is possible. Electrode placement should be under direct vision.

**727, 728   Epicardial pacing.** The spiral-tip, screw-in, pacing electrode has been inserted sub-xiphisternally into the right ventricular myocardium. The pacemaker is in the rectus sheath. The patient was a six-year-old child with heart block following the repair of an atrioventricular cushion defect—hence the cardiac enlargement.

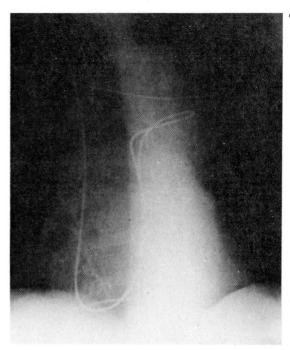

**726**

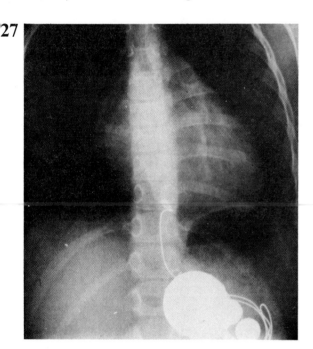

27

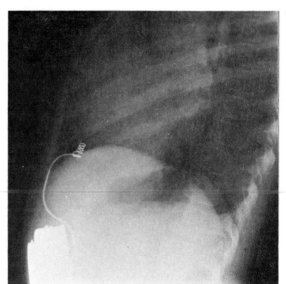

**728**

**729**

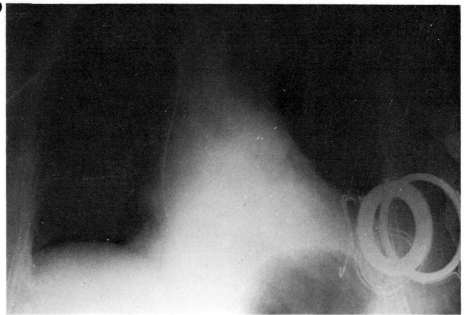

**729  Induction coil pacing.** In this type of pacing an external ring (the thinner one) is connected to a pacemaker which can be worn on a belt or carried in a pocket. This external coil is placed on the skin overlying a second coil which has been buried and which is connected to an electrode (here, epicardial, but alternatively, endocardial). The current passing round the primary coil induces another in the secondary coil and so paces the heart across the intact skin. The primary coil is secured in place by a special harness or more simply with adhesive tape. Note the endocardial catheter within the heart—a temporary electrode used to cover the insertion of the permanent induction coil system.

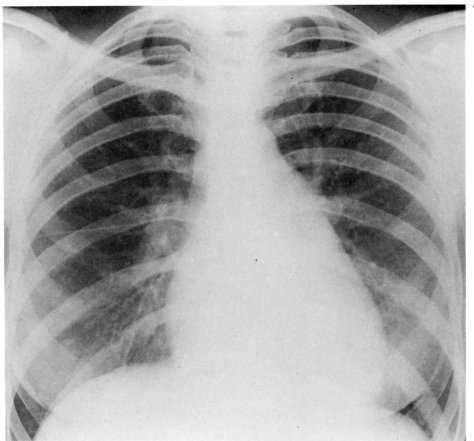

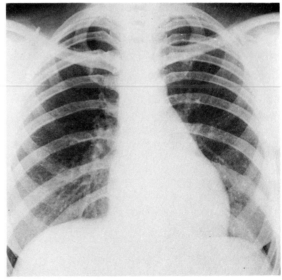

**730, 731  Left atrial myxoma.** Figure **730** shows modest left atrial enlargement, a prominent main pulmonary conus and proximal pulmonary arteries, pulmonary venous congestion, and some interlobar fluid on the right side. The appearances are indistinguishable from ordinary mitral disease and pulmonary hypertension. Figure **731** shows the appearance only two months after the removal of the tumour; there is no definite abnormality.

**732**

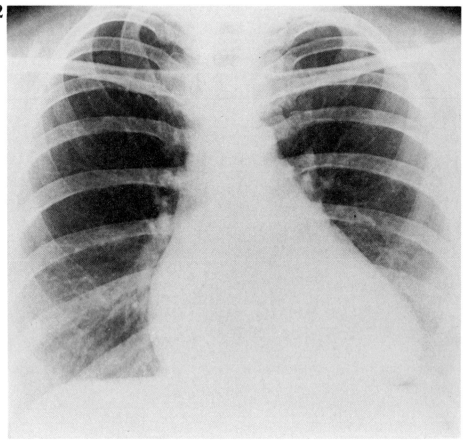

**732–734 Right atrial myxoma.** This, although rarer even than left atrial myxomas may be more readily suspected because isolated tricuspid valve disease is so uncommon. There is cardiac enlargement particularly affecting the right atrium (**732**). Lung vascularity is slightly reduced. The right atrium is almost filled by the tumour (angiogram, **733**). Figure **734** shows the post-operative appearance and emphasises how large the right atrium was beforehand. See electrocardiogram of this patient in **446**.

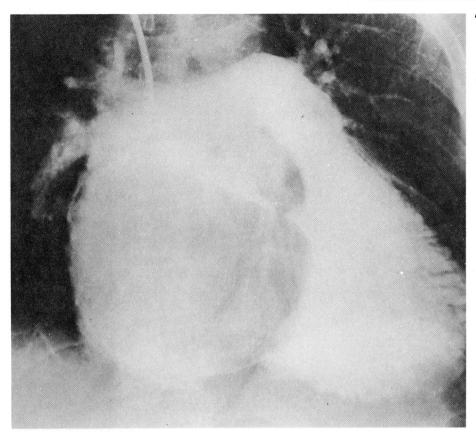

**733**

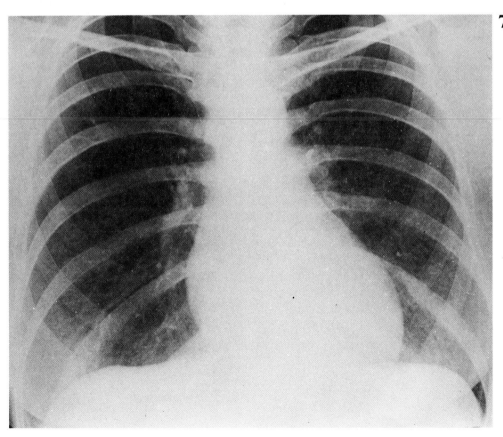

**734**

**735**

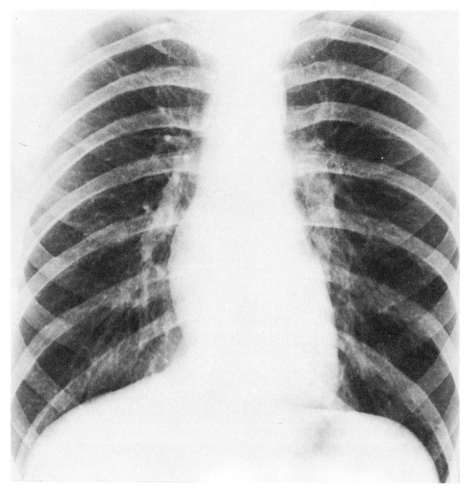

**736**

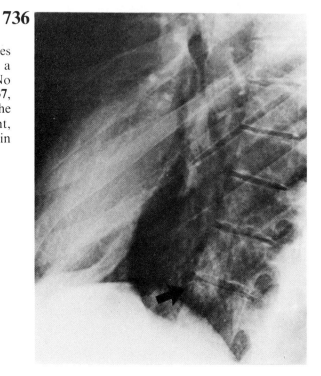

**735–738  Pulmonary arteriovenous fistula.** Figures **735**, **736** show the chest x-ray appearances in a young man with unexplained central cyanosis. No murmur was audible. Pulmonary angiography (**737**, **738**) reveals a large arteriovenous fistula behind the heart in the left lower lobe. With hindsight, abnormal vascularity can be seen in this region in the plain films.

**737**

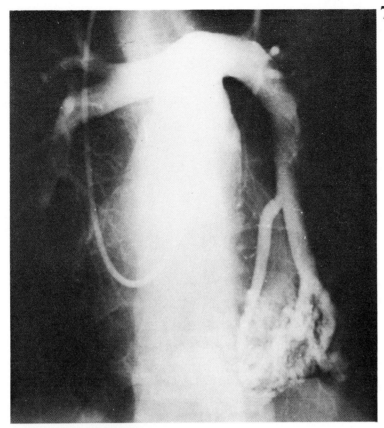

**738**

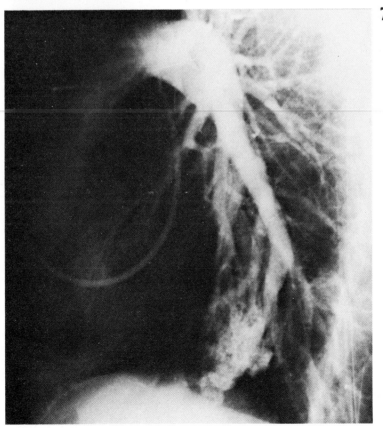

**739**

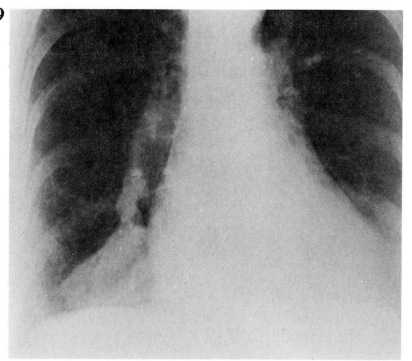

**740**

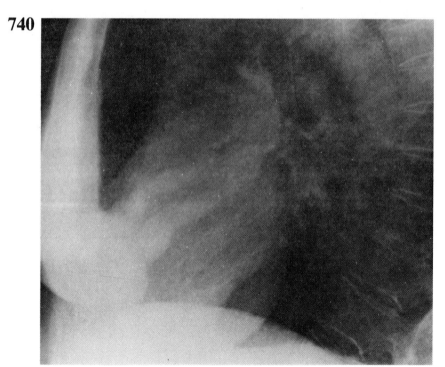

**739, 740  Pulmonary arteriovenous fistula.** Unlike the fistula in **735–738** this pulmonary arteriovenous fistula is readily seen on plain x-rays in the right lower zone. The lateral places it anteriorly. Note the huge vessels feeding and draining it.

**741, 742  Multiple pulmonary arteriovenous fistulae.** The plain x-ray shows several small opacities in the peripheral lung fields, especially on the right, and ill-defined shadowing above the right diaphragm. The pulmonary angiogram reveals these as arteriovenous fistulae. Note the cluster below the level of the right diaphragm.

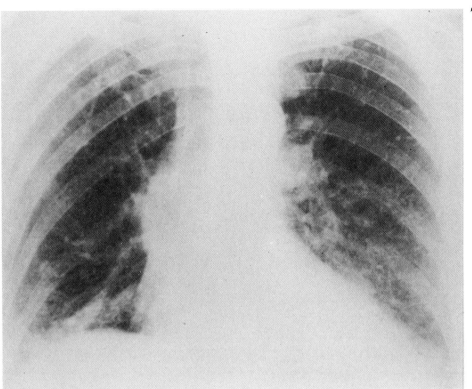

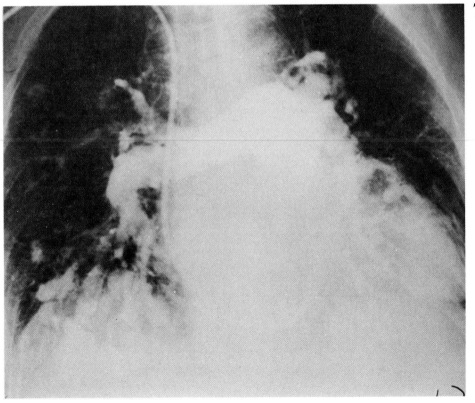

**743**

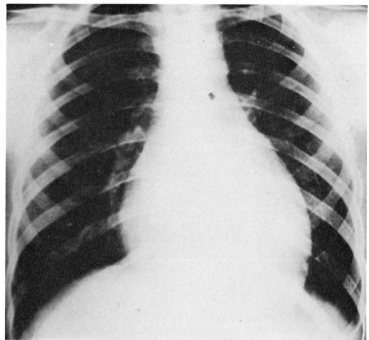

**744**

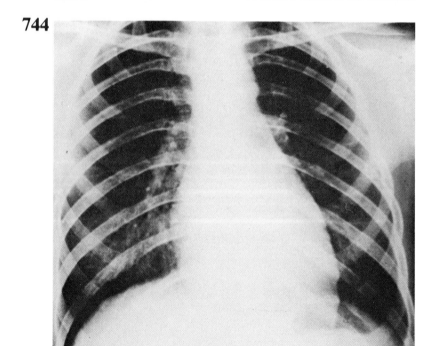

**743, 744 Myxoedema.** The nonspecific cardiac enlargement seen in myoedema may be partly or wholly due to the combination of bradycardia (with its large stroke volume) and pericardial effusion. Figure **743** shows a heart above normal in size in a case before treatment, and **744** the situation after successful therapy with thyroid; the heart is now normal.

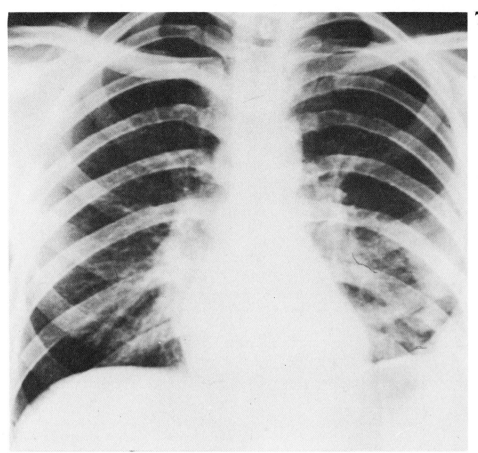

**745    Tricuspid endocarditis.** This may be suspected
in a patient with tricuspid (or pulmonary) valve
disease, with unexplained fever, or frank bacterial
endocarditis, by the appearance of areas of
consolidation due to septic emboli. In **745** the
normal heart shape is accounted for by the absence
of a previous heart lesion in this young man with
acute tricuspid endocarditis; he was a heroin addict.

**746**

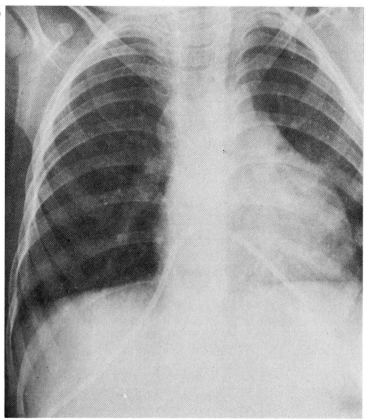

**747**

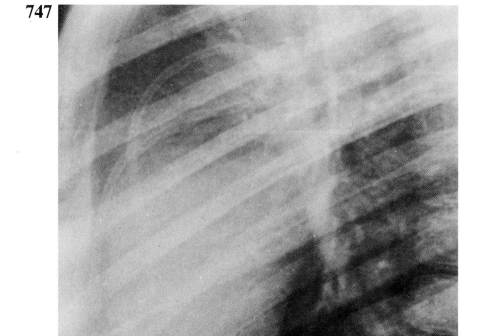

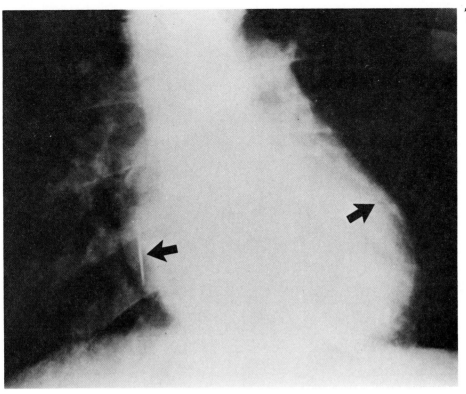

**746, 747  Intracardiac foreign body.** Catheter of a Spitz–Holter valve lost into the vascular system. Initially, it lodged with one end in the right ventricular apex and the other in the liver (**746**). Later, it migrated onwards and became looped in the right ventricle and pulmonary artery (**747**).

**748  Intracardiac foreign body.** A carpenter's nail in the wall of the right atrium. Unlike most intracardiac foreign bodies of this kind, it did not arrive directly through the chest wall, but migrated across the lung after inadvertent, and unnoticed, inhalation. Pericarditis and pericardial constriction resulted—linear calcification at the cardiac apex is just visible.

**749**

**750**

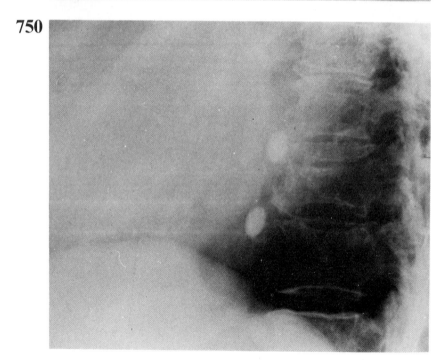

**749, 750 Potassium tablets lodged in the oesophagus.** Slow-release potassium tablets may be held up in the oesophagus and can cause ulceration. Usually, this occurs at the level of the left atrium, particularly when that chamber is enlarged as in mitral valve disease, but in this example, the tablets are lower. They can be seen as rounded opacities on the lateral, but are also just visible at the edge of the spine in the penetrated postero-anterior view (arrows).

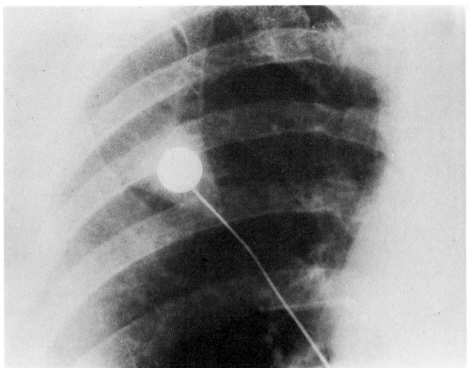

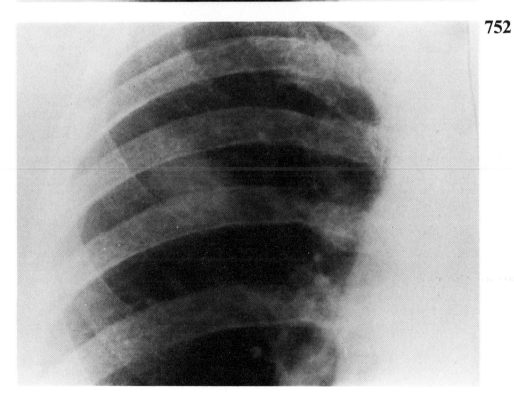

**751, 752 An unlooked-for hazard of cardiac monitoring.** The application of monitoring electrodes to the chest may mask small lesions in the lung, as in this patient with a carcinoma in the right upper zone. The upper film (**751**) shows the electrode in position; after its removal (**752**) the round lesion is revealed.

# INDEX

Aberrant conduction (see also Bundle branch block)
- alternating, in paroxysmal supraventricular tachycardia, 149
- atrial extrasystole and, 108
- atrial fibrillation and, 232–235
- atrial flutter and, 208, 212
- intermittent, in atrial fibrillation, 233, 234
- intermittent, differential diagnosis, 230, 233
- intermittent, in multifocal paroxysmal atrial tachycardia, 147
- intermittent, with reciprocal beats in junctional rhythm, 79
- paroxysmal tachycardia and, 142, 147–149
- QRS pattern, 148
- QRS pattern, varying, 347
- rate dependent, in atrial fibrillation, 234
- rate dependent, in atrial flutter, 212
- rate dependent, at normal heart rates, 342–344
- rate dependent, paradoxical, 345
- rate dependent, in paroxysmal tachycardia, 148, 149
Accelerated idioventricular rhythm, 184–188
Active (negative) pacing electrode, 279
Adolescence
- chest leads, exuberant voltages in, 11
- chest leads, persistent T wave inversion in, 12
- suspended heart syndrome, 15, 468
Adults
- normal heart rate, 17
- normal chest x-ray, 455–458
Agonal rhythm, 192–194
Amyloid disease, 445
Aneurysm
- aortic (see Aortic aneurysm)
- of intercostal arteries, in coarctation, 717
- of right ventricular outflow after correction of Fallot's tetralogy, 637
- of sinus of Valsalva, 565
- ventricular (see Ventricular aneurysm)
Ankylosing spondylitis and aortic regurgitation, 566, 567
Anomalous pulmonary venous drainage (see under Partial and Total pulmonary venous drainage)
Antegrade conduction time
- junctional rhythm, and, 71, 74
- junctional rhythm with capture beats, and, 76–78
Anterior mediastinal window
- aortic aneurysm in, 694
- dermoid cyst in, 493
- obscured by aortic aneurysm, 692
- obscured by enlarged pulmonary artery, 666
Antero-posterior chest dimension, effect on heart size, 477, 478
Antero-posterior chest x-ray, effect on heart size, 463, 469, 470
Antero-septal leads (also see Chest leads)
- QS complexes; significance in left ventricular hypertrophy, 302, 411
- tiny Q waves in, as sign of infarction, 389
Anticlockwise rotation, 7
- and left ventricular hypertrophy, 295
Aorta, hypoplasia (see Marfan's syndrome)
- kyphoscoliosis and, 679, 680
- tortuous, 681–683
Aorta, ascending
- aneurysm (syphilitic), of, 691, 692
- on left cardiac border in corrected transposition, 664
- normal position, 454
- post-stenotic dilatation, of, 554
- prominence in aortic regurgitation, 499, 557
- prominence in Marfan's syndrome, 709–712

- prominence in pulmonary atresia, 638
- prominence in unfolded aorta, 678, 679
- replacement, 710
Aorta, descending
- calcification in, 612
- prominence in unfolded aorta, 678, 679
Aortic aneurysm, 693–696
- coarctation, and, 717
- dissecting, 697–700
- dissecting, mimicked, 701–704
- false, after trauma, 705–708
- fusiform, in syphilis, 691, 692
Aortic arch
- false prominence in kyphoscoliosis, 489
- kinked, 684, 685
- normal position, 454
- right sided, in ventricular septal defect, 622
- right sided, in Fallot's tetralogy, 633
Aortic coarctation (see Coarctation of aorta)
Aortic knuckle
- arch aneurysm and, 695, 696
- calcified, 686
- coarctation and, 713
- double, in dissecting aneurysm, 690, 700
- kinked aortic arch and, 684
- normal position, 454
- small, in atrial septal defect, 642
- small, in atrioventricular canal, 665
Aortic regurgitation
- ankylosing spondylitis and, 566, 567
- ascending aortic prominence in, 499, 557, 559
- cardiomegaly in, 557, 559, 560
- cardiomegaly, absence of, in, 557, 558
- cardiomegaly in acute, 563, 564
- cardiomegaly in, reduction with valve replacement, 559–562
- diastolic overload pattern in, 294, 306
- Marfan's syndrome and, 709, 711, 712
- paraprosthetic, 572, 573
- pulmonary venous congestion in, 557, 563, 564
- sinus of Valsalva aneurysm and, 565
Aortic root, pear-shaped dilatation in Marfan's syndrome, 709
Aortic rupture, false aneurysm in, 707, 708
Aortic stenosis, 554–556
- calcification and, 687–690
- systolic overload pattern and, 294
Aortic valve calcification, 568, 569, 687–690
- and mitral valve calcification, 609
Aortic valve disease (see also Aortic stenosis and Aortic regurgitation)
- bacterial endocarditis and, 563, 564
- cardiac silhouette in, suggesting additional mitral disease, 608
- coarctation and, 715
Aortic valve, position, 568–571, 609, 613–617
Aortic valve replacement, 559–562, 570, 571
- ascending aortic replacement and, 710
- mitral and tricuspid replacement and, 613–617
- prosthetic valve dehiscence, 572, 573
Aorto-pulmonary infilling in patent ductus arteriosus, 667
Asystole, 195, 196
- in hyperkalaemia, 435
Atheroma, calcification and, 687, 688
Athlete's heart, 486
Atrial capture (see Atrial re-entry and capture)
Atrial extrasystoles, 100-112, 122
- aberrant conduction, and, 108

– aberrant conduction of, masking infarction, 351
– blocked, 109
– blocked, mimicking sino-atrial block, 110
– blocked, initiating atrial flutter, 210
– compensatory pause and, 100–102
– coupled, 111, 112
– coupling time in, 104
– early, 103, 109
– early, triggering atrial fibrillation, 235
– early (blocked), triggering atrial flutter, 210
– late, 102
– low, 103, 119
– mimicking junctional extrasystoles, 103, 119
– mimicking ventricular extrasystoles, 108
– multifocal, 104
– P waves in, 100
– PR interval in, 100, 103
– QRS contour in, 100
– QRS contour, variable, 106, 107, 111
– ? sino-atrial, 105
Atrial fibrillation, 215–235
– aberrant conduction in, 232, 235
– aberrant conduction, intermittent and, 233, 234
– aberrant conduction in, mimicking ventricular tachy-cardia, 234
– aberrant conduction in, rate dependent, 344
– aberrant conduction in, paradoxical rate dependent, 345
– atrioventricular dissociation in, 220
– digitalis toxicity in, 220
– Ebstein's anomaly and, 448
– f waves in, 215, 219, 220, 223
– f waves, absence of, 216
– flutter-fibrillation, 221
– heart block and, 219, 229
– heart size, effect on, 481, 482
– idioventricular bradycardia and, 193
– junctional escape beats in, 230, 344
– junctional escape rhythm and, 220, 228
– mimicked by muscle tremor, 37
– mimicking ventricular tachycardia, 172, 234
– onset with atrial extrasystole, 235
– in pericarditis, 416–418
– sick sinus syndrome and, 67
– termination of, 235
– thyrotoxicosis and, 218
– V1 in, 223
– ventricular escape beats in, 231
– ventricular extrasystoles in, 224
– ventricular extrasystoles, bidirectional, in 98, 227
– ventricular extrasystoles, coupled, in, 225, 229
– ventricular extrasystoles, multiform unifocal, in, 226, 228
– ventricular response, irregular, 215
– ventricular response, rapid, mimicking supraventri-cular tachycardia, 218
– ventricular response, regular, in heart block, 219
– ventricular response, regular, in junctional rhythm, 220, 228
– ventricular response, slow, 216, 217, 225–227
– Wolff–Parkinson–White syndrome and, 172
Atrial flutter, 199–214
– 12 lead electrocardiogram, 213, 214
– aberrant conduction in, 208, 212
– aberrant conduction and, mimicking ventricular tachycardia, 212
– carotid sinus massage, effect of, 211
– Ebstein's anomaly and, 448
– F waves, 199, 203, 213, 214, 222
– heart block and, 209
– impure, 221

– onset with blocked atrial extrasystole, 210
– sick sinus syndrome and, 67, 68
– V1 in, 222
Atrial flutter, ventricular response
– 1:1, 208
– 2:1, 200, 201
– 3:1, 207
– 4:1, 203
– 2:1, alternating with 4:1, 204
– 6:1, 206
– 8:1, 206
– 10:1, 206
– irregular, 205
– paired, 204
– varying, 202, 204, 206, 207
Atrial infarction, 413
Atrial pacing, 288
Atrial parasystole, 125
Atrial re-entry and capture
– heart block and, 274
– junctional extrasystoles and, 114, 121, 122
– junctional rhythm and, 72, 73
– junctional tachycardia and, 134, 142
– reciprocal beats (junctional rhythm), 79
– reciprocating tachycardia and, 158–160
– ventricular extrasystoles and, 83
Atrial septal defect, secundum, 642–647
– closure, effect of, 645, 646
– Eisenmenger syndrome and, 623
– Lutembacher syndrome, 648, 649
– partial anomalous pulmonary venous drainage and, 650
– right bundle branch block (incomplete) in, 329
Atrial standstill (see Sinus arrest)
Atrial tachycardia (see Paroxysmal tachycardia)
Atrial T wave, 23
– altered in atrial infarction, 413
Atrially triggered pacing, 287
Atrioventricular block, transient with carotid sinus massage
– in atrial flutter, 211
Atrioventricular canal (see Atrioventricular cushion defect)
Atrioventricular cushion defect
– atrioventricular canal, 665, 666
– multifascicular block in, 340, 341
– ostium primum defect, 642, 643
– repair followed by heart block, 727
Atrioventricular dissociation
– accelerated idioventricular rhythm, and, 186, 187
– atrial fibrillation, and, 220
– junctional rhythm, and, 75–78
– simultaneous junctional and sinus bradycardias, and, 129
– simultaneous atrial and junctional tachycardias, and, 153–155
– ventricular tachycardia, and, 177, 179
Atrioventricular junctional (see Junctional)
Atrioventricular junction
– concealed retrograde conduction, with interpolated junctional extrasystoles, 120
– concealed retrograde conduction, with interpolated ventricular extrasystoles, 89, 90
– concealed retrograde conduction in junctional rhythm, 76–78
Atrioventricular junction, dual conducting pathways manifest in,
– complete heart block, 274
– Lown–Ganong–Levine syndrome, 171
– reciprocal beats, 79, 80
– reciprocating tachycardia, 158, 159, 160
– Wolff–Parkinson–White syndrome, 164, 170

Atrioventricular junction, refractoriness
– with extrasystoles, 100, 103, 109, 110, 210
– with tachyarrhythmias, 152, 160, 233
Atropine
– in sinus bradycardia, 126
– in partial heart block, 256, 257
Axis (see under P, QRS and T)
Axis diagram, 39

Balanced ventricular hypertrophy, 319 (also see Biventricular hypertrophy)
Ball valve prosthesis
– aortic, 561, 562
– aortic, dehisced, 572, 573
– mitral, 603, 604
– mitral, dehisced, 605
– mitral and aortic, 613–615
– mitral, aortic and tricuspid, 616, 617
Balloon septostomy, 676, 677
Banding of pulmonary artery (see Pulmonary artery)
Barium swallow in left atrial enlargement, 504
Bat's wing shadow in pulmonary oedema, 511
Beta blockade in atrial fibrillation, 217
Bidirectional extrasystoles, 95, 98, 227
Bidirectional tachycardia, 151
Bifascicular block, 332–337 (see also Left anterior and posterior hemiblock and Right and Left bundle branch block)
– atrioventricular cushion defects and, 340
– left bundle branch block and PR prolongation, 332
– left ventricular hypertrophy and, 335
– myocardial infarction and, 352, 353
– right bundle branch block and left anterior hemiblock, 334, 335, 340, 352, 353
– right bundle branch block and left posterior hemiblock, 336, 337
– right bundle branch block and PR prolongation, 333, 353
– ? trifascicular block, 353
Bigeminal rhythm
– atrial flutter, and, 204
– coupled atrial extrasystoles, 111, 112
– coupled junctional extrasystoles, 112, 119
– coupled ventricular extrasystoles, 87, 95, 225, 228, 229, 260
– escape capture bigeminy, 70
– partial heart block, 240, 260
Biventricular enlargement
– atrioventricular canal, and, 665, 666
– mitral regurgitation, and, 579, 580, 595–600
– myocarditis, and, 547, 548
– triple valve disease, and, 610–612
– ventricular septal defect, and, 660, 661
Biventricular hypertrophy, 59, 317, 318
Bradycardia
– accelerated idioventricular rhythm, relative, 184–186
– agonal, 192–198
– atrial fibrillation and complete heart block, 219
– atrial flutter with high conduction ratios, 205
– atrial flutter with complete heart block, 209
– carotid sinus massage producing, 66
– complete heart block, 263–275
– congenital heart block, 276
– junctional, 128, 129
– junctional rhythm, 71–75, 220
– reflex, after Valsalva's manoeuvre, 26
– shifting pacemaker in the sinus node, 22
– sinus, 126, 127, 129
– sinus arrhythmia, during marked, 20
Bronchus, left main, elevated in left atrial enlargement, 502

Bundle branch block (see also Left and Right bundle branch block, and Aberrant conduction)
– masking (potential) by Wolff–Parkinson–White syndrome, 165
– mimicked by recording at double speed, 35
– mimicked by Wolff–Parkinson–White syndrome, 165–170
– rate-dependent and paradoxical rate dependent (see Aberrant conduction)

Calcification in
– aortic (false) aneurysm, 705, 706
– aortic atheroma, 612, 687, 688
– aortic knuckle, 686
– aortic valve, 568, 569, 687–690
– dermoid cyst, 491–493
– dissecting aneurysm, 689, 699
– left atrial appendage in mitral valve disease, 585
– left atrial wall in mitral valve disease, 584
– left coronary artery, 518
– left ventricular aneurysm, 525, 526
– mitral ring, 601, 602
– mitral valve, 586, 587, 588, 589
– mitral and aortic valves, 609
– myocardial infarction, 532–534
– patent ductus arteriosus, 624
– pericardial constriction, 541, 542
– syphilitic aortitis, 689, 690
Capture beats (also see Atrial re-entry and capture)
– complete heart block, and, 271, 272
– junctional rhythm, and, 76–78
– ventricular tachycardia, and, 179
Carbon dioxide replacing pericardial fluid, 539, 540
Carcinoma of lung masked by monitoring electrode, 751, 752
Cardiac arrest, 195–197
Cardiac catheter
– in kinked aortic arch, 685
– in left superior vena cava in supracardiac total anomalous pulmonary venous drainage, 655
– in patent ductus arteriosus, 669
– induced extrasystole terminating reciprocating tachycardia, 161
Cardiac massage artefact, 197
Cardiac silhouette
– loss of, with destroyed left lung, 496
– loss of detail in pericardial effusion, 535, 539
– normal, 454–465
– normal, in aortic stenosis, 555
– normal, in Fallot's tetralogy, 636
Cardiomegaly (see under Heart size)
Cardiomyopathy, congestive
– cardiomegaly, 490, 552, 553
– non-specific electrocardiogram, 443
– in rheumatic heart disease, 581, 582
Cardiomyopathy, hypertrophic, 307, 308, 549, 550
Cardiothoracic ratio, 455
Carina (main) widening in left atrial enlargement, 502
Carotid sinus hypersensitivity, 66
Carotid sinus massage
– atrial flutter, and, 211
– causing sinus arrest, 66
– partial heart block, and, 258
– paroxysmal tachycardia, and, 157
Catecholamine release in subarachnoid haemorrhage, 429
Cerebral haemorrhage, ST–T and U wave changes, 433, 434
Chest leads
– anticlockwise rotation, and, 7
– clockwise rotation, and, 6

– dextrocardia, and, 28, 29
– dominant S wave pattern in cor pulmonale, 46, 313
– dominant S wave pattern in right ventricular hypertrophy, 309–313
– high, value of in diagnosis of infarction, 396
– hypercalcaemia, and, 439
– left ventricular hypertrophy, and, 294–302
– normal, in left ventricular hypertrophy, 300, 305
– notched T waves in childhood in, 9
– patterns of right ventricular hypertrophy in, 309–313
– transitional zone in, 6
Childhood
– chest x-ray, normal, in, 463–466
– electrocardiogram, normal, in, 8–11
– heart rate in, 17
– PR interval in, 341
– right ventricular hypertrophy in, 315
Chordal rupture of mitral valve, 593, 594
Clockwise rotation, 6
– and left ventricular hypertrophy, 296, 301, 305
Coarctation of the aorta
– aneurysm of aorta following repair, 705, 706
– chest x-ray, 713–717
– isolated dextrocardia and, 674
– mimicked by kinked aortic arch, 684, 685
Coeur-en-sabot in Fallot's tetralogy, 633, 634
Combined arrhythmias
– bradycardias, 129
– tachycardias, 153–155
Compensatory post-extrasystolic pause
– absence in interpolated extrasystoles, 89, 120
– atrial extrasystoles and, 100–102
– changing heart rate and, 84, 101, 122
– effect on rate-dependent bundle branch block, 343
– inducing demand pacing, 286
– junctional extrasystoles and, 114, 115
– sinus arrhythmia and, 84
– ventricular extrasystoles and, 81
Conduction
– concealed retrograde (see Atrioventricular junction)
– occasional normal in complete heart block, 271, 272
Coronary artery
– calcification in, 518
– left, anomalous origin of, 452
Coronary heart disease (see Myocardial ischaemia and infarction)
Coronary sinus
– inadvertent pacing in, 723, 724
– rhythm, 74
Cor pulmonale
– electrocardiogram mimicking left ventricular hypertrophy, 313
– left axis deviation in, 313
– right ventricular hypertrophy in, 46, 313
– subacute, 422, 423
Corrected transposition (see Transposition)
Cottage loaf shadow in total anomalous pulmonary venous drainage, 654, 655
Coupling (see Bigeminal rhythm)
Coupling time, 87, 91, 93–95, 99, 104, 118, 183
– absence of fixed, in parasystole, 123, 124
– long, in escape beats (see under Junctional and Ventricular escape beats)
Critical rate in rate dependent bundle branch block, 342
Crying, effect on heart size, 484, 485

Delta waves (see Wolff–Parkinson–White syndrome)
Demand pacing (see Pacing)
Dermoid cyst mimicking cardiac enlargement, 491–493
Dextrocardia
– electrocardiogram, 28, 29

– isolated, 673, 674
– mimicked by incorrect lead connection, 31, 32
– mimicking myocardial infarction or ischaemia, 28
– with situs inversus, 672
Diaphragm, high
– effect on cardiothoracic ratio, 471
– left, in dextrocardia, 672
– with obesity, 467
Diastolic film
– effect on heart size, 474
– identified by ball-valve prostheses, 615
Diastolic overload pattern, 306
Digitalis effect, 441
Digitalis
– effect on ventricular rate in atrial fibrillation, 216, 217
Digitalis toxicity causing
– bidirectional tachycardia, 151
– bidirectional ventricular extrasystoles, 95, 98, 227
– coupled ventricular extrasystoles, 87, 225–227
– heart block and coupled ventricular extrasystoles, 229
– junctional rhythm in atrial fibrillation, 220, 228
– linked ventricular extrasystoles, 96, 97
– multiform unifocal ventricular extrasystoles, 93, 95
– paroxysmal atrial tachycardia with block, 143, 144
Diuretics, effect of
– on Kerley's lines, 508, 509
– on pleural effusion in heart failure, 515–517
– on pulmonary venous congestion, 506, 507, 574

Ebstein's anomaly
– chest x-ray, 641
– electrocardiogram, 447, 448
Eisenmenger syndrome, 622–624
Egg shaped heart in transposition of the great arteries, 677, 678
Electrical alternans (see also Bidirectional extrasystoles and tachycardia and Aberrant conduction, alternating)
– in paroxysmal tachycardia, 150
– in pericardial effusion, 417
Electrical positions, 1–6, 15, 24, 25
Encysted effusion in heart failure, 516
Endocardial pacing (see Pacing)
Endocarditis, infective
– aortic regurgitation in, 563, 564
– on prosthetic valve, 572, 573, 605
– tricuspid, 745
Entrance block
– around sino-atrial node in complete heart block with retrograde atrial conduction, 274
– in parasystole, 123
Epicardial pacing (see Pacing)
Escape beats (see under Junctional and Ventricular)
Escape capture bigeminy, 70
Exercise, effect of
– in differential diagnosis of two types of partial heart block, 256, 257
– on junctional escape in sinus arrhythmia, 20
– on non-respiratory sinus arrhythmia, 21
– on sinus arrhythmia, 19
– on sinus bradycardia, 126
– on sickling pattern, 13, 14
– on sinus rhythm, 130
Exercise test, 376
Exit block
– during pacing, 289, 291
– in parasystole, 123
– with competing foci in complete heart block, 268, 269
Expiratory film, effect on heart size, 463, 471, 472
Extrasystoles (see under Atrial, Junctional and Ventricular)

f waves (see Atrial fibrillation)
F waves (see Atrial flutter)
Fallot's tetralogy
– aneurysm of right ventricular outflow tract following repair of, 637
– chest x-ray, 633–636
– unilateral plethora following Waterston's operation, 671
False aneurysm following aortic rupture, 707, 708
Figure-of-eight appearance in supracardiac total anomalous pulmonary venous drainage, 654, 655
Fixed rate pacing (see Pacing)
Food, effect on T waves, 27
Foreign body, intracardiac, 746–748
Fusion beats
– accelerated idioventricular rhythm, and, 184, 185, 188
– pacing, during, 283, 285, 286
– parasystole, and, 123
– sinus and junctional escape beat, 157
– ventricular parasystole, and, 124
– ventricular tachycardia, and, 178, 179
– Wolff–Parkinson–White syndrome complex, 165

Greater fissure thickened in pleural effusion, 516

Haemosiderosis, pulmonary, in mitral valve disease, 590–592
Heart block, complete, 263–276
– atrial fibrillation, and, 219, 229
– atrial flutter, and, 209
– atrial irregularity in, 266, 267
– competition for control by two foci in, 268, 269, 274
– conducted beats in, 271, 272
– congenital, 276, 451
– corrected transposition and, 451
– Ebstein's anomaly and, 448
– intermittent, 285
– irregular idioventricular pacemaker in, 270
– irregular ventricular rate in, 265, 268–272
– mimicked by grade 2 block, 251
– mimicked by partial block and junctional escape, 262
– mimicking partial block, 273
– myocardial infarction, and, 275, 386
– pacing, and, 279–285 (and see Pacing)
– paroxysmal tachycardia, and, 143, 144
– precipitated by an increase in atrial rate in type 2 partial block, 257
– post-operative, 727
– QRS complex in, 263–266
– quinidine, and, 440
– retrograde conduction to atria in, 274
– Stokes–Adams attacks in, 277, 278
– supernormal conduction in, 272
– unstable pacemaker mimicking Wenckebach block, 270
– ventricular extrasystoles, and, 265
Heart block, grade 1, 236–239 (see also PR interval)
– before Stokes–Adams attack, 278
– changing PR interval in, 238, 239
– merging into Wenckebach block, 246
– paroxysmal atrial tachycardia, and, 136
Heart block, grade 2, type 1 (Wenckebach), 240–246 (see also Wenckebach periods)
– 2:1 block in, 243
– atrial rate, effect of increase in, 256
– atrioventricular dissociation with capture beats, and, 78
– changing grade, 246
– escape beats in, 261
– escape beats in, mimicking complete block, 262
– paroxysmal atrial tachycardia, and, 140, 145
Heart block, grade 2, type 2, 247–262

– 2:1, 249, 250
– 3:1, 252–254
– 4:1, 255
– atrial rate, effect of change in, 257, 258
– before Stokes–Adams attack, 277
– escape beats, and, 433
– extrasystole, precipitated by, 259
– mimicked by complete block, 273
– mimicking complete block, 251
– occasional dropped beats only, 247, 248
– P–P intervals in, 249–251
– paroxysmal tachycardia, and, 137, 139, 141
– paroxysmal tachycardia, retrograde conduction in, 142
– ventricular extrasystoles, and, 260
Heart, displaced by
– destroyed lung, 496
– partial absence of pericardium, 543
– scimitar syndrome, 653
Heart failure
– anomalous left coronary artery origin, and, 452
– aortic valve disease, and, 556, 557, 563–565, 711, 712
– cardiomyopathy, and, 552
– coarctation, and, 715
– cor pulmonale subacute and, 422, 423
– endocarditis, followed by, 563–564
– encysted effusion, in, 515–517
– Kerley's lines, in, 508, 556
– left ventricular aneurysm, and, 522
– mitral chordal rupture, and, 593, 594
– mitral regurgitation, and, 603, 605
– mitral regurgitation, iatrogenic, and, 598–600
– muscular dystrophy, and, 551
– myocardial infarction, and, 519, 529, 530
– myocarditis, and, 547
– pleural effusion, in, 514
– prosthetic valve dehiscence, and, 573, 605
– pulmonary oedema, 510–513
– pulmonary venous congestion (see under separate heading)
– sinus of Valsalva aneurysm, and, 565
– transposition of great arteries, and, 676
– ventricular septal defect, and; acquired, 531, congenital, 662
Heart, herniation of, in absent left pericardium, 543
Heart size
– antero-posterior view, effect of, 469, 470
– aortic regurgitation, and, 557–564, 709–712
– aortic regurgitation, acutely acquired, and, 563, 564
– aortic stenosis, and, 554–556
– aortic valve replacement, and, 559–562
– atrial fibrillation, and, 481, 482
– atrial septal defect, and, 642–644
– atrial septal defect, closure and, 646
– atrioventricular canal, and, 665, 666
– coarctation, and, 714, 715
– congestive cardiomyopathy, and, 552, 553
– crying, and, 484, 485
– Ebstein's anomaly, and, 641
– Eisenmenger syndrome, and, 622–624
– Fallot's tetralogy, and, 633–636
– false increase in (see antero-posterior view, crying, flat chest, inadequate inspiration, kyphoscoliosis, mediastinal masses, obesity, pericardial fat pad, sternal depression, straight back syndrome, and systolic/diastolic difference, effect on heart size)
– flat chest, and, 477, 478
– hypertrophic cardiomyopathy, and, 549, 550
– idiopathic dilatation of the pulmonary artery, 627
– inadequate inspiration, and, 471–472
– kyphoscoliosis, and, 487–489

– left ventricular aneurysm, and, 522–524, 529–530
– Lutembacher's syndrome, and, 648
– Maladie de Roger, and, 657
– Marfan's syndrome, and, 709–712
– mediastinal masses, and, 490–493
– mitral regurgitation, and, 579, 580
– mitral regurgitation, acutely acquired, and, 594
– mitral stenosis, and, 576
– mitral valve replacement, and, 604
– mitral valvotomy, and, 577, 578
– mitral valvotomy, unsuccessful, and, 596–598
– multivalvar disease, and, 607–612
– muscular dystrophy, and, 551
– myocarditis, and, 547
– myocardial infarction, failure following, and, 519
– myxoedema, and, 743, 744
– myxoma, left atrial, and, 730
– myxoma, right atrial, and, 732
– patent ductus arteriosus, and, 667, 668
– pericardial effusion, and, 535–540
– pericardial fat, and, 467, 483
– pulmonary atresia, and, 638, 639
– pulmonary embolism, and, 618, 619
– pulmonary hypertension, thromboembolic, and, 620, 621
– pulmonary regurgitation, post-operative, and, 630
– pulmonary stenosis, and, 628–629
– rheumatic cardiomyopathy, and, 581, 582
– sinus of Valsalva aneurysm rupture, and, 565
– sternal depression, and, 475, 476
– straight back syndrome, and, 479, 480
– systolic/diastolic difference in, 473, 474
– total anomalous pulmonary venous drainage, and, 654–656
– transposition of great arteries, and, 676, 677
– tricuspid atresia, and, 640
– tricuspid valve disease, and, 606
– ventricular septal defect, and, 658–662, 664, 673
– ventricular septal defect, acquired, and, 531
– ventricular septal defect, banded and, 663
Heart, unusual mobility of, in absent left pericardium, 545
Hemiblock (see under Left anterior and Left posterior hemiblock)
Hiatus hernia, 490
Homograft, frame mounted, 594
Horizontal heart, 1
– and left ventricular hypertrophy, 297
Hypercalcaemia, 439
Hyperkalaemia, 435
Hypertrophic cardiomyopathy (see under Cardiomyopathy)
Hyperventilation, effect on T waves, 27
Hypocalcaemia, 435, 438
Hypokalaemia, 437
Hypoplasia of right lower lobe in scimitar syndrome, 653
Hypothermia, 427, 428

Indifferent (positive) pacing electrode, 279
Idioventricular bradycardia
– in agonal rhythm, 192, 193, 195, 196
– severe hypothermia, 428
Idioventricular pacemaker in complete heart block
– competing, 268, 269, 274
– unstable, 270
Idioventricular rhythm, accelerated, 184–188
Indeterminate axis, 52, 53
Induction coil pacing (see Pacing)
Infants
– normal heart rate in, 17
– thymic shadow, 464

Infarction (see Myocardial and Pulmonary infarction)
Inferior leads
– doubtful Q waves, in, 25, 401, 402
– in left ventricular hypertrophy, 298
Intermediate electrical position, 3
Interpolated extrasystoles (see under type)
Intracardiac electrocardiogram, 30

J waves in hypothermia, 427, 428
James tract, in Lown–Ganong–Levine syndrome, 171
Junction, atrioventricular (see Atrioventricular junction)
Junctional bradycardia, 128
– combined with sinus bradycardia, 129
– dissociated and agonal, 194
– hyperkalaemia, and, 435
– hypothermia, and, 427
– irregular, 129
– sick sinus syndrome, and, 67
Junctional escape
– atrial fibrillation, and, 230, 344
– escape capture bigeminy, and, 70
– partial heart block, and, 261, 262, 433
– QRS contour variation of, 20, 261
– sinus arrest, and, 63, 65
– sinus arrhythmia, and, 20, 21
– sinus rhythm, and, 112
Junctional extrasystoles, 113–122
– compensatory pause, and, 114, 115
– coupled, 119
– coupling time in, 118
– interpolated, 120
– mimicking atrial extrasystoles, 103, 119
– multifocal, 118
– P waves, and, 114, 115
– post-extrasystolic T wave change, 117
– QRS contour of, 113–116, 118, 120, 122
– reciprocal beat, and, 121
Junctional rhythm, 71–80
– atrial fibrillation, and, 220, 228
– atrioventricular dissociation, 75–78
– capture beats, and, 76–78
– coronary sinus rhythm, 74
– coupled atrial extrasystoles, and, 112
– Ebstein's anomaly, and, 448
– mimicking myocardial infarction, 410
– P waves, and, 71–74
– paroxysmal atrial tachycardia, blocked, and, 143
– reciprocal beats, and, 79
– retrograde block, and, 71–73
Junctional tachycardia (see under Paroxysmal tachycardia)

Kent, bundle of, 158, 164, 167, 168
Kerley's lines, 556, 575, 576, 598–600, 603
– disappearance of with diuretics, 508, 509
Kyphoscoliosis
– aortic unfolding, and, 679, 680
– heart silhouette, and, 487–489

Laevocardia, isolated, 673
Lateral chest film, diagnostic value of, in,
– ankylosing spondylitis, 567
– aorta, tortuous, 683
– aorta, unfolded, 680
– aortic aneurysm, 692, 694, 706
– aortic arch, kinked, 685
– aortic atheroma, 688
– aortic dissection, 698
– aortic valve calcification, 569, 609
– aortic valve position, 569, 571–573, 609, 614, 615, 617
– aortic valve replacement, 562, 614, 615, 617

– calcific constrictive pericarditis, 542
– coronary sinus pacing, 724
– dermoid cyst, 493
– diagram of, 454
– encysted effusion, 516
– flat chest, 478
– foreign body, 747, 750
– kyphoscoliosis, 488
– large left to right shunts, 661, 664
– left atrial enlargement, 454, 503, 649
– left ventricular aneurysm, 523, 526
– left ventricular enlargement, 500, 560, 569, 580, 612
– mediastinal masses, 493
– mitral valve calcification, 587, 589, 602, 609
– mitral valve position, 587, 589, 602, 609, 614, 615, 617
– mitral valve replacement, 614, 615, 617
– pacing catheter position, 719, 722, 724
– prosthetic valve function, 571–573, 614, 615
– pulmonary arterio-venous fistulae, 736, 740
– pulmonary artery, post-stenotic dilatation of, 632
– right ventricular enlargement, 454, 498, 580, 612, 621, 643, 661
– sternal depression, 476
– straight back, 480
– syphilitic aortitis, 690
– tricuspid valve position, 617
Left anterior hemiblock (also see Left axis deviation)
– anomalous origin of left coronary artery, and, 452
– atrioventricular cushion defects, and, 340, 341
– bifascicular block, and, 334, 335, 340
– congestive cardiomyopathy, and, 443
– isolated, 47, 48, 330
– left bundle branch block, and, 322, 324, 325
– left ventricular hypertrophy, and, 304, 305
– masking myocardial infarction (potentially), 353
– mimicked by myocardial infarction, 353, 390, 393
– mimicked by Wolff–Parkinson–White syndrome, 168, 169
– myocardial ischaemia, and, 356, 400
– myocardial infarction, and, 49, 352, 353
– right bundle branch block, and, 334, 335, 338, 339
– tricuspid atresia, and, 449
– trifascicular block, and, 338, 339, 341
Left atrial appendage
– amputation in mitral valvotomy, 578, 596
– calcified, 585
– herniated, 543
– large, mimicking pulmonary artery dilatation, 494, 495
– mitral stenosis, and, 574, 577
– position of, 454
Left atrial calcification, 584
Left atrial enlargement
– atrial septal defect, absence of, 642
– atrioventricular canal, and, 665
– barium swallow demonstrating, 504
– carinal splaying in, 454, 502
– congestive cardiomyopathy, and, 552, 553
– double shadow at right cardiac border in, 501
– giant, 583
– lateral view, and, 503
– left main bronchus, and, 502
– Lutembacher's syndrome, and, 648, 649
– mimicked by dermoid cyst, 491
– mitral stenosis, absence in, 575
– mitral valve disease, and, 501–504, 574, 577, 579, 582, 586–589, 593, 602, 603, 607, 608, 610–612
– mitral valve surgery, and, 578, 596–600, 604
– myxoma, left atrial, and, 730
– patent ductus arteriosus, and, 668
– penetrated PA view in, 501, 502
– ventricular septal defect, and, 660

Left atrial hypertrophy (see P mitrale)
Left atrial myxoma, 730, 731
Left atrium, position in cardiac silhouette, 454
Left axis deviation (see also Left anterior hemiblock)
– calculation of, 39
– cor pulmonale, and, 313
– examples, 47–49
– myocardial infarction, and, 353, 393
– pre-existing, effect of left bundle branch block on, 323, 324
– Q waves in inferior leads, and, 308, 353, 393
– Wolff–Parkinson–White syndrome, and, 168, 169
Left bundle branch block (see also Aberrant conduction)
– bifascicular block, and, 332
– completeness of, 322, 325, 326
– criteria, 320
– incomplete, 325, 327
– left axis deviation, and, 322, 324, 325
– mimicking myocardial infarction, 320
– myocardial infarction, and, 350
– myocardial infarction, masking of by, 320, 351
– Q waves, pathological, in, 350
– QRS axis and, 320, 322–325
– QRS complex, in, 320–327
– ST segments in, 320
– T waves in, 320, 321
– trifascicular block, and, 339
Left cardiac border
– convex, in corrected transposition, 664, 673
– Fallot's tetralogy, and, 633–636
– herniated left atrial appendage, and, 543
– left ventricular hypertrophy, and, 499, 500
– myocardial infarction, step shadow, 519
– pericardium, absent left, in, 543–546
– pleuro-pericardial adhesions, 548
– pulmonary bay, in, 633, 634
– right ventricular outflow tract aneurysm after repair of Fallot's tetralogy, 637
– right ventricular hypertrophy, and, 497, 498
– tricuspid atresia, and, 640
– ventricular aneurysm, and, 520–528
Left posterior hemiblock
– bifascicular block, and, 336, 337
– criteria of, 331
– diagnosis in presence of right bundle branch block, 336, 337
– mimicking right ventricular hypertrophy, 331, 337
– myocardial ischaemia, and, 376
Left subclavian artery, dilated in coarctation, 713
Left superior vena cava
– isolated, 626
– in supracardiac total anomalous pulmonary venous drainage, 654, 655
Left ventricle
– inert segment in myocardial infarction, 412
– position in cardiac silhouette, 454
Left ventricular aneurysm (see Ventricular aneurysm)
Left ventricular enlargement
– absence in aortic stenosis, 554
– absence in aortic regurgitation, 558
– aortic valve disease, and, 556, 557, 559, 560, 563, 565, 569, 709, 711–712
– aortic valve replacement, reduction after, 561, 562, 564
– atrioventricular canal, and, 665, 666
– congestive cardiomyopathy, and, 552, 553
– diagnosis of, 499, 500
– hypertrophic cardiomyopathy, and, 549, 550
– mitral regurgitation, and, 579, 580, 602
– multivalvar disease, and, 608, 610–612
– muscular dystrophy, and, 551

– myocardial infarction, ? ventricular aneurysm, and, 528, 529
– myocarditis, and, 547
– patent ductus arteriosus, and, 668
– ventricular septal defect, and, 660, 661
Left ventricular hypertrophy
– absence of changes in chest leads, 300, 305
– absence of changes in limb leads, 296, 299, 301
– anomalous origin of left coronary artery, and, 452
– antero-septal myocardial infarction, and, 302, 411
– anticlockwise rotation, and, 295
– apparent, in youth, 11
– balanced ventricular hypertrophy, 319
– bifascicular block, and, 335
– clockwise rotation, and, 296, 301, 305
– criteria of, 294
– diastolic overload pattern, 294
– diastolic overload, acute, 306
– horizontal heart, and, 297
– hypertrophic cardiomyopathy, and, 307, 308
– inferior leads showing pattern of, 294, 296, 298
– late changes, 296–298
– left anterior hemiblock, and, 304, 305, 324
– mimicked in cor pulmonale, 313
– mimicking myocardial infarction, 297, 302
– mimicking myocardial ischaemia, 298
– myocardial infarction, and, 411
– Q waves, septal, in, 296, 302, 304
– QS complexes in, 302, 411
– QRS complex, prolonged, in, 296, 304, 324
– QRS vector, in, 299–301
– right axis deviation, and, 307, 317, 318
– right bundle branch block, and, 303
– right ventricular hypertrophy, and, 317–319
– ST segment, high take-off, in, 297, 298
– semihorizontal heart, and, 295
– semivertical heart, and, 294, 298
– strain pattern in, 296–298
– systolic overload pattern in, 294, 296
– T wave changes in, 294–298
– tricuspid atresia, and, 449
– vertical heart, and, 299
Limb leads
– left ventricular hypertrophy, and, 296, 299–301, 305
– normal, in myocardial infarction, 387
– Q waves in, 25, 400, 401
Low voltage curves in
– amyloid disease, 445
– chest leads in dextrocardia, 28
– congestive cardiomyopathy, 443–445
– Ebstein's anomaly, 447
– myxoedema, 424
– obesity, 16
– pericardial constriction, 416
– pericardial effusion, 417
– right atrial myxoma, 446
Lower lobe venous constriction in pulmonary venous congestion, 505
Lown–Ganong–Levine syndrome, 171
– possible, 112
Lung fields
– crying, and, 484, 485
– pulmonary arteriovenous fistulae in, 736, 739–742
– systemic vascular supply in Fallot's tetralogy, 633, 634, 636
– vascularity (see Pulmonary oligaemia and plethora)
Lutembacher's syndrome, 453, 648, 649

Mahaim fibres, 170
Maladie de Roger, 657
Marfan's syndrome, 709–712

Mediastinal mass
– effect on heart size, 490–493
– mimicked by left ventricular aneurysm, 527
Mediastinal widening in
– aortic hypoplasia, 709, 711, 712
– aortic rupture, 707, 708
– aortic tortuosity, 681, 682
– crying, and, 484, 485
– dissecting aneurysm, and, 697
– false, in antero-posterior film, 701–704
Mesocardia, 675
Mitral regurgitation
– acute, with prosthetic valve dehiscence, 605
– cardiac silhouette in, 579, 580
– chordal rupture, causing, 593, 594
– diastolic overload in, 294, 306
– following mitral valvotomy, 596–600
– pulmonary hypertension, and, 580
– senile mitral calcification, and, 601, 602
Mitral stenosis, 574–576, 577
– Lutembacher's syndrome, 648, 649
Mitral valve
– calcification, 586–589
– calcification and aortic valve calcification, 609
– calcification in ring, 601, 602
– chordal rupture of, 306, 593, 594
– position, 587, 589, 602, 609, 614, 615, 617
Mitral valve disease, 505, 603 (and see Mitral regurgitation and Mitral stenosis)
– aortic valve disease, and, 608
– calcification in left atrium, and, 584, 585
– cardiomyopathy, and, 581, 582
– giant left atrium in, 583
– Kerley's lines, and, 598–600
– pulmonary bone formation, and, 592
– pulmonary haemosiderosis, and, 590, 591
– tricuspid valve disease, and, 607
– triple vessel disease, 610–612
Mitral valve replacement
– aortic replacement, and, 613–615
– aortic and tricuspid replacement, and, 616, 617
– heart size, and, 604
– mechanical prosthetic, 603, 604, 613–615
– prosthetic dehiscence, 605
Mitral valvotomy, 577, 578
– unsuccessful, 595–600
Mobitz block (see under grade 2 heart block, types 1 and 2)
Monitoring electrode masking lung lesion, 751, 752
Mural thrombus, calcified
– mitral valve disease, and, 584, 585
– myocardial infarction, and, 532–534
– ventricular aneurysm, and, 525, 526
Muscular dystrophy, cardiac involvement, 551
Myocardial damage
– in left bundle branch block, 321
Myocardial infarction
– acute pericarditis, distinction from, 414
– anomalous origin of left coronary artery, and, 452
– bifascicular block, and, 352, 353
– calcification in, 532–534
– changes limited to chest leads, 387, 388, 399, 400
– disappearance of changes of, 407–409
– earliest changes of, 380, 382–384, 386
– extension of, 380, 381, 384, 385, 397, 398
– following ischaemia, 374, 375
– full-thickness, 387 (and see under sites)
– full thickness, association with ventricular aneurysm, 412
– heart block, and, 275, 386
– heart failure following, 519

– high chest leads in diagnosis of, 396
– inert segment in, 412
– infant's electrocardiogram, and, 452
– left axis deviation in inferior, 353, 393
– left bundle branch block, and, 350
– left ventricular hypertrophy, and, 411
– localised, 387, 388, 399
– masked by aberrant conduction, 351
– masked by Wolff–Parkinson–White syndrome, 165
– mimicked by amyloid disease, 445
– mimicked by dextrocardia, 28
– mimicked in hypertrophic cardiomyopathy, 307, 308
– mimicked by junctional rhythm, 410
– mimicked by left bundle branch block, 320
– mimicked by left ventricular hypertrophy, 298, 302
– mimicked by pericarditis, 380
– mimicked by Prinzmetal angina, 378
– mimicked by subarachnoid haemorrhage, 429, 430
– mimicked by Wolff–Parkinson–White syndrome, 167–170
– partial thickness, 381 (and see under sites)
– pathological Q waves, absence of, in partial-thickness, 381
– pathological Q waves, in full-thickness infarction, 387
– pathological Q waves, false, in junctional rhythm, 410
– pathological Q waves in limb leads, and, 401
– pathological Q waves, in old infarction (see under sites)
– pathological Q waves, possible, 389, 402
– QRS complex, voltage increase with ST segment shift, 386
– QS complexes in, 400
– QT prolongation, 381
– R waves, broad anteroseptal, in true posterior, 384, 395, 396
– R waves, loss of, 389, 407
– R waves, voltage increase in true posterior, 405
– right axis deviation, and, 391
– right bundle branch block, and, 348, 349, 352
– ST elevation in, 380, 382–384, 387, 390–397
– ST elevation, marked, effect on QRS voltage, 386
– ST elevation, minimal, 394, 395, 397
– ST elevation, normal progression of, 380, 381, 384, 385, 388, 389
– ST elevation, persistent, in ventricular aneurysm, 412
– ST elevation, suspicious, 388, 389
– ST segment, reciprocal depression, 380–382
– step shadow in, 519
– subendocardial, 366
– T waves, inverted, 371, 387, 400, 403, 404, 407–409
– T waves, progression of, 381
– T waves, upright, in early hours, 380, 382–384
– ventricular aneurysm (see under title)
– ventricular septal defect, acquired, 531
– versus myocardial ischaemia, 363, 364, 366, 367, 371, 406
Myocardial infarction, sites
– anterior and inferior, 390, 404
– antero-lateral, 383, 391
– antero-lateral and inferior, 398
– antero-septal, 382, 387–389, 399, 400, 411
– high lateral, 396
– inferior, 380, 392, 397, 403, 406
– inferior, lateral, and true posterior, 395
– inferior and true posterior, 384, 405, 406
– inferolateral, 375, 381, 393, 394, 398
– true posterior, 384, 396, 405
Myocardial ischaemia
– causing extrasystole, 362
– diffuse, versus ventricular aneurysm, 529, 530
– exercise test, 376
– followed by myocardial infarction, 374, 375

– grouping of changes, 355, 357 (and see sites)
– left anterior hemiblock, and, 356, 400
– left posterior hemiblock, and, 376
– mimicked by congestive cardiomyopathy, 443, 444
– mimicked by dextrocardia, 28
– mimicked by digitalis effect, 441
– mimicked by hyperkalaemia, 435
– mimicked by hypocalcaemia, 438
– mimicked by hypokalaemia, 437
– mimicked by left bundle branch block, 320
– mimicked by left ventricular hypertrophy, 298
– mimicked by myocarditis, 442
– mimicked by myxoedema, 424
– mimicked by pericarditis, 415, 416, 418
– mimicked by persistent T wave inversion into adult life, 12
– mimicked by physiological stimuli, 27
– mimicked by post paroxysmal tachycardia changes, 162, 163
– mimicked by pulmonary embolism, 419, 421
– mimicked by quinidine, 440
– mimicked by ST–T changes of sinus tachycardia, 131
– mimicked by subarachnoid haemorrhage, 429
– mimicked by suspended heart syndrome, 15
– mimicked by Wolff–Parkinson–White syndrome, 165
– minor signs of, 355, 356
– normal electrocardiogram in, 354
– Prinzmetal angina, 379
– QRS axis shift, 361, 365
– ST segment, depression, 365, 374, 376
– ST segment, horizontal, 355, 356, 359, 376
– ST–T angulation, 355, 373
– T waves flattened, 359, 360
– T waves inverted, 356, 360, 361, 363–365, 367, 376
– T waves, tall, 362, 373, 406
– U wave inversion, 358, 376
Myocardial ischaemia, sites
– anterior, 366, 368
– high lateral, 371
– inferior, 369
– infero-lateral, 367, 370, 374
– lateral and posterior, 406
– true posterior, 372, 373
Myocarditis
– cardiomegaly in, 547, 548
– superficial, in pericarditis, 417, 418
– T wave changes in, 442
Myxoedema, 424–426, 743, 744
Myxoma
– left atrial, 730, 731
– right atrial, 446, 732–734

Neonate
– electrocardiogram, 10
– heart silhouette, 463
– normal heart rate, and, 17
– paroxysmal tachycardia in, 146
– right ventricular dominance in, 314
– thymic 'sail' shadow in, 463
Nodal (see Junctional)
Normal cardiac silhouette
– adults, 456–462
– children, 463–466
– diagram, 454
Normal electrocardiogram, 1–7
– children and, 8–11
– incomplete right bundle branch block, and, 329
– myocardial ischaemia, and, 354
– pericardial constriction, and, 416
– sickling pattern, 13

Obesity, 16, 467
Oligaemia (see Pulmonary oligaemia)
Ossification in pulmonary haemosiderosis, 592
Ostium primum defect (see Atrioventricular cushion defect)

P waves
– absent in atrial fibrillation, 215
– absent in junctional rhythm, 71
– absent in sino-atrial block, 60, 64
– absent in sinus arrest, 62, 63
– atrial extrasystoles, and, 100, 104, 119
– atrial parasystole, and, 125
– axis, 39
– axis shift, in atrial infarction, 413
– intracardiac electrocardiogram, and, 30
– inverted, in atrial extrasystoles, 114
– inverted, in atrioventricular dissociation with retrograde conduction, 80
– inverted, in complete heart block with retrograde conduction, 274
– inverted, in coronary sinus rhythm, 74
– inverted, in dextrocardia, 28
– inverted, in junctional extrasystoles, 114, 121
– inverted, in junctional rhythm, 72, 79
– inverted, in junctional rhythm, mimicking Q waves, 410
– inverted, in leads I and VL in transposition of arm leads, 31
– inverted, in paroxysmal junctional tachycardia, 134
– inverted, in reciprocating tachycardia, 158–160
– inverted, in retrograde atrial activation from ventricular extrasystole, 83
– junctional extrasystoles, and, 113–115, 118, 119
– mimicked by notched bifid T waves in children, 9
– mitrale (see P mitrale)
– obscured by AC interference, 38
– obscured by muscle tremor, 37
– pacing, and, 282
– paroxysmal tachycardia, and, 133, 135, 143, 144, 147
– pulmonale (see P pulmonale)
– 'sandwiched', in escape capture bigeminy, 70
– shifting pacemaker in the sinus node, and, 22
– sino-atrial extrasystoles, and, 105
– tiny, in digitalis-induced paroxysmal tachycardia, 143, 144
– varying or altered morphology (see under atrial extrasystoles, Atrial infarction, atrial parasystole, Atrial re-entry, Atrial tachycardia, junctional extrasystoles, Junctional rhythm, Junctional tachycardia, P mitrale, P pulmonale, shifting pacemaker in the sinus node, subarachnoid haemorrhage, wandering pacemaker)
– ventricular extrasystoles, and, 81, 82, 83
– wandering pacemaker, and, 69
P in QRST
– blocked atrial extrasystoles, and, 108, 109, 110
– atrial extrasystoles, and, 103, 106–108, 111
– atrial tachycardia with block, 137–145
– complete heart block, and, 263–276
– interpolated extrasystoles, and, 90
– junctional extrasystoles, and, 114, 115
– junctional rhythm, and, 72, 73, 75–80
– junctional tachycardia, and, 134, 153, 154
– pacing, and, 282
– partial heart block, and, 237–262
– simultaneous tachycardias, and, 153, 154
– sinus tachycardia, and, 130
– supraventricular tachycardia, and, 135, 157
– ventricular extrasystoles, and, 81–83
– ventricular tachycardia, and, 177, 180

P–P interval
– fixed in partial heart block, 250
– varying in complete heart block, 266, 267, 273
– varying in partial heart block, 249, 251, 261
– varying in paroxysmal atrial tachycardia, 152
– varying in sinus arrhythmia, 18
– varying in sinus tachycardia, 130
PR interval, artificial, in atrially triggered pacing, 287
PR interval, changing, in
– atrial infarction, 413
– grade 1 heart block, 238, 239
– irregular atrial tachycardia, 152
– multifocal atrial extrasystoles, 104
– multifocal atrial tachycardia, 147
– shifting pacemaker in the sinus node, 22
– supraventricular tachycardia with alternating aberration, 149
– Wenckebach periods, 240–246
PR interval, normal, in
– children, 341
– grade 2, type 2 heart block, 249, 252, 255
– paroxysmal atrial tachycardia with partial block, 137
– sino-atrial extrasystole, 105
– sinus arrhythmia, 18
– Wolff–Parkinson–White syndrome, 170
PR interval, prolonged
– atrial extrasystoles, and, 100, 103, 104, 106, 107, 111
– atrioventricular cushion defect, and, 341
– bifascicular block, and, 332, 333
– concealed retrograde conduction, and, 76–78, 89, 90, 120
– Ebstein's anomaly, and, 448
– grade 1 heart block, 236, 237
– grade 2, type 1 heart block, 244
– grade 2, type 2 heart block, 247, 248, 253, 254
– junctional extrasystole, interpolated, and, 120
– junctional rhythm with capture beats, and, 76–78
– mimicked by inadvertent recording at 50mm/sec, 35
– paroxysmal atrial tachycardia with partial block, and, 138
– trifascicular block, and, 338
– ventricular extrasystole, interpolated, and, 89, 90
PR interval, shortened
– atrial extrasystoles and, 103
– coronary sinus rhythm, and, 74
– following dropped beat in atrial tachycardia with partial block, 141
– following dropped beat in partial heart block, 247, 248
– junctional extrasystoles, and, 119
– Lown–Ganong–Levine syndrome, and, 171
– post-extrasystolic beat after blocked atrial extrasystoles, and, 210
– subarachnoid haemorrhage, and, 432
– tachycardia, and, 341
– Wolff–Parkinson–White syndrome, and, 164
PR interval in Wenckebach periods
– abnormal incremental behaviour, 241
– normal incremental behaviour, 240
– paradoxically long last, 242
PR segment depression
– acute pericarditis, and, 413
– atrial T wave, 23
– atrial infarction, and, 413
P mitrale, 54, 55
– 12 lead electrocardiogram, 56
– apparent in constrictive pericarditis, 416
– biphasic appearance in V1, 56
– Lutembacher's syndrome, and, 453
– P pulmonale, and, 59, 417, 453
P pulmonale, 57
– 12 lead electrocardiogram, 58

– cor pulmonale, and, 313, 422, 423
– Ebstein's anomaly, and, 447
– Lutembacher's syndrome, and, 453
– mimicked by superimposition of P on T, 10
– mimicked in subarachnoid haemorrhage, 429, 431
– P mitrale, and, 59, 417, 453
– right atrial myxoma, and, 446
– tricuspid atresia, and, 449
Pacemaker, shifting, in the sinus node, 22
Pacing (and see Pacing faults)
– artefact, alteration with respiration, 293
– artefact, with bipolar catheter, 280
– artefact, direction, 279
– artefact, with unipolar catheter, 279
– atrial, 288
– atrial loop, importance of, 718, 720, 721
– atrially triggered, 287
– competition with sinus rhythm, and, 283
– complexes, 281
– demand (inhibited), 285
– electrode, 279, 280
– endocardial, 279, 280, 718–724
– epicardial, 727–729
– fixed rate, 282–284
– induction coil, 729
– paroxysmal reciprocating tachycardia, control of, 160
– subxiphisternal approach, 727, 728
– temporary, 729
– ventricular extrasystoles, and, 284
Pacing faults
– artefact of inconstant size, 290
– artefact unrelated to QRS, 283, 284, 289–291
– broken connection or electrode, 290
– electrode contact lost, 289, 291, 292
– electrode in coronary sinus, 723, 724
– exit block, 289, 291
– failure of demand pacing, 292
– generator failure, 289
– perforation of heart, 725
– sinus rhythm, return of, 283
– unstable position of electrode, 720–724, 726
Paradoxical rate-dependent bundle branch block, 345
Parasystole
– accelerated idioventricular rhythm, and, 185, 188
– atrial, 125
– ventricular, 123, 124
Paroxysmal tachycardia
– aberrant conduction, and, 142, 148, 149, 157
– atrial, 133, 145
– atrial, with complete block, 143, 144
– atrial, with partial block, 136–141, 145, 159
– bidirectional, 151
– brief burst of, 145
– carotid sinus massage in, 157
– corrected transposition, and, 450
– Ebstein's anomaly, and, 447, 448
– electrical alternation in, 150
– infancy, and, 146
– irregular, 152
– junctional with retrograde block, 142
– junctional with retrograde conduction, 134
– Lown–Ganong–Levine syndrome, and, 171
– multifocal, 147
– reciprocating, 158–161
– reciprocating, terminated by pacing, 160
– reciprocating, terminated by extrasystole, 161
– ST–T changes following, 162, 163
– simultaneous atrial and junctional, 153–155
– supraventricular, 135, 146, 148, 149 (and see Atrial, Junctional and Reciprocating tachycardia)
– very rapid, 146

– ventricular (see Ventricular tachycardia)
– Wolff–Parkinson–White syndrome, and, 172
Partial anomalous pulmonary venous drainage, 650–653
Patent ductus arteriosus, 667–669
– calcification in, 624
– Eisenmenger syndrome, and, 624
Penetrated postero-anterior view, value of, in,
– aortic calcification, 568
– coarctation of aorta, 717
– constrictive pericarditis, 542
– left atrial enlargement, 502
– mitral calcification, 586, 588
Pericardial effusion, 535–540
– aspiration of, 540
– atrial fibrillation, and, 418
– electrical alternans in, 417
– low voltage electrocardiogram in, 418
– mimicked by Ebstein's anomaly, 641
– myxoedema, and, 743
Pericardial fat, 467, 483
Pericarditis
– acute, 414
– constrictive, 416, 541, 542
– healed, 415
– mimicked by sickling pattern, 13
– mimicking acute myocardial infarction, 380
– mimicking myxoedema, 424
Pericardium, absent, 543–546
Pleural effusion, 514–517
– encysted, 515, 516
– significance in ruptured aorta, 707
Pleuro-pericardial adhesion, 548
Pneumothorax, in diagnosis of absent pericardium, 546
Portal venous obstruction in infradiaphragmatic total anomalous pulmonary venous drainage, 656
Post-extrasystolic pause (see Compensatory pause)
Post-extrasystolic T wave changes, 84–86, 117, 122
Post-mortem complexes, 197, 198
Post-stenotic dilatation (see Coarctation, Aortic stenosis, Pulmonary stenosis)
Potassium, serum (see Hyper and Hypokalaemia)
Potassium tablets in oesophagus, 749, 750
Pre-excitation, 164
Prinzmetal angina, 377–379
Prosthetic valve (see under individual valve)
Pulmonary arterio-venous fistulae, 735–742
Pulmonary artery banding, 662, 663
Pulmonary artery, dilatation
– atrial septal defect, and, 642, 644, 645, 647
– atrioventricular cushion defect, and, 665, 666
– Eisenmenger syndrome, and, 622–624
– idiopathic, 627
– mimicked by dermoid cyst, 492, 493
– mimicked by large left atrial appendage, 494, 495
– mimicked by left ventricular aneurysm, 527
– normal, 459–462
– patent ductus arteriosus, and, 667, 668
– pulmonary hypertension, and, 497, 498, 576, 597–600, 620, 621
– post-stenotic, 628–630
– thrombosis-in-situ, and, 625
Pulmonary artery, electrocardiogram within, 30
Pulmonary artery, position of
– on cardiac silhouette, 454
– in transposition, 673
Pulmonary atresia, 638, 639
Pulmonary embolism, 419–421, 618, 619
Pulmonary haemosiderosis, 590–592
Pulmonary hypertension
– cor pulmonale, and, 46, 313, 422, 423
– Eisenmenger syndrome, 622–624

– electrocardiogram, and, (see Right ventricular hypertrophy)
– hyperkinetic, in left to right shunts (see lesions)
– mitral valve disease, and, 59, 576, 579, 580, 595–600, 603
– pulmonary oligaemia, and, 620
– right ventricular enlargement, and, 497, 498, 620, 621
– thromboembolic, 620, 621
– thrombosis-in-situ, in, 625
– tricuspid incompetence, and, 576, 598–600, 607
– triple valve disease, and, 610–612
Pulmonary infarction, 619
– in tricuspid endocarditis, 745
Pulmonary oedema, 510–512, 575
– with prosthetic valve dehiscence, 605
– unilateral, 513
Pulmonary oligaemia
– Ebstein's anomaly, and, 641
– Fallot's tetralogy, and, 633–636
– normal upper lobe, lost, in pulmonary venous congestion, 505
– pulmonary atresia, and, 638, 639
– pulmonary embolus, and, 618
– pulmonary hypertension, and, 620–625
– pulmonary stenosis, and, 628–630
– right atrial myxoma, and, 732
– transposition and pulmonary stenosis, and, 676
– tricuspid atresia, and, 640
Pulmonary plethora
– atrial septal defect, and, 642, 644, 646
– atrioventricular canal, and, 665, 666
– partial anomalous venous drainage, and, 650
– patent ductus arteriosus, and, 667, 668
– sinus of Valsalva aneurysm rupture into right heart, 565
– total anomalous pulmonary venous drainage, and, 654
– transposition of great arteries, and, 676, 677
– unilateral, 670, 671
– ventricular septal defect, and, 658–662, 664
– ventricular septal defect, acquired, and, 531
Pulmonary regurgitation (post-operative), 630
Pulmonary stenosis
– electrocardiogram, 314 (and see Right ventricular hypertrophy)
– Fallot's tetralogy, and, 633
– mild versus idiopathic dilatation of the pulmonary artery, 627
– moderate-severe, 628, 629
– post-stenotic dilatation in, 628, 629, 631, 632
– tricuspid atresia, and, 640
– transposition of great arteries, and, 676
– valvotomy, results of, 630
Pulmonary vascular pattern, reversed, in pulmonary venous congestion, 505
Pulmonary venous congestion
– aortic valve disease, and, 557, 563, 564
– diuretics, effect of, 506, 507, 517, 552, 574, 577
– haemosiderosis in, 590–592
– heart failure, and, 515
– Lutembacher's syndrome, and, 648
– mitral valve disease, and, 505, 574–577
– mitral valve replacement, loss of, after, 604
– multivalvar disease, and, 610–612
– myocarditis, and, 547
– myxoma, left atrial, and, 730
– total anomalous pulmonary venous drainage, and, 656
– upper lobe veins in, 505–507
– vascular pattern, reversed, in, 505

Q waves (see also QS complexes)
– abolition of, on inspiration, 25
– absence of, in partial thickness infarction, 381
– absence of, in acute pericarditis, 414
– amyloid disease, and, 445
– anomalous origin of left coronary artery, and, 452
– bifascicular block, and, 352
– corrected transposition, and, 450, 451
– disappearance of after infarction, 407–409
– hypertrophic cardiomyopathy, and, 307, 308
– left bundle branch block, and, 350
– left posterior hemiblock, and, 331
– left ventricular hypertrophy, and, 302, 411
– masked by aberrant conduction, 351
– mimicked by delta waves, 167–169
– mimicked by junctional P waves, 410
– mirror image appearance as R waves, 384, 385, 395, 396
– myocardial infarction, full thickness, and, (see under Myocardial infarction)
– pathological (see significance)
– pulmonary embolism, and, 419, 420
– right bundle branch block, and, 348, 349
– right ventricle, over, in right ventricular hypertrophy, 310
– significance of, 25, 302, 350, 389, 401, 402
– ventricular aneurysm, and, 412
QRS axis (mean)
– —90° to —180°, 50, 51
– adults, 39–44
– alteration with age, 39
– children, 8, 10, 11, 39
– diagram, 39
– indeterminate, 52, 53
– initial forces in left posterior hemiblock, 336, 337
– initial forces in right bundle branch block, 328, 336, 346
– left (see Left axis deviation)
– left bundle branch block, and, 320, 322–325
– right (see Right axis deviation)
– right bundle branch block, and, 328, 346
– shift in acute myocardial ischaemia, 361, 365
– shift in acute pulmonary embolism, 419, 420
– shift with Wolff–Parkinson–White syndrome, 169
– terminal forces in right bundle branch block, and, 328
QRS complex, altered contour, normal duration
– atrial extrasystoles, and, 104, 106, 107, 111
– electrical alternation, 95, 98, 150, 151
– height decreased artefactually, 26
– height increased by F waves, 204, 207, 209
– height increased by P waves, 75, 76, 262, 264, 386
– intracardiac electrocardiogram, 30
– junctional escape beats, 20, 230, 261, 433
– junctional extrasystoles, 113, 116, 118, 120, 121, 122
– respiratory variation, 24–26
– Wolff–Parkinson–White syndrome, 164–169
QRS complex voltage
– decreased (see under Low voltage curves)
– increased in left bundle branch block, left ventricular hypertrophy, myocardial infarction, adolescence and childhood (see under these headings)
– unimpressive, in balanced ventricular hypertrophy, 319
QRS complex, widened, in
– accelerated idioventricular rhythm, 184–188
– atrial extrasystoles with aberrant conduction, 108
– atrial fibrillation with aberrant conduction, 232–234
– atrial fibrillation with complete heart block, 219
– atrial fibrillation and parasystole, 124
– atrial fibrillation and ventricular escape beats, 231
– atrial fibrillation and ventricular extrasystoles, 224–228, 229
– atrial flutter with complete heart block, 209
– bundle branch block, 320–328, 332–339
– complete heart block, 264–275
– hyperkalaemia, 435
– hypothermia, 427, 428

INDEX

– left ventricular hypertrophy, 296, 304, 324
– parasystole (ventricular), 123, 124
– paroxysmal supraventricular tachycardia with aberration, 148, 149
– partial heart block, 240–262
– quinidine intoxication, 440
– ventricular escape, 64, 231
– ventricular extrasystoles, 81–99
– ventricular pacing, 279–285, 286
– ventricular tachycardia, 173–183
QS complexes
– amyloid disease, and, 445
– left ventricular hypertrophy, and, 302, 411
– myocardial infarction, examples, 391, 396, 400
– subarachnoid haemorrhage, and, 429
– ventricular aneurysm, and, 412
QT interval, prolongation in
– cerebral haemorrhage, 433, 434
– hypocalcaemia, 435, 438
– hypothermia, 427
– mimicked by T–U changes in hypokalaemia, 437
– myocardial infarction, 381
– myxoedema, 424–426
– post-extrasystolic beat, 86
– quinidine intoxication, 440
QT interval, shortening, in hypercalcaemia, 439
Quinidine intoxication, 440

R waves, small, in left chest leads in
– dextrocardia, 28
– myocardial infarction, 391
– right ventricular hypertrophy, 309–315
– ventricular aneurysm, 412
R waves, small in right chest leads in
– left bundle branch block, 320, 327
– left ventricular hypertrophy, 302, 411
– myocardial infarction, 389, 399, 400, 407
R waves, tall, in left chest leads in
– left bundle branch block, 320–327
– left ventricular hypertrophy, 294–299
R waves, tall, in right chest leads in
– mirror image Q waves in hypertrophic cardio-myopathy, 307
– mirror image Q waves in true posterior myocardial infarction, 384, 385, 395, 396, 405
– right ventricular hypertrophy, 309, 310, 314, 315
– right bundle branch block and right ventricular hypertrophy, 316
rS pattern in right ventricular hypertrophy, 46, 58, 311, 312, 313
RSR complex in right bundle branch block, 328, 329
R on T phenomenon
– causing ventricular tachycardia and fibrillation, 183
– in fixed rate pacing with sinus rhythm, 283
– in fixed rate pacing with ventricular extrasystoles, 284
– ventricular extrasystole, and, 99
Rate change (see P–P interval)
– partial heart block, and, 237–239, 241, 256–258
– post-extrasystolic compensatory pause, effect on, 84, 101, 122
– rate-dependent bundle branch block, and, 212, 342–345
– timing of Wenckebach periods, and, 241
Rate-dependent aberration, 342–344
– paradoxical, 345
Rate, synchronisation tendency in combined supraventricular tachycardias, 155
Reciprocal beats, 79, 80, 83, 121
– interpolated extrasystoles, and, 83
– mimicked in escape capture bigeminy, 70
Reciprocating tachycardia, 158–161, 171

Recording fault
– AC interference, 38
– arm leads reversed in error, 31, 32
– double speed recording, 35
– failure to switch from VF position, 33, 34
– muscle tremor, 27, 37
– normal lead placement in dextrocardia, 28
– variable baseline, 36
Repetitive tachycardia, 156, 159, 181, 182
Respiration
– heart size, and, 471, 472
– pacing artefact, and, 293
– Q waves, and, 25
– QRS contour, and, 24–26
– sinus arrhythmia, and, 18, 20
– T waves, and, 27
– Valsalva manoeuvre, and, 26
Retrograde block to atria
– accelerated idioventricular rhythm, and, 184–188
– complete heart block, and, 263–273, 275, 276
– junctional extrasystoles, and, 115, 121
– junctional rhythm, and, 75–78
– pacing, and, 279–284
– partial, in junctional rhythm, 73, 80
– paroxysmal junctional tachycardia, and, 142, 153–155
– ventricular tachycardia, and, 173–182
Retrograde conduction to atria
– junctional extrasystoles, and, 114, 121
– junctional rhythm, and, 71, 72, 79
– mimicked in escape capture bigeminy, 70
– partial, in junctional rhythm, 73, 80
– paradoxical, in complete heart block, 274
– paroxysmal junctional tachycardia, and, 134
– ventricular extrasystoles, and, 83
Rib notching in coarctation, 716
Rib obliquity
– in kyphoscoliosis, 487, 489
– in sternal depression, 475
Right atrial enlargement
– atrial septal defect, and, 642
– criteria, 497, 498
– Ebstein's anomaly, and, 641
– functional tricuspid regurgitation, and, 576
– right atrial myxoma, and, 732, 733
– tricuspid valve disease, and, 606, 607
Right atrial myxoma, 446, 732–734
Right atrium
– anomalous vein joining, 650, 651
– foreign body in, 748
– position on cardiac silhouette, 454
Right axis deviation
– absence of, in neonatal tricuspid atresia, 449
– calculation of, 39
– children, and, 11
– cor pulmonale, and, 313
– examples, 45, 46, 50, 51
– hypertrophic cardiomyopathy, and, 307
– left posterior hemiblock, and, 331, 336, 337
– myocardial infarction, and, 391, 396
– neonates, and, 10
– probable, 50, 51
– right bundle branch block (initial forces) and, as sign of right ventricular hypertrophy, 453
– right bundle branch block (later forces) and, 328, 346
– right bundle branch block and left posterior hemiblock, 336, 337
– right ventricular hypertrophy, and, 50, 51, 59, 309, 311, 312, 314, 315, 453
– right ventricular hypertrophy in presence of left ventricular hypertrophy, sign of, 317, 318

Right bundle branch block
– atrioventricular cushion defects, and, 340, 341
– bifascicular block, and, 333–337, 340, 341, 353
– complete, criteria, 328
– complete, in atrial septal defect, 341, 453
– complex, in Ebstein's anomaly, 447, 448
– incomplete, 329
– incomplete, in atrial septal defect, 329, 340
– incomplete, and left ventricular hypertrophy, 303
– incomplete, and pulmonary embolism, 419, 420
– indeterminate axis, and, 52, 53
– intermittent, 346
– left axis deviation (left anterior hemiblock) and, 334, 335, 338–341
– left axis deviation (myocardial infarction) and, 352, 353
– left posterior hemiblock, and, 336, 337
– masking right ventricular hypertrophy, 316
– myocardial infarction, and, 348, 349, 352, 353
– pathological Q waves, and, 348, 349
– pattern favouring aberration, 148, 234
– QRS axis, and, 328, 336, 337, 346
– right ventricular hypertrophy, and, 50, 310, 316, 334, 451, 453
– trifascicular block, and, 338, 339, 341
Right cardiophrenic angle, acute, in pericardial effusion, 535
Right ventricle
– electrocardiogram within, 30
– foreign body in, 746, 747
– position on cardiac silhouette, 454
Right ventricular activation, unopposed in right bundle branch block, 328
Right ventricular dominance
– absent, in tricuspid atresia, 449
– normal, in neonate, 10
Right ventricular enlargement
– atrial septal defect, and, 643
– atrioventricular cushion defect, and, 665, 666
– criteria, 497, 498
– pulmonary hypertension, and, 580, 596–600, 610–612, 620, 621
– pulmonary stenosis, and, 628
– tricuspid valve disease, and, 607
– ventricular septal defect, and, 660, 661
Right ventricular hypertrophy
– apparent, in childhood, 11
– balanced ventricular hypertrophy, and, 319
– child with, 315
– criteria for, 309, 310
– examples, 51, 58, 309–313, 315
– hypertrophic cardiomyopathy, and, 308
– left ventricular hypertrophy, and, 59, 317, 318
– masked by right bundle branch block, 316
– mimicked by left posterior hemiblock, 331, 337
– mimicked by mirror image Q waves in hypertrophic cardiomyopathy, 307
– mimicked by mirror image Q waves in true posterior infarction, 396, 405
– mimicking left ventricular hypertrophy, 313
– neonate with, 314
– P pulmonale, and, 309–311, 315
– qR complex in V1, and, 310
– rS pattern in chest leads, 46, 58, 311–313
– right axis deviation, and, 46, 309, 311, 312, 315
– right axis deviation (initial forces) as evidence of, in presence of right bundle branch block, 453
– right bundle branch block, and, 50, 310, 316, 334, 451, 453
– strain, pattern in, 309, 310
Right ventricular pacing
– acceptable catheter position, 718, 719
– poor catheter position, 720–722, 726

S wave in left chest leads
– absence in anticlockwise rotation, 7
– appearance in pulmonary embolism, 419, 420
– clockwise rotation, and, 6
– right bundle branch block, and, 328, 329
– right ventricular hypertrophy, and, 308–315, 317
S wave in right chest leads, in left ventricular hypertrophy, 294
ST–T changes, grouping suggestive of myocardial ischaemia, 355, 357
ST segment depression (see also T wave inversion)
– acute aortic or mitral regurgitation, and, 306
– digitalis effect, and, 441
– hypokalaemia, and, 437
– hypothermia, and, 427, 428
– left ventricular diastolic overload, and, 306
– left ventricular strain, and, 296–298
– masked by AC interference, 38
– mimicked by variable baseline, 36
– minor, but significant, 369, 374, 397
– mirroring ST elevation in true posterior region, 405
– myocardial ischaemia, and, 365, 369, 370
– paroxysmal tachycardia, producing, 162, 163
– positive exercise test, and, 376
– progressive in early infarction, 380, 381
– reciprocal, absence of, in acute pericarditis, 414
– reciprocal, absence of, in sickling pattern, 13
– reciprocal, in acute infarction, 380–382
– reciprocal, in Prinzmetal angina, 377, 378
– right ventricular hypertrophy, and, 309, 310
– sinus tachycardia, and, 131
ST segment elevation
– acute pericarditis, and, 414
– amyloid disease, and, 445
– anomalous origin of left coronary artery, and, 452
– left bundle branch block, and, 320
– left ventricular hypertrophy, and, 297, 298
– marked, masking P waves, 386
– myocardial infarction, and, 380–398
– persistent, in amyloid disease, 445
– persistent, in left ventricular aneurysm, 412
– Prinzmetal angina, and, 377, 378
– return to baseline after infarction, 412
– right bundle branch block and infarction, and, 348
– sickling pattern, and, 13
– subarachnoid haemorrhage, and, 429
ST segment, horizontal
– in hypocalcaemia, 438
– in myocardial ischaemia, 355, 356, 359, 373, 376
– in subendocardial infarction, 366
Sail shadow, 463
Scimitar syndrome, 652, 653
Semihorizontal heart, 2
– and left ventricular hypertrophy, 295
Semivertical heart, 4
– and left ventricular hypertrophy, 294, 298
Septal Q waves
– absence of in left bundle branch block, 320, 324, 325, 327, 339
– absence over left ventricle in corrected transposition, 450
– hypertrophic cardiomyopathy, and, 307, 308
– left ventricular hypertrophy, and, 296, 302, 304
Sick sinus syndrome, 67, 68
Sickling pattern, 13, 14
– mimicked by acute pericarditis, 414
Silhouette
– normal cardiac, 454
– sign, 496, 514

Sino-atrial block, 60
– junctional escape beats, and, 65
– mimicked by blocked atrial extrasystoles, 110
– partial, 61
– ventricular escape beats, and, 64
– versus sinus arrest, 62, 64
Sinus arrest, 62
– accelerated idioventricular rhythm, and, 184, 185
– carotid sinus hypersensitivity, causing, 66
– junctional escape, and, 63, 65
– junctional rhythm, and, 71, 128
– hyperkalaemia, and, 435
– hypothermia, and, 428
– quinidine intoxication, and, 440
– sick sinus syndrome, and, 67
– versus sino-atrial block, 62, 64
Sinus arrhythmia, 18
– abolition on exercise, 19
– effect on post-extrasystolic pause, 84
– grade 1 heart block, and, 239
– marked, with junctional escape, 20
– non-respiratory, 21
Sinus bradycardia, 126, 127, 129
– agonal, 194
– athletes, and, 486
– dissociated, with junctional rhythm, 129
– hypothermia, and, 427
– irregular, slow, in escape capture bigeminy, 70
– mimicked by incorrect speed of recording, 35
– myxoedema, and, 424
– sick sinus syndrome, and, 67, 68
Sinus node
– depression of automaticity by atrial extrasystole, 102
– discharge with atrial extrasystoles, 100
– discharge in atrial parasystole, 125
– extrasystole, 105
– irregular discharge in complete heart block, 265–267
– irregular discharge in partial heart block, 249, 251, 261
– shifting pacemaker in, 22
– vagal tone acting on, 18
Sinus rhythm, 17
Sinus tachycardia, 130–132
– acute pulmonary embolism, and, 419, 420
– effect on PR interval, 341
– reflex, in Valsalva's manoeuvre, 26
Sinus of Valsalva aneurysm, rupture of, 565
Situs inversus, 672, 673
Situs solitus, 674
Spitz–Holter catheter, as intracardiac foreign body, 746, 747
Stencilled cardiac silhouette
– in Ebstein's anomaly, 641
– in pericardial effusion, 535
Step shadow in acute myocardial infarction, 519
Sternal bowing in hyperkinetic pulmonary hypertension, 661, 666
Sternal depression, 475, 476
Stokes–Adams attacks, 66, 277, 278
Stomach bubble in dextrocardia and laevocardia, 672–674
Straight back syndrome, 479, 480
Strain pattern
– in left ventricular hypertrophy, 296–298
– in right ventricular hypertrophy, 309, 310
Stroke volume
– aortic regurgitation, and, 561, 562
– athletes, and, 486
– myxoedema, and, 743
– systolic/diastolic difference due to, 473, 474
Subacute bacterial endocarditis
– acute aortic regurgitation, and, 563, 564

– prosthetic valve dehiscence, and, 572, 573, 605
Sub-aortic stenosis, 554 (and see Hypertrophic cardio-myopathy)
Subarachnoid haemorrhage, 429–432
Superior vena cava
– anomalous vein joining, 650, 651
– electrocardiogram within, 30
– position on cardiac silhouette, 454
– prominence in right atrial enlargement, 497, 498
Supernormal conduction phase, 272
Supine position, effect on heart size, 463
Supraventricular tachycardia, 135, 146 (see also Paroxysmal tachycardia)
– aberrant conduction, and, 148, 149
– corrected transposition, and, 450
– Ebstein's anomaly, and, 448
– repetitive, 156
– sick sinus syndrome, and, 67
Suspended heart, 15, 468
Syphilitic aortitis, 689–692
Systemic-pulmonary vessels
– Fallot's tetralogy, and, 636
– pulmonary atresia, and, 639
Systolic film, 473, 614

T wave
– atrial, 23
– axis, 39
– bifid, in children, 9
– labile, 27
– mimicked by U wave in cerebral haemorrhage, 433, 434
– mimicked by U wave in hypokalaemia, 437
– P wave in (see under P wave)
T waves, flat or inverted
– aberrant conduction, and (see under that heading)
– adolescence, and, 12
– anomalous origin of left coronary artery, and, 452
– cerebral haemorrhage, and, 433, 434
– childhood, and, 8
– congestive cardiomyopathy, and, 443
– constrictive pericarditis, and, 416
– dextrocardia, and, 28
– differential diagnosis of, 27, 357
– digitalis effect, and, 441
– food, and, 27
– hyperventilation, and, 27
– hypocalcaemia, and, 438
– hypothermia, and, 427, 428
– intracardiac electrocardiogram, and, 30
– left bundle branch block, and, 320–327
– left ventricular hypertrophy, and, 295–298
– myocardial ischaemia, and, 356–375
– myocardial infarction, and, 380–412
– myocarditis, and, 442
– myxoedema, and, 424–426
– paroxysmal tachycardia, and, 162, 163
– pericardial effusion, and, 417, 418
– pericarditis, and, 415
– positive exercise test, and, 376
– post-extrasystolic, 84, 85, 117, 122
– pulmonary embolism, and, 419–421
– quinidine intoxication, and, 440
– right bundle branch block, and, 328
– right ventricular hypertrophy, and, 309, 310
– sinus tachycardia, and, 131
– subarachnoid haemorrhage, and, 429–431
– suspended heart, and, 15
– symmetrical 'arrow head', 363, 364, 371, 387, 404, 415
– ventricular extrasystoles, and, 81–99
– ventricular tachycardia, and, 173–183
– Wolff–Parkinson–White syndrome, and, 164–170, 172

T waves, upright and/or taller than expected
– acute myocardial ischaemia, and, 362, 372, 373
– acute pericarditis, and, 414
– early left ventricular hypertrophy, and, 294
– early myocardial infarction, and, 380, 382–384
– hypercalcaemia, and, 439
– hyperkalaemia, and, 435
– left bundle branch block, and, 321
– mirror image, in acute ischaemia, 362
– mirror image, in left bundle branch block, 320
– mirror image, in left ventricular hypertrophy, 297, 298
– mirror image, in Prinzmetal angina, 377, 378
– mirror image, in true posterior infarction, 405, 406
– post-extrasystolic, 86
Thrombosis-in-situ in severe pulmonary hypertension, 625
Thymic shadow in infancy, 463, 464
Thyroid, effect on electrocardiogram in myxoedema, 425, 426
Total anomalous pulmonary venous drainage, 654–656
Transposition of the great arteries, 676, 677
– corrected, 450, 451, 664, 673
– tricuspid atresia, and, 640
Trauma
– aortic rupture, 707, 708
– cardiac perforation with pacing catheter, 725
– nail in myocardium, 748
Tricuspid atresia, 449, 640
Tricuspid valve disease, 576, 598–600, 606, 607
Trifascicular block, 338, 339, 341, 353
Triple valve disease, 610–612
Triple valve replacement, 616, 617

U waves
– cerebral haemorrhage, and, 433, 434
– inverted in myocardial ischaemia, 358, 376
– mistaken for T waves in hypokalaemia, 437
– post-extrasystolic alteration in, 86
– prominent in children, 9
– prominent in hypokalaemia, 437
Upper lobe pulmonary vein distension (see Pulmonary venous congestion)

V4R in corrected transposition, 450
Vagal tone
– grade 2 heart block, and, 258
– rhythmic alteration unrelated to respiration, 21
– sinus arrest, and, 20
– sinus arrhythmia, and, 18
Valsalva manoeuvre, 26
Valve replacement (see under particular valve)
Vanishing tumour of lung, 515–517
Vascular pedicle, narrow
– in corrected transposition, 664, 673
– in Ebstein's anomaly, 641
– in transposition of great arteries, 676, 677
Ventricular aneurysm
– appearance of, 520, 521
– calcified, 525, 526, 532, 533
– differential diagnosis, of, 529, 530, 552, 553
– electrocardiogram, 412
– heart failure, and, 522, 523, 529, 530
– high lateral, 527
– large, 522, 523
– possible, 529, 530
– resected, 524
Ventricular escape beats
– in atrial fibrillation, 231
– in sino-atrial block, 64
Ventricular escape rhythm
– in accelerated idioventricular rhythm, 186

– in complete heart block, 269
Ventricular extrasystoles, 81–99
– atrial fibrillation, and, 98, 224–229
– atrial fibrillation, and, differential diagnosis, 230
– bidirectional, 95
– bidirectional, linked, 98, 227
– chordal rupture of mitral valve, and, 306
– compensatory pause following, 81, 84, 122
– complete heart block, and, 229, 265
– coupling time of, 87, 91, 93–95, 99
– coupling with, 87, 95, 225–229, 260
– digitalis, and, 93, 98, 225–229
– effect of, in rate-dependent bundle branch block, 343
– iatrogenic (see Pacing)
– increase in aberrant conduction after, 326
– interpolated, 89, 90
– junctional rhythm, and, 228
– late, mimicry of, 165
– left ventricular origin of, 92
– mechanically induced, 197, 278
– mimicked by atrial extrasystoles with aberrant conduction, 108
– multifocal, 91, 94, 96–98, 122
– multifocal, linked, 96, 97, 227
– multifocal, linked, as ventricular tachycardia, 180
– multifocal uniform, 94
– multiform, unifocal, 93, 95, 226, 228
– myocardial ischaemia, and, 362, 377
– P waves in, 81–83
– pacing, and, 284
– partial heart block, and, 259, 260
– post-extrasystolic T wave changes, 84–86, 122
– precipitating accelerated idioventricular rhythm, 186
– precipitating demand pacing, 286
– precipitating partial heart block, 259
– Prinzmetal angina, and, 377
– QRS contour in, 81, 91–98
– R on T phenomenon, 99
– R on T phenomenon, causing ventricular tachycardia and fibrillation, 183
– reciprocal beats, and, 83
– retrograde conduction to atria, and, 83
– right ventricular, 92
– Stokes–Adams attack, and, 278
– T wave in, 81
– terminating accelerated idioventricular rhythm, 186
– terminating reciprocating tachycardia, 160, 161
– unifocal, 87, 88, 90, 224
– unifocal multiform (see multiform unifocal)
– very premature, 99
Ventricular fibrillation
– coarse, 190
– fine, 191
– following asystole, 195
– following R on T phenomenon, 183
– mimicked by coarse f waves in V1, 223
– mimicked by F waves in V1, 222
– with quinidine intoxication, 440
Ventricular flutter, 189
– mimicry of, 222, 223
Ventricular hypertrophy (see also under Left, Right, Balanced, and Biventricular hypertrophy)
– athletes, and, 486
– masked by Wolff–Parkinson–White syndrome, 165–168
– mimicked in marked ST segment shifts in acute myocardial infarction, 386
– mimicked by Wolff–Parkinson–White syndrome, 167–168
Ventricular inversion in corrected transposition, 450

Ventricular septal defect
– acquired, after myocardial infarction, 531
– banded, 662, 663
– corrected transposition, and, 664, 673
– Eisenmenger syndrome, and, 622
– effect of closure, 659
– large, 660, 661, 662
– moderate-sized, 658
– right aortic arch in, 622
– small (Maladie de Roger), 657
– unilateral plethora in, 670
Ventricular standstill (see Asystole, Stokes–Adams
  attacks, Sinus arrest, Ventricular fibrillation)
– in partial heart block, 261
Ventricular tachycardia, 173–180 (see also Accelerated
  idioventricular rhythm)
– differential diagnosis, 148, 149, 172, 174–179, 212, 234
– extrasystolic sequence as, 180
– following R on T phenomenon, 183
– fusion beats in, 178, 179
– independent atrial activity in, 177, 179
– mimicked by atrial fibrillation with aberrant conduction, 234
– mimicked by atrial flutter with aberrant conduction,
  212
– mimicked by supraventricular tachyarrhythmias and
  Wolff–Parkinson–White syndrome, 172
– P waves in, 177, 179, 180
– repetitive, 181, 182
Vertical heart 5
– and left ventricular hypertrophy, 298, 299

Wandering pacemaker, 69
Waterston's operation, unilateral plethora in, 671
Wenckebach periods (see also Partial heart block, grade
  2, type 1)
– atrial rate, changing, effect of, 241
– atrioventricular dissociation with antegrade conduction, and, 78
– commencement, 246
– cycle length in, 240, 242, 243, 245
– description, 61, 240–242
– junctional escape beats, and, 261, 262
– mimicked by unstable pacemaker in complete heart
  block, 270
– PR intervals in, 240, 242
– paroxysmal tachycardia, and, 140, 145
– prolonged cycles, 245
– QRS timing in, 240–242
– retrograde conduction in junctional rhythm, and, 80
– sino-atrial block, and, 61
Wolff–Parkinson–White syndrome, 164–170, 172 (and
  see Lown–Ganong–Levine syndrome)
– alternating, 165, 169
– corrected transposition, and, 450
– Ebstein's anomaly, and, 447
– intermittent, 166
– masking bundle branch block, myocardial infarction
  myocardial ischaemia, or ventricular hypertrophy, 165
– mimicking bundle branch block, myocardial infarction,
  myocardial ischaemia, or ventricular hypertrophy,
  165–170
– mimicking late ventricular extrasystole, 165
– normal PR interval, and, 170
– producing left axis deviation, 168, 169
– QRS complex as fusion beat, 165
– reciprocating tachycardia, and, 158
– tachyarrhythmias in, 172
– type A, 167, 169
– type B, 168